W.B. SAUNDERS COMPANY
A Division of Elsevier Inc.

1600 John F. Kennedy Boulevard • Suite 1800 • Philadelphia, Pennsylvania 19103

http://www.theclinics.com

THE PEDIATRIC CLINICS OF NORTH AMERICA
June 2005
Editor: Carin Davis

Volume 52, Number 3
ISSN 0031-3955
ISBN 1-4160-2750-5

The Pediatric Clinics of North America (ISSN 0031-3955) is published bi-monthly by W.B. Saunders Company, Corporate and Editorial offices: 1600 JFK Boulevard, Suite 1800, Philadelphia, PA 19103-2822. Accounting and Circulation offices: 6277 Sea Harbor Drive, Orlando, FL 32887-4800. Periodicals postage paid at Orlando, FL 32862, and additional mailing offices. Subscription prices are $135.00 per year (US individuals), $246.00 per year (US institutions), $177.00 per year (Canadian individuals), $320.00 per year (Canadian institutions), $200.00 per year (international individuals), $320.00 per year (international institutions), $68.00 per year (US students), $100.00 per year (Canadian students), and $100.00 per year (foreign students). To receive student/resident rate, orders must be accompanied by name of affiliated institution, date of term, and the signature of program/residency coordinator on institution letterhead. Orders will be billed at individual rate until proof of status is received. Foreign air speed delivery is included in all Clinics subscription prices. All prices are subject to change without notice. POSTMASTER: Send address changes to *The Pediatric Clinics of North America*, W.B. Saunders Company, Periodicals Fulfillment, Orlando, FL 32887-4800. **Customer Service: 1-800-654-2452 (US). From outside of the US, call 1-407-345-4000.** E-mail: hhspcs@harcourt.com.

The Pediatric Clinics of North America is also published in Spanish by McGraw-Hill Inter-americana Editores S.A., Mexico City, Mexico; in Portuguese by Reichmann and Affonso Editores, Rua Comandante Coelho 1085, CEP 21250, Rio de Janeiro, Brazil; and in Greek by Althayia SA, Athens, Greece.

The Pediatric Clinics of North America is covered in *Index Medicus, Excerpta Medica, Current Contents, Current Contents/Clinical Medicine, Science Citation Index, ASCA, ISI/BIOMED,* and *BIOSIS.*

Printed in the United States of America.

GUEST EDITOR

CHARLES G. PROBER, MD, Professor of Pediatrics, Medicine, Microbiology & Immunology; Associate Chair of Pediatrics, Stanford University School of Medicine; and Scientific Director, Glaser Pediatric Research Network, Stanford, California

CONTRIBUTORS

MANUEL R. AMIEVA, MD, PhD, Assistant Professor, Department of Pediatrics, Division of Infectious Diseases, and Department of Microbiology & Immunology, Stanford University School of Medicine, Stanford, California

JOHN S. BRADLEY, MD, Children's Hospital and Health Center, San Diego, California

KAREN R. BRODER, MD, National Immunization Program, Centers for Disease Control and Prevention, Atlanta, Georgia

SUSANA CHÁVEZ-BUENO, MD, Pediatric Infectious Diseases Fellow, Department of Pediatrics, Division of Pediatric Infectious Diseases, University of Texas Southwestern Medical Center of Dallas, Dallas, Texas

AMANDA C. COHN, MD, Office of Workforce and Career Development, National Immunization Program, Centers for Disease Control and Prevention, Atlanta, Georgia

MICHAEL A. GERBER, MD, Professor, Department of Pediatrics, University of Cincinnati College of Medicine, and Division of Infectious Diseases, Cincinnati Children's Hospital Medical Center, Cincinnati, Ohio

KATHLEEN GUTIERREZ, MD, Assistant Professor, Department of Pediatrics, Division of Pediatric Infectious Disease, Stanford University School of Medicine, Stanford, California

DAVID W. KIMBERLIN, MD, Associate Professor, Department of Pediatrics, Division of Pediatric Infectious Diseases, The University of Alabama at Birmingham, Birmingham, Alabama

SARAH S. LONG, MD, Professor, Department of Pediatrics, Drexel University College of Medicine; Chief, Section of Infectious Diseases, St. Christopher's Hospital for Children, Philadelphia, Pennsylvania

GEORGE H. McCRACKEN, Jr, MD, Professor, Department of Pediatrics, Division of Pediatric Infectious Diseases, University of Texas Southwestern Medical Center of Dallas, Dallas, Texas

H. CODY MEISSNER, MD, Division of Pediatric Infectious Disease, Tufts–New England Medical Center, Tufts University School of Medicine, Boston, Massachusetts

TROY D. MOON, MD, MPH, Fellow in Infectious Diseases, Department of Pediatrics, Tulane University School of Medicine, New Orleans, Louisiana

RICHARD A. OBERHELMAN, MD, Associate Professor, Department of Tropical Medicine, Tulane School of Public Health and Tropical Medicine, New Orleans, Louisiana

STEPHEN I. PELTON, MD, Professor, Departments of Pediatrics and Epidemiology, Boston University Schools of Medicine and Public Health; and Director, Division of Pediatric Infectious Diseases, Boston Medical Center, Boston, Massachusetts

LARRY K. PICKERING, MD, National Immunization Program, Centers for Disease Control and Prevention, Atlanta, Georgia

ALICE L. PONG, MD, Children's Hospital and Health Center, San Diego, California

WILLIAM J. STEINBACH, MD, Department of Pediatrics, Division of Pediatric Infectious Diseases, and Department of Molecular Genetics and Microbiology, Duke University Medical Center, Durham, North Carolina

CONTENTS

that mandates new insights for achieving a successful outcome. 2004 guidelines by the American Academy of Pediatrics for the treatment of acute otitis media provide one perspective that proposes a rethinking of the routine use of antimicrobial therapy with the hope of preventing further increases in bacterial resistance among otopathogens. The goals of this article are to incorporate the advances in diagnosis, treatment, prevention, and management of sequelae into strategies that optimize the outcome of acute otitis media and limit further emergence of resistant otopathogens.

Diagnosis and Treatment of Pharyngitis in Children **729**
Michael A. Gerber

Acute pharyngitis is one of the most common illnesses for which children visit primary care physicians. Most cases of acute pharyngitis in children are caused by viruses and are benign and self-limited. Group A beta-hemolytic streptococcus is the most important of the bacterial causes of acute pharyngitis. Strategies for diagnosis and treatment of acute pharyngitis are directed at distinguishing children with viral pharyngitis, who would not benefit from antimicrobial therapy, from children with group A beta-hemolytic streptococcal pharyngitis, for whom antimicrobial therapy would be beneficial. Making this distinction is crucial in attempting to minimize the unnecessary use of antimicrobial agents in children.

Important Bacterial Gastrointestinal Pathogens in Children: A Pathogenesis Perspective **749**
Manuel R. Amieva

This article focuses on the five most common bacterial enteropathogens of the developed world—*Helicobacter pylori, Escherichia coli, Shigella, Salmonella*, and *Campylobacter*—from the perspective of how they cause disease and how they relate to each other. Basic and recurring themes of bacterial pathogenesis, including mechanisms of entry, methods of adherence, sites of cellular injury, role of toxins, and how pathogens acquire particular virulence traits (and antimicrobial resistance), are discussed.

Bone and Joint Infections in Children **779**
Kathleen Gutierrez

Bone and joint infections are a significant cause of morbidity in infants and young children. Although many principles regarding pathogenesis, diagnosis, and treatment of infection have remained constant over the years, other aspects of this important pediatric diagnosis are continuing to evolve. This article reviews current information regarding pathogenesis, epidemiology, and microbiology of pediatric bone and joint infections and the clinical presentation, diagnosis, and treatment of these infections.

FORTHCOMING ISSUES

August 2005

Pediatric Hospital Medicine
Vincent Chiang, MD, and
Lisa Zaoutis, MD, *Guest Editors*

October 2005

Internation Adoption
Dana Johnson, MD,
Lisa Albers, MD,
Elizabeth Barnett, MD, and
Jerri Ann Jenista, MD, *Guest Editors*

December 2005

Pediatric Endocrinology
Mark Sperling, MD, *Guest Editor*

RECENT ISSUES

April 2005

Pediatric Rheumatology
Ronald M. Laxer, MD, FRCPC, *Guest Editor*

February 2005

College Health
Donald E. Greydanus, MD, FAAP, FSAM,
Mary Ellen Rimsza, MD, FAAP, and
Dilip R. Patel, MD, FAAP, FACCPDM,
FACSM, FSAM, *Guest Editors*

December 2004

From Fetus to Young Adult: Contemporary Topics in Pediatric Cardiovascular Disease
Gil Wernovsky, MD, FACC, FAAP, *Guest Editor*

PEDIATRIC CLINICS OF NORTH AMERICA JUNE 2005

GOAL STATEMENT

The goal of *Pediatric Clinics of North America* is to keep practicing physicians and residents up to date with current clinical practice in pediatrics by providing timely articles reviewing the state-of-the-art in patient care.

ACCREDITATION

The *Pediatric Clinics of North America* is planned and implemented in accordance with the Essential Areas and Policies of the Accreditation Council for Continuing Medical Education (ACCME) through the joint sponsorship of the University of Virginia School of Medicine and Elsevier. The University of Virginia School of Medicine is accredited by the ACCME to provide continuing medical education for physicians.

The University of Virginia School of Medicine designates this educational activity for a maximum of 90 category 1 credits per year, 15 category 1 credits per issue, toward the AMA Physician's Recognition Award. Each physician should claim only those credits that he/she actually spent in the activity.

The American Medical Association has determined that physicians not licensed in the US who participate in this CME activity are eligible for AMA PRA category 1 credit.

Category 1 credit can be earned by reading the text material, taking the CME examination online at http://www.theclinics.com/home/cme, and completing the evaluation. After taking the test, you will be required to review any and all incorrect answers. Following completion of the test and evaluation, your credit will be awarded and you may print your certificate.

FACULTY DISCLOSURE

Disclosure of faculty financial affiliations: As a provider accredited by the Accreditation Council for Continuing Medical Education (ACCME), the Office of Continuing Medical Education of the University of Virginia School of Medicine must ensure balance, independence, objectivity, and scientific rigor in all its individually sponsored or jointly sponsored educational activities. All authors/editors participating in a sponsored activity are expected to disclose to the readers any significant financial interest or other relationship (1) with the manufacturer(s) of any commercial product(s) and/or provider(s) of commercial services discussed in an educational presentation and (2) with any commercial supporters of the activity (significant financial interest or other relationship can include such things as grants or research support, employee, consultant, stock holder, member of speakers bureau, etc.) The intent of this disclosure is not to prevent authors/editors with a significant financial or other relationship from writing an article, but rather to provide readers with information on which they can make their own judgments. It remains for the readers to determine whether the author's/editor's interest or relationships may influence the article with regard to exposition or conclusion.

The authors/editors listed below have identified no professional or financial affiliations related to their presentation: Manuel R. Amieva, MD, PhD; Karen R. Broder, MD; Susana Chavez-Bueno, MD; Amanda C. Cohn, MD; Carin Davis, Acquisitions Editor; Michael A. Gerber, MD; Kathleen Gutierrez, MD; David W. Kimberlin, MD; Sarah S. Long, MD; George H. McCraken, Jr., MD; H. Cody Meissner, MD; Troy D. Moon, MD, MPH; Richard A. Oberhelman, MD; Larry K. Pickering, MD; Alice L. Pong, MD; and, Charles G. Prober, MD.

The authors listed below have identified the following professional or financial affiliation related to their presentations:

John S. Bradley, MD has received research support from BMS, Johnson and Johnson, Elan, Astra Zeneca, GlaxoSmithKline, Pfizer, and Merck; he also serves on Advisory Boards for AstraZeneca and Johnson and Johnson.

Stephen I. Pelton, MD has a research grant from Wyeth Vaccines and serves on the Vaccine Advisory Board. Other disclosures: Sanofi-Aventis - Research Grant and Vaccine Advisory Board; Novartis - Research Grant GlaxoSmithKline - Advisory Board for Respiratory Tract Infection and new antibiotic development.

William J. Steinbach, MD serves on Pfizer and Astellas US speakers' bureaus.

Disclosure of Discussion of non-FDA approved uses for pharmaceutical products and/or medical devices: The University of Virginia School of Medicine, as an ACCME provider, requires that all authors identify and disclose any "off label" uses for pharmaceutical and medical device products. The University of Virginia School of Medicine recommends that each physician fully review all the available data on new products or procedures prior to instituting them with patients.

All authors who provided disclosures have indicated that they will not be discussing off-label uses except the following:

John S. Bradley, MD has indicated that virtually all conditions listed do not have FDA-approved indications for infants and children.

Kathleen Gutierrez, MD is discussing Linezolid that is not labeled for use in bone infections. The recommended dose of oral drugs used for treatment of bone and joint infection (cephalexin, dicloxacillin) is higher than the usual recommended dose.

David W. Kimberlin, MD indicates that most antiviral drugs are not licensed for use in children. In this article on antivirals in pediatrics, he cites references in which particular antiviral agents were evaluated in children. Since many of these are not FDA-approved for children, this constitutes discussion of "off-label" uses.

William J. Steinbach, MD indicates that dosing in children is not fully established; his viewpoint is expressed.

TO ENROLL

To enroll in the *Pediatric Clinics of North America* Continuing Medical Education program, call customer service at **1-800-654-2452** or visit us online at www.theclinics.com/home/cme. The CME program is available to subscribers for an additional fee of $195.00.

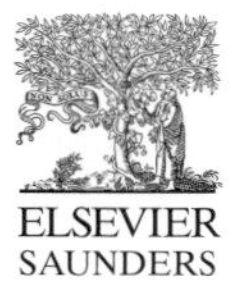

ELSEVIER
SAUNDERS

PEDIATRIC CLINICS
OF NORTH AMERICA

Pediatr Clin N Am 52 (2005) xi–xiii

Preface

Pediatric Infectious Diseases

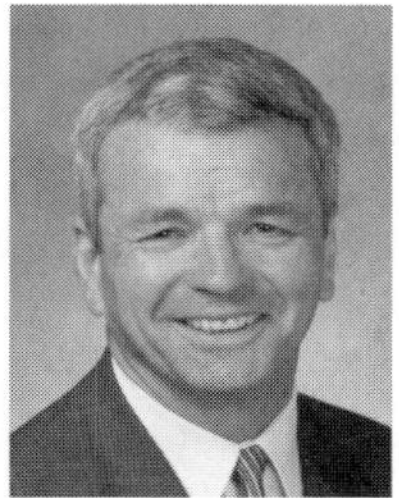

Charles G. Prober, MD
Guest Editor

I am pleased to introduce this issue of the *Pediatric Clinics of North America* dedicated to infectious diseases. Each of the 12 articles was selected because of the importance of the subject matter from the pediatric practitioner's perspective. I am indebted to all of the authors who have done a marvelous job in summarizing a large body of material in a succinct, relevant, and accessible fashion.

Because pediatricians know better than any other group of physicians that "an ounce of prevention is worth a pound of cure," the first article in this issue deals with immunization. Drs. Cohn, Broder, and Pickering, all from the Centers for Disease Control and Prevention, provide a spectacular summary of the state of immunization in the United States. In addition to developing a more full appreciation of the tremendous accomplishments of the national immunization program, the reader will learn a great deal about immunization policies, safeguards, challenges, and emerging strategies.

The second article of this issue, authored by Cody Meissner, underscores the impact of respiratory viruses on infants and young children. Dr. Meissner reminds us of the enormous burden of pediatric illness attributable to respiratory syncytial virus and influenzaeviruses and warns us of the coming influenza pandemic. This article also summarizes the important role of parainfluenza viruses, adenoviruses, rhonoviruses, and the recently recognized human metapneumovirus in childhood respiratory diseases.

doi:10.1016/j.pcl.2005.04.001 *pediatric.theclinics.com*

Articles three and four provide a wealth of information on the diagnosis and management of two of the most common infections managed in pediatricians' offices: otitis media and pharyngitis. Dr. Pelton provides a thoughtful point of view on the diagnosis, management, and outcome of acute otitis media in the current era of universal conjugated pneumococcal vaccination. Dr. Gerber carefully leads us through the approach to the diagnosis and treatment of pharyngitis in children. Much has changed (eg, strategies for diagnostic testing), but much remains the same (eg, antimicrobial therapy for streptococcal infection).

Gastrointestinal pathogens are an important cause of morbidity and mortality among children around the world. Dr. Amieva's article on important bacterial gastropathogens teaches us how appreciating basic pathogenesis facilitates understanding the clinical courses of different illnesses and leads to the development of prudent management strategies.

Articles six and seven deal with serious infections in childhood that usually lead to hospitalization. Dr. Gutierrez's article on bone and joint infections represents a succinct and timely analysis of the pathogenesis, epidemiology, clinical manifestations, diagnosis, management, and outcome of osteomyelitis and septic arthritis in children. The increasing prevalence of community-acquired methicillin-resistant staphylococci, noted by Dr. Gutierrez in reference to bone and joint infections, also is critical to appreciate in managing other infections that might be caused by *Staphylococcus aureus* (eg, skin and soft tissue infections). Drs. Chavez-Bueno and McCracken's article on bacterial meningitis provides a wealth of information regarding this severe and potentially life-threatening infection. The shifting epidemiology of bacterial meningitis following the introduction of effective vaccination programs against *Haemophilus influenzae* type b, *Streptococcus pneumoniae*, and most recently *Neisseria meningitidis* is most noteworthy. Optimal empiric antimicrobial therapy and the role of corticosteroids are other aspects of this article that are of particular interest to the reader.

Dr. Sarah Long brings her incredible wealth of clinical experience to a topic that challenges (and frustrates) many practitioners and infectious disease consultants: prolonged, recurrent, and periodic fever syndromes. Dr. Long offers a logical framework for the evaluation and management of children with these often enigmatic illnesses. Subtle clinical clues are emphasized and a measured diagnostic approach proposed.

The last four articles provide up-to-date, user-friendly summaries of antimicrobial therapy in infants and children. Dr. Kimberlin provides a valuable overview of the 18 non-HIV antiviral agents currently licensed in the United States and the 16 HIV drugs. A brief summary of each agent includes the spectrum of activity, drug resistance, pharmacokinetics and adverse effects, and clinical use. An overview of the factors governing prudent antibiotic selection accompanied by thoughtful recommendations for the therapy of children with suspected or proved bacterial infections can be found in the article authored by Drs. Ping and Bradley. Dr. Steinbach's article deals with the expanding array of antifungal drugs available for the therapy of the increasing array of fungal infections, especially prevalent in children with compromised immunity. Unfortunately, as is true of many biologics used in children, much of the data on the pharmacology, toxicity, and use of these drugs is derived from studies conducted in adults. The shortfalls of data specific to infants and children is emphasized by Dr. Steinbach, and interim dosing recommendations are provided. Recommendations for antiparasitic therapy in children are contained in the article by Drs. Moon and Oberhelman. The detailed table outlining the drugs of choice for common parasitic infections worldwide will be of particular value to practitioners who provide care to international patients or those returning from parts of the world where parasitic infections are endemic. Few of us can recall the drugs of choice and dosages of these valuable medication; this article does it all.

In summary, the authors of this issue of the *Pediatric Clinics of North America* offer a wealth of information relevant to the recognition and management of infections commonly encountered in pediatric practice. These articles will serve as an excellent reference for years to come.

Charles G. Prober, MD
Division of Infectious Disease
Department of Pediatrics
Stanford University School of Medicine
Stanford University Medical Center, G312
300 Pasteur Drive
Stanford, CA 94305-5208, USA
E-mail address: cprober@stanford.edu

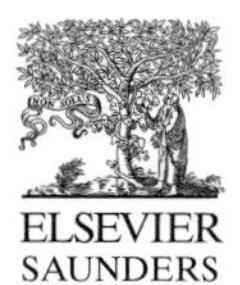

ELSEVIER
SAUNDERS

Pediatr Clin N Am 52 (2005) 669–693

PEDIATRIC CLINICS
OF NORTH AMERICA

Immunizations in the United States: A Rite of Passage

Amanda C. Cohn, MD, Karen R. Broder, MD, Larry K. Pickering, MD*

National Immunization Program, Centers for Disease Control and Prevention, 1600 Clifton Road, NE Mailstop E05, Atlanta, GA 30333, USA

> We must plan for the future, because people who stay in the present will remain in the past.
>
> —Abraham Lincoln

In 1796, when Jenner showed successful inoculation of humans with cowpox to protect them from the devastation of smallpox, a revolution in science and medicine began [1]. More than 2 centuries later, immunizations were hailed as one of "ten great public health achievements" of the twentieth century [2,3]. Today, vaccination is a cornerstone of pediatric preventive health care and a rite of passage for nearly all of the approximately 11,000 infants born daily in the United States.

Immunizations have had a profound impact on the health of children, adolescents, and adults in the United States (Table 1). The most extraordinary success of immunizations was the worldwide eradication of smallpox. Declared in 1980, smallpox eradication was achieved through an unprecedented collaborative international initiative, led by the World Health Organization, establishing an example for other vaccine-preventable diseases [1]. Vaccination since has led to elimination of wild-type poliomyelitis and indigenous measles in the United States, both major causes of pediatric morbidity and mortality in the prevaccine era [4,5].

An integral part of achieving these successes was establishment of a federal immunization infrastructure, which followed the introduction of polio vaccination in the 1950s [3]. Immunization programs, legislation, and funding mecha-

* Corresponding author.
E-mail address: LPickering@cdc.gov (L.K. Pickering).

doi:10.1016/j.pcl.2005.03.001 ***pediatric.theclinics.com***

Table 1
Reported morbidity of selected vaccine-preventable diseases and vaccine coverage levels—US twentieth century and 2003

Disease	US, 20th century annual morbidity [3]	US, 2003 morbidity*	Vaccine coverage levels, 2003[†]	Healthy People 2010 Coverage level goals
Diphtheria	175,885	1	85%[‡] (≥4 doses)	90%
Tetanus	1314	20	85%[‡] (≥4 doses)	90%
Pertussis	147,271	11,647	85%[‡] (≥4 doses)	90%
Poliomyelitis (paralytic)	16,316	0	92%[§] (≥3 doses)	90%
Measles	503,282	56	93%[‖] (≥1 dose)	90%
Mumps	152,209	231	93%[‖] (≥1 dose)	90%
Congenital rubella	823	1	93%[‖] (≥1 dose)	90%
Varicella		20,948	85% (≥1 dose)	90%

* MMWR Morb Mortal Wkly Rep 2004;53:687–96, number of reported cases.
† MMWR Morb Mortal Wkly Rep 2004;53:658–61, number of reported cases.
‡ Administered as diphtheria and tetanus toxoids and acellular pertussis (DTaP) vaccine.
§ Inactivated polio vaccine.
‖ Administered as measles, mumps, and rubella (MMR) vaccine.

nisms are now in place to ensure that immunizations are accessible to all children. As a result, coverage levels for most routinely recommended childhood vaccines in the United States are approaching or have surpassed the US Department of Health and Human Services Healthy People 2010 goal of 90% coverage [6].

Immunizations have changed the scope of pediatric practice in the United States. Pediatric residents now infrequently encounter varicella, which in the 1990s was commonplace. Likewise, although *Haemophilus influenzae* type b (Hib) was the leading cause of meningitis in young children before availability of Hib vaccines in 1985, most newly trained pediatricians will never see a case of invasive Hib [7]. This article reviews the US immunization program with an emphasis on its role in ensuring that vaccines are effective, safe, and available and highlights several new vaccines and recommendations that will affect the health of children and adolescents and the practice of pediatric medicine in future decades.

United States immunization program

Childhood and adolescent immunization schedule

The Centers for Disease Control and Prevention (CDC), American Academy of Family Physicians, and American Academy of Pediatrics (AAP) annually publish a childhood and adolescent immunization schedule. The Advisory Committee on Immunization Practices (ACIP), with input from many liaison organizations, periodically reviews the schedule to ensure consistency with new vaccine developments and policies [8]. The first combined immunization schedule was published in 1995 and recommended six vaccines containing antigens against nine infectious diseases [9]: diphtheria and tetanus toxoids and whole-cell pertussis vaccine (DTP); tetanus and diphtheria toxoids (Td); measles, mumps, and rubella vaccine (MMR); Hib; oral polio vaccine (OPV); and hepatitis B virus vaccine. Ten years later in February 2005, there were ten vaccines against 13 infections in this schedule: diphtheria and tetanus toxoids and acelluar pertussis vaccine (DTaP), Td, MMR, Hib, inactivated polio vaccine (IPV), hepatitis B virus vaccine, varicella vaccine, pneumococcal conjugate vaccine (PCV7), inactivated influenza vaccine, and meningococcal conjugate vaccine (MCV4). The 2005 schedule includes the conjugated meningococcal vaccine, which was licensed by the US Food and Drug Administration (FDA) on January 14, 2005 [8].

Immunization policy

Before a vaccination becomes part of routine clinical pediatric practice, three steps need to be taken: (1) the FDA must license the vaccine, (2) the ACIP and the Committee on Infectious Diseases of the AAP and AAFP must recommend the vaccine for use, and (3) the vaccine must be subsidized to cover children without private health insurance. Numerous government and partner organizations participate in bringing a vaccine from the bench into the clinic. Table 2 provides links where information about these organizations can be obtained.

Table 2
Websites for vaccine-related programs and organizations

	Website
Government programs	
National Immunization Program	www.cdc.gov/nip
National Vaccine Program Office	www.hhs.gov/nvpo/
Vaccines for Children	www.cdc.gov/nip/vfc/default.htm
Vaccine Injury Compensation Program	www.hrsa.gov/osp/vicp/INDEX.HTM
Advisory Committee on Immunization Practices	www.cdc.gov/nip/ACIP/default.htm
Nongovernment organizations	
National Network for Immunization Information	www.immunizationinfo.org/
Immunization Action Coalition	www.immunize.org
National Partnership for Immunization	www.partnersforimmunization.org
AAP: Immunization Initiatives	www.cispimmunize.org/
Vaccine schedule information	
CDC Recommended Childhood and Adolescent Immunization Schedule	www.cdc.gov/nip/recs/child-schedule.htm#mmwr
AAP Recommended Childhood and Adolescent Immunization Schedule	www.cispimmunize.org/
Vaccine safety information	
Vaccine Adverse Event Reporting System	www.vaers.org
Institute of Medicine Immunization Safety Review	www.iom.edu/project.asp?id=4705
Clinical Immunization Safety Assessment Network	www.vaccinesafety.net/CISA/index.htm

Abbreviations: AAP, American Academy of Pediatrics; CDC, Center for Disease Control and Prevention.

Table 3
Clinical trials by phase in development of a vaccine

Clinical trials	Approximate duration in years	Study population	Criteria evaluated
Phase I	1.5	20–100	Assess safety
Phase II	2	100–1000	Expand safety data and determine optimal dose or schedule
Phase III	3.5	1000 – ≥10,000	Establish efficacy and determine safety
FDA consideration	1.5	Review process, license granted	All clinical trial data
Phase IV	Many	100,000 – millions	Monitor safety and effectiveness

Before FDA licensure, a new vaccine goes through 10 to 15 years of preclinical testing and clinical trials, costing pharmaceutical companies millions of dollars in new development costs. Before testing the vaccine in humans, a company files an Investigational New Drug application with the FDA followed by three phases of clinical trials that are performed to study vaccine safety, immunogenicity, and efficacy (Table 3) [10]. After completion of the prelicensure clinical trials, the manufacturer files a Biologics Licensure Application (BLA), and the FDA, with input from its advisory committee, determines if data support vaccine safety, immunogenicity, and efficacy (Fig. 1) [11]. After licensure, monitoring for rare adverse events continues for some vaccines through formal phase IV trials conducted by the FDA and manufacturer.

After FDA licensure of a new vaccine, information about the vaccine is reviewed by the ACIP. The ACIP comprises 15 voting members appointed by the Secretary of the Department of Health and Human Services. In addition, several professional medical and public health groups and industry representatives participate in ACIP discussions. To formulate recommendations, the ACIP establishes subject-specific working groups to review and synthesize data months to

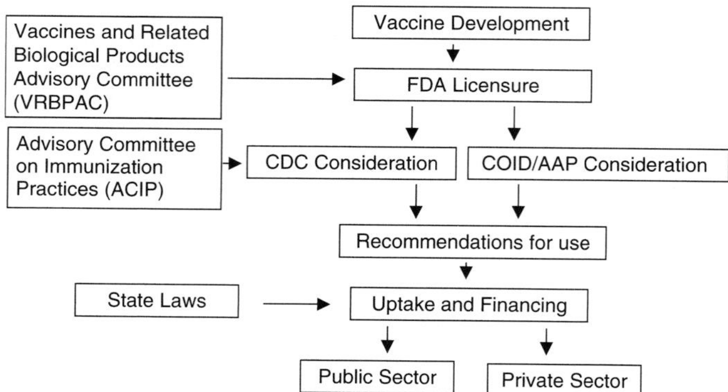

Fig. 1. Development of pediatric vaccine recommendations and policies. (*From* Pickering LK, Orenstein WA. Development of pediatric vaccine recommendations and policies. Semin Pediatr Infect Dis 2002;13:148–54; with permission.)

years before a recommendation is released. ACIP recommendations are subject to the approval of the CDC director (www.cdc.gov/nip/ACIP/charter). The American Academy of Family Physicians and the Committee on Infectious Diseases of the AAP also develop recommendations for vaccine use, which usually are the same as ACIP recommendations.

Ensuring that all US children and adolescents, regardless of health insurance status or income level, have access to recommended immunizations requires a complex system of financing comprised of private and public funding mechanisms (Table 4). In 2002, 57% of US children received vaccines purchased through the public sector, and 43% received vaccines purchased through the private sector. Most of the public-purchase vaccines are financed through the Vaccines for Children (VFC) program, an entitlement program established in 1994 as part of the Social Security Act [11,12]. Other government funding mechanisms include Section 317 of the Public Health Service Act of 1962, a federal grant program, and state and local government funding. These programs provide support for states to provide immunizations to children who do not qualify for the VFC program but who are not covered by private insurance. Fourteen states, referred to as "universal" purchase states, use a combination of federal and state funding to purchase and distribute vaccines recommended for children to all immunization providers in private and public sectors. The remaining 36 states purchase vaccines for uninsured and underinsured chil-

Table 4
Major government financing programs for childhood immunization

Variable	Vaccines for Children program	Section 317	State/local government
Type of program	Entitlement funded through Medicaid trust fund	Annual discretionary appropriation by Congress	Appropriations through state or local legislatures
Eligibility	Age <19 y and membership in ≥1 of the following categories: Medicaid-eligible; uninsured; Alaska Native or Native American; or underinsured at a federally qualified health center	No federal eligibility restrictions	Varies by state or local area
Financing of new vaccines and recommendations	Vote of ACIP and establishment of a federal contract; funds must be approved by the Office of Management and Budget and the Department of Health and Human Services	Funding must be sought from Congress	Funding must be sought from state legislatures
Proportion of childhood vaccine market purchased	41%	11%	5%

Abbreviation: ACIP, Advisory Committee on Immunization Practices.
Data from Hinman AR, Orenstein WA, Rodewald L. Financing immunizations in the United States. Clin Infect Dis 2004;38:1440–6.

dren who are not eligible for VFC. In addition, insurance provides vaccines for children in the private sector.

Immunization program challenges

As the number of vaccines has increased and the scope of the immunization program has expanded, new challenges have emerged. The increasing cost of vaccines, vaccine shortages, and immunization safety are important concerns the immunization program will continue to address in coming years.

The rising cost of fully immunizing a child in the United States is due to the increasing number of vaccines and the increasing price of existing vaccines. The estimated cost of completing the childhood immunization series through 6 years of age in 1987 was $33.70 per child at the government-purchasing rate. The cost of immunizing a child through 6 years of age in 2003 was $436 per child for all vaccines, not including influenza vaccine [12]. Increasingly, state and local health departments are required to make difficult choices about which vaccines to purchase using public funds, including Section 317 grant funds. The recommendation in 2000 to vaccinate routinely with PCV7 doubled the cost of immunizing a child. Section 317 and state funding have not been adequate to cover PCV7 for underinsured children in many states, including 7 of the 14 universal purchase states. The addition of new, effective childhood and adolescent vaccines to the schedule has the potential to create serious funding challenges in the future.

Despite the increasing costs of immunization programs, numerous studies have shown that vaccination continues to be a cost-effective public health intervention. These studies show the need to continue to identify adequate funding sources to support immunization recommendations [13–16]. An Institute of Medicine (IOM) report on vaccine financing released in 2004 concluded, "alternatives to current vaccine pricing and purchasing programs are required to sustain stable investment in development of new vaccine products and attain their social benefits for all" [17].

In addition to the increasing cost of vaccines, an unparalleled number of vaccine shortages in the United States has had a substantial impact on vaccine delivery. From 2000 through 2005, vaccine shortages and changes in routine recommendations occurred for 9 of the 12 diseases for which childhood and adolescent vaccination is recommended (Fig. 2) [18–23]. The shortages affected millions of children and health care providers, even triggering suspension of vaccine school entry requirements [24,25]. Two vaccine shortages (PCV7 and tetanus and diphtheria toxoids [Td]) lasted nearly 2 years, one (PCV7) occurred twice [26], and one (inactivated influenza vaccine, 2004–05 season) halved the US influenza vaccine supply virtually overnight [17,22].

The causes of these widespread vaccine shortages are multifactorial. One important long-term factor is the decrease in number of vaccine manufacturers of childhood vaccines routinely recommended in the United States. In 1977, a federal immunization working group expressed concern about the stability of the US vaccine supply in the setting of "a steady attrition of specific

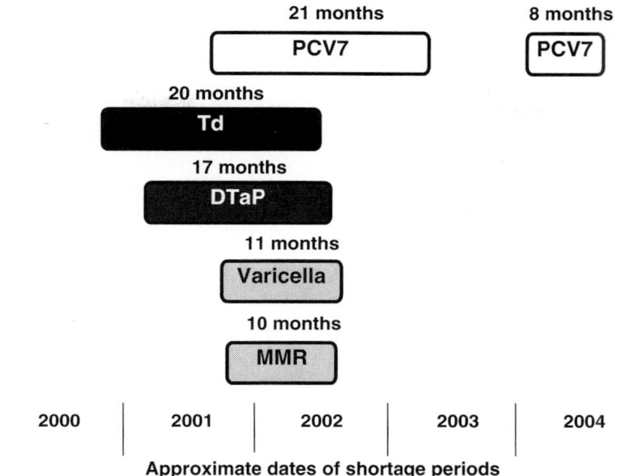

Fig. 2. Shortages of vaccines in the US childhood and adolescent immunization schedule, 2000–2004, not including influenzae vaccine shortage.

pharmaceutical manufacturers from the entire field of biologics" [17]. In 1993, six manufactures produced the six vaccines. In 2005, although four vaccines (PCV7, varicella, influenza, and MCV4) have been added to the recommended schedule, the number of manufacturers decreased to five. In addition, there are single manufacturers for four of the childhood and adolescent vaccines (MMR, varicella, PCV7, and MCV4). In response to concerns over fragility of the US vaccine supply, the General Accounting Office and National Vaccine Advisory Committee conducted in-depth reviews of the vaccine shortages and concluded that future disruptions in vaccine supply are likely to continue, and proposed solutions [17,27].

Vaccines are administered routinely to healthy children and must uphold a scrupulously high safety standard; however, no vaccine is completely safe. In 1986, the National Childhood Vaccine Injury Act was passed creating a compensation program for families affected by childhood vaccine–associated adverse events. Several other government programs and committees to ensure the safety of the vaccine supply also were created by this Act (Table 5).

As many vaccine-preventable diseases approach or reach elimination in the United States, continuing to balance the risks and benefits of each vaccine becomes increasingly important [28]. OPV, formerly recommended for routine use in the United States, was associated with vaccine-associated paralytic poliomyelitis (1 case among 2.4 million vaccine doses distributed). This rare adverse event was no longer considered acceptable after elimination of polio in the United States [29]. In 2000, the ACIP recommended using IPV for all doses of polio vaccine. Public perceptions of vaccine safety are a challenge to the continued success of the vaccination program. New parents and younger physicians grew up without appreciation of the morbidity and mortality of

Table 5
National Childhood Vaccine Injury Act, 1986

National Vaccine Injury Compensation Program	Limits manufacturer liability Provides payments to families of children who sustain documented injuries after routine immunization
National Vaccine Program	Develops and coordinates a comprehensive national vaccine plan
Advisory Commission on Childhood Vaccines	Advises Secretary of Health and Human Services on injury compensation program
National Vaccine Advisory Committee	Advises Secretary of Health and Human Services on national vaccine policy
Federal Excise Tax on Childhood Vaccines	1987 amendment to Compensation Act Proceeds used to finance payments to families of children affected by a vaccine-associated adverse event

Data from Schwartz B, Orenstein WA. Vaccination policies and programs: the federal government's role in making the system work. Prim Care 2001;28:697–711.

several vaccine-preventable diseases. Risk or perception of risk for adverse events becomes an important concern. Two current prominent public vaccine safety concerns are the perceived causal association between MMR and autism and thimerosal-containing vaccines and autism. As a result of heightened concerns about safety, in 2000 the CDC and National Institutes of Health commissioned the IOM of the National Academy of Science to convene an

Box 1. Institute of Medicine Immunization Safety Review Committee reports and dates of release, 2001–2004*

1. Measles-mumps-rubella vaccine and autism—April 2001
2. Thimerosal-containing vaccines and neurodevelopmental disorders—October 2001
3. Multiple immunizations and immune dysfunction—February 2002
4. Hepatitis B vaccine and demyelinating neurologic disorders—May 2002
5. SV40 contamination of polio vaccine and cancer—October 2002
6. Vaccinations and sudden unexpected death in infancy—March 2003
7. Influenza vaccines and neurologic complications—October 2003
8. Vaccines and autism—May 2004

* *Data from* http://www.iom.edu/search_results.asp?qs=immunization%20safety%20review%20committee%20reports.

Immunization Safety Review Committee [30]. Between 2001 and 2004, this independent expert committee published eight reports related to immunization safety concerns. The committee has made recommendations in the areas of public health response, policy review, research, and communications (Box 1). With respect to autism, the IOM concluded that the body of epidemiologic evidence favors rejection of a causal relationship between the MMR vaccine and autism. The committee also concluded that there is no relationship between thimerosal-containing vaccines and autism [30]. None of the eight IOM reports recommended a policy review of the current vaccine recommendations or change in the immunization schedule.

To help ensure safety of vaccines, a robust infrastructure consisting of several systems has been established to monitor vaccine safety after vaccine licensure. The Vaccine Adverse Event Reporting System, operated jointly by CDC and FDA, is a national passive surveillance system used to detect early warning signals and generate hypotheses about possible new vaccine adverse events or changes in frequency of recognized events [31]. Intussusception associated with receipt of rotavirus vaccine, leading to the withdrawal of the vaccine from the market in 1999, was an adverse event detected by the Vaccine Adverse Event Reporting System [31,32]. A third system is the Vaccine Safety Datalink, which consists of large linked databases from health maintenance organizations. Associations between serious medical events and immunizations can be evaluated through the Vaccine Safety Datalink. The newest system is the Clinical Immunization Safety Assessment Centers network, which consists of selected clinical academic medical centers in partnership with CDC to study the pathophysiology of vaccine reactions and develop clinical management protocols for affected patients [34]. These systems are crucial to the vitality and strength of the US immunization program.

Adolescent vaccination considerations

Since its inception, the major focus of the US immunization program has been on vaccinating infants and young children. Of the 10 vaccines routinely recommended for children and adolescents, only two, Td vaccine and the MCV4, are recommended for all adolescents [8]. In 1996, as a result of growing concern about morbidity associated with vaccine-preventable diseases in the hard-to-reach adolescent population, the ACIP recommended expanding efforts to immunize adolescents (11–21 years old) by establishing a routine vaccination visit at 11 to 12 years old [35]. In addition to providing Td and previously missed vaccinations, the report emphasized that this visit should be used to provide other important preventive health services. The anticipated addition of several new adolescent vaccines to the recommended schedule has stimulated a reappraisal of the approaches that most effectively and efficiently would increase the proportion of adolescents who receive newly recommended vaccines and develop ways to integrate these approaches with other adolescent health, education, and development programs.

Vaccines in the spotlight

Similar to all aspects of clinical medicine, immunization recommendations continuously change as new vaccines are licensed and new information becomes available. Since 1990, several new vaccination recommendations were implemented for existing and new vaccines. Notable examples are PCV7 and the hepatitis B vaccine; new recommendations for both have affected children and health care providers. Several vaccines with expected FDA licensure in the near future likely will alter the US immunization program and preventive health care practices (Table 6). Vaccines with a pediatric or adolescent focus under review by the ACIP are relevant to the prevention of pertussis, human papillomavirus (HPV), influenza, varicella, and rotavirus. This section presents a summary of these vaccines in addition to information on PCV7, hepatitis B vaccine, and MCV4. The potential impact of vaccines on the distant horizon also will be highlighted. Emphasis is on how recent and upcoming policy decisions might affect children and adolescents, health care providers, and society during the next decade.

Table 6
Selected pediatric vaccines in phase II and phase III clinical trials, 2004

Vaccine	Type	Age group	Development phase	Potential impact
Diphtheria, tetanus, pertussis	Diphtheria and tetanus toxoids and pertussis vaccine	Adolescents	Submitted to FDA	Decrease burden of disease in adolescents Might reduce overall burden of pertussis disease and protect unvaccinated infants from disease
Rotavirus	Live, attenuated, oral	Infants	Phase III	Reduce morbidity and mortality due to diarrhea and dehydration associated with rotavirus
Human papillomavirus	Virus-like particle vaccine	Adolescents	Phase III	Reduce rates of cervical cancer Reduce number of colposcopy and cervical biopsy procedures
MMR, varicella (MMRV)	Live, attenuated, combination	Anytime MMR given	Phase III	Decrease number of injections
DTaP, Hib, IPV, Hep B	Hexavalent combination	Infants	Phase II	Decrease number of injections
DTaP, Hib, polio	Combination	Infants	Phase III	Decrease number of injections

Data from http://www.phrma.org/newmedicines/resources/2004-06-13.131.pdf.

Pneumococcal conjugate vaccine

PCV7 was recommended for routine use in infants in the United States beginning in 2000. Before introduction of PCV7, *Streptococcus pneumoniae* (pneumococcus) was a leading cause of infectious morbidity in young children in the United States, annually causing approximately 17,000 cases of invasive disease in children younger than 5 years old, including 700 cases of meningitis and 200 deaths. In addition, the burden of pneumonia without bacteremia, otitis media, and sinusitis was substantial [36].

After introduction of routine PCV7 vaccination, the incidence of invasive pneumococcal disease declined dramatically, especially in children younger than 2 years old [37–39]. Active US population–based surveillance data show that within 2 years of PCV7 licensure, the rate of invasive pneumococcal disease in children younger than 2 years old declined by 69% [39]. In tandem with the decrease in invasive disease, data suggest the incidence of pneumococcal non-invasive disease, including otitis media, also decreased [40,41]. In addition to decreasing the burden of pediatric pneumococcal disease, PCV7 may have an impact on reducing pediatric antibiotic prescriptions and procedures such as blood cultures in young, febrile children [42].

The decline in invasive pneumococcal disease is beyond what would be expected from childhood vaccination, given vaccine efficacy and PCV7 coverage data, suggesting that herd immunity may play a role in protecting unimmunized people from invasive disease [37]. Reduced nasopharyngeal carriage of vaccine-containing serotypes in vaccinated children is believed to contribute to development of herd immunity against pneumococcus. Rates of invasive pneumococcal disease seem to be declining among some unvaccinated groups after implementation of universal infant PCV7 vaccination. In addition, postlicensure surveillance data suggest a decrease in antibiotic-resistant strains of *S. pneumoniae* [37,39].

Because PCV7 includes only 7 of the more than 90 serotypes of pneumococcus, there is theoretical concern that serotype replacement might occur in highly vaccinated populations. One study noted an increase in the proportion of cases of invasive pneumococcal disease resulting from nonvaccine serotypes, but the total number of cases was not changed [38]. This study supports the need for continued pneumococcal surveillance in the post-PCV7 era [43].

Hepatitis B

Hepatitis B vaccine holds a unique place in the US immunization schedule because they are the only vaccines licensed for neonates and the only licensed vaccine that prevents cancer. The continued evolution of hepatitis B vaccine recommendations reflects many of the challenges associated with vaccines that will be licensed in the near future.

Before 1982, an estimated 200,000 to 300,000 people in the United States were infected annually with hepatitis B virus, including approximately 20,000 children [44]. Although most vaccine-preventable diseases are spread via contact or airborne droplets, hepatitis B infection is spread via exposure to infected blood or blood products, sexual contact, and injection devices. Much of the transmission of hepatitis B in adults is silent; there is no accompanying rash or symptoms. Although adults have a 10% chance of developing chronic hepatitis B virus infection, infants infected perinatally who do not receive hepatitis B immunoglobulin and vaccine at birth have a 90% chance of developing chronic infection. Twenty-five percent of these infections lead to hepatocellular carcinoma [45].

The complexity of hepatitis B transmission required a vaccination strategy to protect infants and high-risk adults from infection. The first ACIP hepatitis B recommendation in 1982 was to vaccinate groups known to be at high risk for hepatitis B virus infection, such as health care workers, men who have sex with men, and intravenous drug users [46]. In 1984, the ACIP expanded recommendations to include infants born to mothers who were hepatitis B surface antigen (HBsAg) positive. Recognition of the difficulty in identifying mothers infected with hepatitis B led to a recommendation in 1988 to test all women for HBsAg during the prenatal period. Vaccinating high-risk groups continued to be difficult because no foundation existed to vaccinate adolescents and adults who already were participating in high-risk activities. In 1991, a universal infant vaccination strategy was instituted to achieve the goal of reducing transmission of hepatitis B virus [46]. It is recommended that the first dose be given at or before 2 months of age with a preference for all infants to receive the first dose at birth. Neonatal vaccination works by protecting the infant from contracting hepatitis after vertical or horizontal exposure. Giving all infants the birth dose protects infants whose mothers were not tested for HBsAg during pregnancy. Infant vaccination eventually will provide protection against hepatitis B virus to adolescents who may engage in high-risk activities before exposure. From 1990 to 2002, rates of hepatitis B virus infection in children and adolescents younger than 20 years old declined more than 88% in the United States [47].

Meningococcal vaccines

From 2000 to 2002, approximately 2400 to 3000 cases of invasive meningococcal disease occurred annually in the United States [48]. The case-fatality ratio for meningococcal disease is approximately 10%, and severe sequelae (eg, neurologic disability, limb loss) occur in approximately 10% of survivors [49]. Nasopharyngeal carriage of *Neisseria meningitidis* occurs in approximately 5% to 10% of the US population [48]. Transmission is through direct contact with respiratory tract droplets of infected individuals. Infants younger than 1 year of age have the highest rates of meningococcal disease, with an annual incidence of 6.5 cases per 100,000 population during 2002 [50]. During the 1990s, incidence rates of meningococcal disease increased among adolescents and young adults [49]. Evidence also showed that college freshmen living in dormitories have a modestly increased risk of meningococcal disease (4.6 cases per 100,000) compared with other persons the same age [49].

A meningococcal polysaccharide (MPS) vaccine containing the antigens of serogroups A, C, Y, and W135 has been used in the United States since licensure in 1981. This vaccine protects against the serogroups that cause approximately two thirds of meningococcal disease that occurs in persons 18 to 23 years old in the United States. More than half of cases in infants are due to serogroup B, however, for which a licensed vaccine does not exist in the United States [49]. Similar to other polysaccharide vaccines, MPS induces a T cell–independent immune response resulting in poor long-term immunity and inconsistent immunogenicity in children younger than 2 years old. An additional shortcoming is that MPS does not reduce nasopharyngeal carriage or induce herd immunity [48]. Before February 2005, MPS vaccine was recommended for groups at high risk for meningococcal disease and for outbreak control. Educating college freshmen about the potential for the MPS vaccine to prevent severe infection also was recommended. Some states required proof of vaccination or vaccine waiver for entry into colleges and universities [49].

Employing the same technology used to develop PCV7, a meningococcal serogroup C conjugate vaccine was licensed in the United Kingdom in 1999. The vaccine was introduced into the routine infant schedule, with catch-up vaccination for older children and adolescents. In the 2 years after introduction of infant meningococcal conjugate vaccine, the incidence of serogroup C meningococcal disease declined by 87% in vaccinated persons and at least 34% in unvaccinated persons, suggesting the vaccine produced herd immunity [48].

In the United States, a quadrivalet meningococcal conjugate vaccine (serogroups A, C, Y, and W-135) (MCV4) was licensed on January 14, 2005, for use in persons 11 to 55 years old. During prelicensure clinical trials, immune responses to MPS and MCV4 were similar in adolescents and adults. Because MCV4 induces T cell–mediated immunity, the duration of protection is thought to be longer than immunity produced by MPS. On February 10, 2005, the ACIP voted to recommend that MCV4 be administered universally to adolescents ages 11 to 12 and around 15 years of age, and college freshmen living in dormitories; a VFC resolution also was passed. With the addition of MCV4 to the immunization schedule, a new era of adolescent vaccination was launched. In the United States, meningococcal conjugate vaccines for use in children younger than 11 years of age are under study.

Pertussis vaccine

Pertussis remains endemic in the United States despite high immunization coverage rates of infants and young children [51]. Immunity to pertussis wanes approximately 5 to 10 years after vaccination, and loss of immunity seems to play a major role in the continued circulation of pertussis [52]. In 2003 and 2004, 11,647 and more than 18,000 cases of pertussis were reported to the CDC, respectively [53]. Much of the reported increase is thought to be due to increasing physician recognition of pertussis as a nonspecific, persistent cough illness in adolescents and adults, coupled with increasing use of polymerase chain reaction testing for diagnosis of all age groups. How much of the reported increase is due to enhanced surveillance or improved diagnostic methodology is unclear. One study suggested that a true increase in the incidence of pertussis disease occurred in young infants in the United States between 1980 and 1999 [54].

The burden of pertussis disease in adolescents is substantial. Of the reported cases of pertussis in the United States in 2003, 39% were in adolescents; the true number of cases is likely to be much higher (CDC, unpublished data). Although pertussis is rarely life-threatening in adolescents, the morbidity and societal costs associated with adolescent pertussis disease are important [55]. In a Canadian study, 47% of adolescents with pertussis reported a cough duration of at least 9 weeks [56]. Paroxysms, shortness of breath, posttussive vomiting, and difficulty sleeping occur commonly in adolescents with pertussis disease [55,56]. To reduce pertussis disease in adolescents, some countries have recommended an adolescent booster dose. In summer 2004, two manufacturers submitted BLAs to the FDA for use of adolescent and adult pertussis vaccines in the United States (tetanus toxoid, reduced diphtheria toxoid and acellular pertussis vaccine adsorbed (Tdap). The BLA indication for one vaccine includes persons 10 to 18 years old, and the other includes persons 11 to 64 years old.

Policymakers are reviewing several strategies for pertussis vaccination in adolescents and adults. A cost-benefit analysis in the United States found universal vaccination for persons 10 to 19 years old to be the most economic strategy [57]. The expected impact of adolescent pertussis vaccination would be to reduce the risk of pertussis in vaccinated adolescents. Ideally, another public health goal of pertussis vaccination is to reduce transmission to infants younger than 6 months old who have not completed the primary vaccination series and are at highest risk of death from pertussis. The role of an adolescent vaccination program in reducing transmission to infants is unknown. Vaccinating mothers and other close family members of young infants, referred to as a "cocoon strategy," is one method under consideration to decrease pertussis transmission to infants. One study suggested that adult family members are the most frequently identified source for pertussis transmission to infants [58]. Universal replacement of the Td booster given every 10 years with Tdap is another strategy being discussed. Finally, vaccinating women during pregnancy and vaccinating neonates against pertussis have been raised as potential strategies to improve control of pertussis, although pertussis vaccines for these indications are unlikely to be licensed in the United States in the near future [59,60].

Human papillomavirus vaccine

More than 200 types of papillomaviruses have been recognized on the basis of DNA sequence analyses [61]. Papillomaviruses are ubiquitous, have been detected in a wide variety of animals and humans, and are specific to their respective hosts. HPV is associated with a variety of clinical conditions that range from benign skin and mucous membrane lesions to cancer. Most HPV infections are benign. Clinical manifestations with the most frequently associated HPV type are as follows: skin warts (types 1, 2, 3, and 10), recurrent respiratory papillomatosis (types 6 and 11), condyloma acuminata (types 6 and 11), and cervical cancer (types 16, 18, 31, 33, and 45). Based on the association of HPV with cervical cancer and precursor lesions, HPVs can be grouped into low-risk and high-risk HPV types [61]. In the United States and Europe, HPV 16 accounts for approximately 50% of the cases of cervical cancer, with types 18, 31, and 45 accounting for an additional 25% to 30% of cases [62].

HPV is one of the most common causes of sexually transmitted diseases in men and women worldwide, causing almost all of the morbidity and mortality associated with cervical cancer [61]. Epidemiologic studies have shown that the risk of contracting genital HPV infection and cervical cancer is related directly to sexual activity. Several specific factors increase the risk of becoming infected with HPV, including multiple sexual partners at any time, having sex with a person who has had multiple sexual partners, sexual activity at an early age, presence of other sexually transmitted diseases, and HPV type.

Vaccination against high-risk HPV types could reduce substantially the incidence of cervical cancer. Administration of HPV-16 vaccine has been shown to reduce the incidence of HPV-16 infection and HPV-related cervical intraepithelial neoplasia [63]. In addition, a bivalent HPV vaccine was efficacious in preventing persistent cervical infections with HPV-16 and HPV-18 and associated cytologic abnormalities and lesions [64]. Currently, two HPV vaccines are in the final stages of phase III testing. One vaccine contains HPV types 16, 18, 6, and 11, and the second HPV vaccine contains types 16 and 18. Applications for licensure are expected to be filed with the US FDA in late 2005 or 2006.

Rotavirus vaccine

Rotavirus is a common cause of gastrointestinal tract illness in young children. By 5 years of age, nearly all children test seropositive for rotavirus, indicating previous infection. In the United States, rotavirus disease leads to an estimated 600,000 clinic visits, 50,000 to 60,000 hospital admissions, and 20 to 40 deaths annually [33].

The first rotavirus vaccine was licensed in the United States in 1998 and was removed from the market and from the immunization schedule in 1999 because of an association with intussusception. This vaccine was a tetravalent rhesus human reassortant vaccine [65,66]. Currently, several other rotavirus vaccines are in different stages of development. Two late-stage vaccines have completed phase III clinical trials. One vaccine is derived from a monovalent human strain, and the other is a pentavalent bovine-human reassortant vaccine. Large-scale phase III trials did not show an association of these vaccines with intussusception, but postlicensure monitoring is planned. In January 2005, Mexico became the first country to make a new rotavirus vaccine available. The company has filed license applications in more than 20 other countries outside the United States. The manufacturer of the second rotavirus vaccine plans to release it first in the United States after licensure by the US FDA. After licensure in the United States, educational efforts that address identifiable barriers to achieving practitioner advocacy and patient acceptance will be necessary to ensure implementation of rotavirus vaccine recommendations [67]. Ensuring physician acceptance of the vaccine is critical to achieving high coverage levels [67].

Varicella vaccine

Varicella vaccine, licensed for use in the United States in 1995, is a live, attenuated virus vaccine developed from the vesicles of a healthy infected child with chickenpox. This vaccine is recommended as a single dose for children 12 months to 12 years old. Susceptible persons 13 years old or older should receive two doses administered 4 weeks apart. Before varicella vaccine became widely used, varicella was one of the most recognizable rashes seen by pediatricians and was associated with 11,000 hospitalizations and 100 deaths in the United States each year [68]. In 2003, the vaccine had 85% coverage levels, resulting in a significant decrease in mortality, morbidity, and hospitalizations attributable to varicella [68].

Breakthrough varicella infections in vaccinated children occur in 15% of children exposed to varicella. Breakthrough infections usually are mild (<50 lesions), however, with few complications [69]. Vaccinated children with mild disease were only one third as contagious as children with moderate-to-severe disease, whether they were vaccinated or unvaccinated. Vaccine effectiveness for prevention of moderate disease (>50 lesions and complications requiring a visit to a clinician) was 92% [69]. A second dose of varicella vaccine has been approved by the FDA and is being considered for the routine childhood vaccination schedule.

The impact of varicella vaccine on the incidence of zoster infections in adults in the United States is unknown. Varicella vaccine may protect children receiving the vaccine from zoster when they become adults. Studies suggest, however, that continued exposure to varicella protects latently infected adults [70]. Vaccination in children could lead to an increase in zoster incidence in unvaccinated adults because exposure to varicella-infected children has declined, but zoster surveillance is limited. A vaccine to prevent herpes zoster in adults is under investigation.

Influenza vaccines

Since the worldwide influenza pandemic of 1918 that caused an estimated 25 to 50 million deaths, the control of influenza circulation has been a major challenge to clinicians and public health experts. The threat of an unpredictable influenza pandemic and the concern about avian influenza heighten the importance of preventing morbidity and mortality caused by epidemics of influenza disease in the United States, which cause more than 250,000 hospitalizations and more than 36,000 deaths annually [71]. Implementing the expansion of influenza vaccine recommendations to 6- to 23-month-old children and prioritizing vaccine during influenza vaccine shortages are important issues the US immunization program faces regarding influenza prevention.

Influenza virus contains eight major proteins, including hemagglutinin (HA), which controls viral penetration and attachment, and neuraminidase (NA), which controls viral particle release and spread. Influenza strains are identified by type (A, B, and C) and by subtype categorized by HA and NA. There are 15 different HA and 9 different NA subtypes. Major changes in HA and NA, called *antigenic shifts,* are associated with emergence of novel influenza viruses to which little or no immunity exists in the exposed population. Antigenic shifts were the cause of the three influenza pandemics in the twentieth century (Table 7) [72]. Minor changes in HA and NA, called *antigenic drifts,* define the influenza viruses that circulate each year. Influenza vaccines are developed yearly based on antigenic drifts. Worldwide surveillance established by the World Health Organization allows predictions to be made regarding antigenic drifts, which enables vaccine to be updated before the start of an influenza season. Recommendations for which influenza strains should be included in the vaccine are made in early spring before influenza season. Three influenza types are formulated and combined to make a new trivalent vaccine each year.

Two types of influenza vaccines are licensed for use in the United States. One is an inactivated vaccine recommended for persons ≥ 6 months of age in high-risk groups and their close contacts. The second is a cold adapted, live, nasally administered vaccine licensed for healthy people 5 to 49 years of age, including close contacts of high-risk persons. The ACIP and AAP recommended in 2004 to expand influenza vaccine recommendations to include all children 6 to 23 months old and household contacts of children up to 23 months old as well as to continue immunization of all children in high-risk groups. This recommendation was made based on epidemiologic data showing that healthy children in this age group are at high risk of hospitalization from influenza, and that deaths in this age group occur [73–76]. More than 150 reports of pediatric influenza-associated deaths during the 2003–04 influenza season stimulated the addition

Table 7
Influenza pandemics in the twentieth century

			Approximate deaths	
Year	Pandemic name	Strain	US	Worldwide
1918	Spanish flu	H1N1	675,000	25–50 million
1957	Asian flu	H2N2	70,000	>1 million
1968	Hong Kong flu	H2N2	34,000	>1 million

of influenza-associated pediatric mortality to the Council of State and Territorial Epidemiologists list of nationally notifiable diseases [77].

The influenza vaccine is unique to the recommended childhood and adolescent immunization schedule because it is the only vaccine that requires a visit during a certain time of year and that requires annual immunization. Even if the circulating strains of virus are the same as the year before, an annual booster is necessary to retain immunity. In addition, children 6 months to 8 years old are recommended to have two doses of influenza vaccine administered 1 month apart if they previously have never been vaccinated for influenza [76]. Adding influenza into the childhood schedule is challenging for public health officials and primary care physicians developing programs to attain high coverage rates in children 6 to 23 months old.

Vaccines on the horizon

Vaccine development is expanding to include products against cancers, chronic diseases, and other infectious diseases. Vaccines against inflammatory diseases for which an infectious cause has not been identified, such as multiple sclerosis and rheumatoid arthritis, are being developed as therapeutic vaccines. Scientists effectively are using new biologic tools to improve existing vaccines. New technologies also are being used to improve vaccine delivery systems, producing better combination, oral, and intranasal vaccines.

The science behind new vaccines continues to advance at a remarkable pace, driven by an evolving understanding of the cellular and molecular processes involved in different responses of the immune system [78]. Many infectious organisms have evolved over thousands of years to evade this immune response. Adjuvants to vaccines are now being used not only to create an immune response, but also to focus the immune response down a desired path [79]. DNA vaccines, plasmids of DNA encoding the desired antigen, also are being developed with the intention of simplifying vaccine production and eliminating the possible risk of organism reversion [78]. As was true during the time of Jenner, vaccines continue to push the frontiers of science and medicine.

In 2000, the IOM published a report prioritizing development of vaccines to be used in the United States. The IOM committee considered vaccines that could be licensed within 20 years directed against conditions of domestic health importance [80]. Health benefits of these vaccines were measured by a standard health outcome measure, quality-adjusted life years gained. These vaccines were placed into categories of most favorable to least favorable (Box 2). Since publication of this report, PCV7 has been licensed for infants beginning at 2 months of age (most favorable category), and HPV vaccine (more favorable category) and rotavirus vaccine administered to infants (favorable category) are on the near horizon as discussed in this article. Since release of this report, several organisms not included on the IOM list have emerged or became larger public health threats, including West Nile virus, metapneumovirus, methicillin-resistant *Staphylococcus aureus*, the coronavirus associated with severe acute respiratory syndrome

Box 2. Institute of Medicine report on vaccines for the twenty-first century

Most favorable: vaccination strategy would save money

- Cytomegalovirus vaccine administered to 12-year-olds
- Influenza virus vaccine administered to the general population (once per person every 5 years)
- Insulin-dependent diabetes mellitus therapeutic vaccine
- Multiple sclerosis therapeutic vaccine
- Rheumatoid arthritis therapeutic vaccine
- Group B streptococcus vaccine given to women during first pregnancy and to high-risk adults
- *Streptococcus pneumoniae* vaccine given to infants and 65-year-olds

*More favorable: vaccination strategy would incur small costs (<$10,000) for each QALY**

- *Chlamydia* vaccine administered to 12-year-olds
- *Helicobacter pylori* vaccine administered to infants
- Hepatitis C vaccine administered to infants
- Herpes simplex virus vaccine administered to 12-year-olds
- HPV vaccine administered to 12-year-olds
- Melanoma therapeutic vaccine
- *Mycobacterium tuberculosis* vaccine administered to high-risk populations
- *Neisseria gonorrhoeae* vaccine administered to 12-year-olds
- Respiratory syncytial virus vaccine administered to infants and 12-year-olds

Favorable: vaccination strategy would incur moderate costs (>$10,000 but <$100,000) per QALY gained

- Parainfluenza virus vaccine administered to infants and women during their first pregnancy
- Rotavirus vaccine administered to infants
- Group A streptococcus vaccine administered to infants
- Group B streptococcus vaccine given to high-risk adults and low utilization in 12-year-olds or women during their first pregnancy

Less favorable: vaccination strategy would incur significant costs (>$100,000–>$1 million per QALY gained)

- *Borrelia burgdorferi* vaccine given to resident infants born in and immigrants of any age to geographically defined high-risk areas
- *Coccidioides immitis* vaccine given to resident infants born in and immigrants of any age to geographically defined high-risk areas
- Enterotoxigenic *Escherichia coli* vaccine administered to infants and travelers
- Epstein-Barr virus vaccine administered to 12-year-olds
- *Histoplasma capsulatum* vaccine given to resident infants born in and immigrants of any age to geographically defined high-risk areas
- *Neisseria meningitidis* type b vaccine given to infants
- Shigella vaccine given to infants and travelers or travelers only

* Quality-adjusted life year (QALY) takes into account quantity and quality of life generated by health care interventions. QALY is calculated by placing a weight on time in different health states. The cost per QALY is the cost required to generate 1 year of perfect health.
Data from www.iom.edu/vaccinepriorities.

(SARS), and avian influenza virus (H5N1). The ongoing outbreak of H5N1 influenza in Asia, associated with high mortality rates, has stimulated research of a vaccine that has the potential to thwart a possible major influenza pandemic. Circulating H5N1 viruses may adapt to humans through genetic mutation or reassortant with human influenza strains, allowing for human-to-human transmission, facilitated by the fact that most humans lack preexisting immunity owing to lack of previous exposure [81]. These emerging infectious diseases and the need to prevent them add further complexity to immunization schedules of the future.

Summary

Until the twentieth century, approximately half of children in the United States died as a result of childhood illness. Until the 1920s, infectious diseases were the leading cause of death in the United States. In the first edition of the *Red Book* published by the AAP in January 1938, 18 chapters dealt with infectious diseases, ranging from the common cold to smallpox. Except for pertussis, diphtheria, and tetanus, and smallpox, active immunization was not available for the other 14 conditions in this edition. Currently, active immunization exists for 12 of the 18 diseases contained in the eight pages of the 1938 *Red Book,* and one disease, smallpox, has been eradicated. Since then, many other infectious disease have emerged or reemerged, including SARS, HIV, West Nile virus, metapneumovirus, avian influenza, and methicillin-resistant *S. aureus*. Many of these conditions are expected to be controlled in the future by immunizations.

As the recommended childhood and adolescent immunization schedule continues to expand, the US immunization program will be challenged to integrate novel immunization strategies into the current immunization infrastructure. The impact of future vaccines in the United States will be more difficult to calculate because they will prevent fewer deaths than vaccines in the past. The cost of these vaccines will continue to increase, and funding support will be challenged. The risk of adverse vaccine events will have to be weighed against the risk of the disease if not vaccinated. Pediatric health care providers face a growing complexity of problems in children, including injury, obesity, asthma, and mental health and behavioral disorders. As the cost and complexity of the childhood and adolescent immunization schedule increase, considering the role of immunizations within the context of other preventive health interventions and overall societal values becomes increasingly important. Immunizations are one of the most effective clinical preventive services in pediatric practice [15]. Despite the challenges facing the US immunization program, immunizations will likely remain on the list of great public health accomplishments of the twenty-first century, and the legacy of Jenner will continue.

Acknowledgments

The authors acknowledge the valuable contributions of Ms. Stephanie Renna, CDC, who provided editorial assistance, and Dr. Benjamin Schwartz, National Vaccine Program Office, Dr. Renee Renfus, Children's Medicine P.C., Lawrenceville, Georgia, and M. Rutman, who reviewed the manuscript. The authors also acknowledge the following individuals at the CDC for their assistance and support: Drs. R. Chen, M. Cortese, D. Fishbein, K. Kretsinger, D. Guris, J. Moran, T. Murphy, P. Nuorti, S. Reef, M. Roper, M. McCauley, and B. Slade.

References

[1] Fenner F, Henderson DA, Arita I, et al. Smallpox and its eradication. Geneva: WHO; 1998. Available at: http://www.who.int/emc/diseases/smallpox/Smallpoxeradication.html. Accessed February 2005.

[2] Centers for Disease Control and Prevention. Ten great public health achievements, United States. MMWR Morb Mortal Wkly Rep 1999;48:241–3.

[3] Centers for Disease Control and Prevention. Impact of vaccines universally recommended for children–United States, 1990–1998. MMWR Morb Mortal Wkly Rep 1999;48:243–8.

[4] Orenstein WA, Papania MJ, Wharton ME. Measles elimination in the United States. J Infect Dis 2004;189(Suppl 1):S1–3.
[5] Strebel PM, Sutter RW, Cochi SL, et al. Epidemiology of poliomyelitis in the United States one decade after the last reported case of indigenous wild virus-associated disease. Clin Infect Dis 1992;14:568–79.
[6] US Department of Health and Human Services. Healthy people 2010: national health promotion and disease prevention objectives. Washington (DC): US Public Health Service; 2000.
[7] Bisgard KM, Kao A, Leake J, Strebel PM, Perkins BA, Wharton M. *Haemophilus influenzae* invasive disease in the United States, 1994–1995: near disappearance of a vaccine-preventable childhood disease. Emerg Infect Dis 1998;4:229–37.
[8] Centers for Disease Control and Prevention. Recommended childhood and adolescent immunization schedule—United States, 2005. MMWR Morb Mortal Wkly Rep 2005;53:Q1–4.
[9] Centers for Disease Control and Prevention. Recommended childhood immunization schedule–United States, January 1995. Advisory Committee on Immunization Practices, American Academy of Pediatrics, American Academy of Family Physicians, National Immunization Program, CDC. MMWR Morb Mortal Wkly Rep 1995;43:959–60.
[10] Pickering LK, Orenstein WA. Development of pediatric vaccine recommendations and policies. Semin Pediatr Infect Dis 2002;13:148–54.
[11] Schwartz B, Orenstein WA. Vaccination policies and programs: the federal government's role in making the system work. Prim Care 2001;28:697–711.
[12] Hinman AR, Orenstein WA, Rodewald L. Financing immunizations in the United States. Clin Infect Dis 2004;38:1440–6.
[13] Lieu TA, Cochi SL, Black SB, et al. Cost-effectiveness of a routine varicella vaccination program for US children. JAMA 1994;271:375–81.
[14] Lieu TA, Ray GT, Black SB, et al. Projected cost-effectiveness of pneumococcal conjugate vaccination of healthy infants and young children. JAMA 2000;283:1460–8.
[15] Coffield AB, Maciosek MV, McGinnis JM, et al. Priorities among recommended clinical preventive services. Am J Prev Med 2001;21:1–9.
[16] Sharfstein J, Wise P. Cost-effectiveness of hepatitis B virus immunization. JAMA 1996;275:908.
[17] National Vaccine Advisory Committee. Strengthening the supply of routinely recommended vaccines in the United States: recommendations from the National Vaccine Advisory Committee. JAMA 2003;290:3122–8.
[18] Centers for Disease Control and Prevention. Shortage of tetanus and diphtheria toxoids. MMWR Morb Mortal Wkly Rep 2000;49:1029–30.
[19] Centers for Disease Control and Prevention. Update on the supply of tetanus and diphtheria toxoids and of diphtheria and tetanus toxoids and acellular pertussis vaccine. MMWR Morb Mortal Wkly Rep 2001;50:189–90.
[20] Centers for Disease Control and Prevention. Notice to readers: decreased availability of pneumococcal conjugate vaccine. MMWR Morb Mortal Wkly Rep 2001;50:783–4.
[21] Centers for Disease Control and Prevention. Shortage of varicella and measles, mumps and rubella vaccines and interim recommendations from the Advisory Committee on Immunization Practices. MMWR Morb Mortal Wkly Rep 2002;51:190–7.
[22] Centers for Disease Control and Prevention. Experiences with obtaining influenza vaccination among persons in priority groups during a vaccine shortage—United States, October–November, 2004. MMWR Morb Mortal Wkly Rep 2004;53:1153–5.
[23] Centers for Disease Control and Prevention. Notice to readers: pneumococcal conjugate vaccine shortage resolved. MMWR Morb Mortal Wkly Rep 2003;52:446–7.
[24] Stokley S, Santoli JM, Willis B, Kelley V, Vargas-Rosales A, Rodewald LE. Impact of vaccine shortages on immunization programs and providers. Am J Prev Med 2004;26:15–21.
[25] Freed GL, Davis MM, Clark SJ. Variation in public and private supply of pneumococcal conjugate vaccine during a shortage. JAMA 2003;289(5):575–8.
[26] Centers for Disease Control and Prevention. Limited supply of pneumococcal conjugate vaccine: suspension of recommendation for fourth dose. MMWR Morb Mortal Wkly Rep 2004;53:108–9.

[27] United States General Accounting Office. Report to congressional requesters: childhood vaccines: ensuring an adequate supply poses continuing challenges. 2002. Available at: http://www.gao.gov/new.items/d02987.pdf. Accessed Janurary 2005.

[28] Chen RT, Davis R, Sheedy KM. Safety of immunizations: vaccine. In: Plotkin SA, Orenstein WA, editors. Vaccines. Philadelphia: WB Saunders; 2004. p. 1557–77.

[29] Centers for Disease Control and Prevention. Poliomyelitis prevention in the United States: updated recommendations of the Advisory Committee on Immunization Practices (ACIP). MMWR Morb Mortal Wkly Rep 2000;49(RR-5):1–22.

[30] Institute of Medicine. Immunization safety review: committee reports. Washington, DC: National Academy of Sciences; 2004. Available at: www.iom.edu/project.asp?id=4705. Accessed February 2005.

[31] Varricchio F, Iskander J, Destefano F, et al. Understanding vaccine safety information from the Vaccine Adverse Event Reporting System. Pediatr Infect Dis J 2004;23:287–94.

[32] Centers for Disease Control and Prevention. Withdrawal of rotavirus vaccine recommendation. MMWR Morb Mortal Wkly Rep 1999;48:1007.

[33] Centers for Disease Control and Prevention. Rotavirus vaccine for the prevention of rotavirus gastroenteritis among children: recommendations of the Advisory Committee on Immunization Practices (ACIP). MMWR Morb Mortal Wkly Rep 1999;48(RR-2):1–23.

[34] Chen RT, Davis RL, Sheedy KM. Safety of immunizations. In: Plotkin SA, Orenstein WA, editors. Vaccines. Philadelphia: WB Saunders; 2004. p. 1557–82.

[35] Centers for Disease Control and Prevention. Immunization of adolescents: recommendations of the Advisory Committee on Immunization Practices, the American Academy of Pediatrics, the American Academy of Family Physicians, and the American Medical Association. MMWR Morb Mortal Wkly Rep 1996;45:1–16.

[36] Centers for Disease Control and Prevention. Preventing pneumococcal disease among infants and young children: recommendations of the Advisory Committee on Immunization Practices (ACIP). MMWR Morb Mortal Wkly Rep 2000;49(No. RR-9):1–38.

[37] Black S, Shinefield H, Baxter R, et al. Postlicensure surveillance for pneumococcal invasive disease after use of heptavalent pneumococcal conjugate vaccine in Northern California Kaiser Permanente. Pediatr Infect Dis J 2004;23:485–9.

[38] Kaplan SL, Mason Jr EO, Wald ER, et al. Decrease of invasive pneumococcal infections in children among 8 children's hospitals in the United States after the introduction of the 7-valent pneumococcal conjugate vaccine. Pediatrics 2004;113:443–9.

[39] Whitney CG, Farley MM, Hadler J, et al. Decline in invasive pneumococcal disease after the introduction of protein-polysaccharide conjugate vaccine. N Engl J Med 2003;348:1737–46.

[40] Poehling KA, Lafleur BJ, Szilagyi PG, et al. Population-based impact of pneumococcal conjugate vaccine in young children. Pediatrics 2004;114:755–61.

[41] Fireman B, Black SB, Shinefield HR, Lee J, Lewis E, Ray P. Impact of the pneumococcal conjugate vaccine on otitis media. Pediatr Infect Dis J 2003;22:10–6.

[42] Lee KC, Finkelstein JA, Miroshnik IL, et al. Pediatricians' self-reported clinical practices and adherence to national immunization guidelines after the introduction of pneumococcal conjugate vaccine. Arch Pediatr Adolesc Med 2004;158:695–701.

[43] O'Brien KL, Santosham M. Potential impact of conjugate pneumococcal vaccines on pediatric pneumococcal diseases. Am J Epidemiol 2004;159:634–44.

[44] Armstrong GL, Mast EE, Wojczynski M, Margolis HS. Childhood hepatitis B virus infections in the United States before hepatitis B immunization. Pediatrics 2001;108:1123–8.

[45] Poland GA, Jacobson RM. Clinical practice: prevention of hepatitis B with the hepatitis B vaccine. N Engl J Med 2004;351:2832–8.

[46] Centers for Disease Control and Prevention. Hepatitis B vaccination—United States, 1982–2002. MMWR Morb Mortal Wkly Rep 2002;51:549–52.

[47] Centers for Disease Control and Prevention. Acute hepatitis B among children and adolescents—United States, 1990–2002. MMWR Morb Mortal Wkly Rep 2004;53:1015–8.

[48] Raghunathan PL, Bernhard SA, Rosenstein NE. Opportunities for control of meningococcal disease in the US. Annu Rev Med 2004;55:333–53.

[49] Centers for Disease Control and Prevention. Prevention and control of meningococcal disease and meningococcal disease and college students: recommendations of the Advisory Committee on Immunization Practices (ACIP). MMWR Morb Mortal Wkly Rep 2000;49(RR-7):1–20.
[50] Centers for Disease Control and Prevention. Active Bacterial Core Surveillance Report, Emerging Infections Program Network. Available at: http://www.cdc.gov/ncidod/dbmd/abcs/reports.htm#pubs. Accessed February 2005.
[51] Centers for Disease Control and Prevention. Pertussis United States, 1997–2000. MMWR Morb Mortal Wkly Rep 2002;51:73–6.
[52] Guris D, Strebel PM, Bardenheier B, et al. Changing epidemiology of pertussis in the United States: increasing reported incidence among adolescents and adults, 1990–1996. Clin Infect Dis 1999;28:1230–7.
[53] Centers for Disease Control and Prevention. Final: 2003 reports of notifiable diseases. MMWR Morb Mortal Wkly Rep 2004;53:687–96.
[54] Tanaka M, Vitek CR, Pascual FB, Bisgard KM, Tate JE, Murphy TV. Trends in pertussis among infants in the United States, 1980–1999. JAMA 2003;290:2968–75.
[55] Lee GM, Lett S, Schauer S, et al. Societal costs and morbidity of pertussis in adolescents and adults. Clin Infect Dis 2004;39:1572–80.
[56] De Serres G, Shadmani R, Duval B, et al. Morbidity of pertussis in adolescents and adults. J Infect Dis 2000;182:174–9.
[57] Purdy KW, Hay JW, Botteman MF, Ward JI. Evaluation of strategies for use of acellular pertussis vaccine in adolescents and adults: a cost-benefit analysis. Clin Infect Dis 2004;39:20–8.
[58] Bisgard KM, Pascual FB, Ehresmann KR, et al. Infant pertussis: who was the source? Pediatr Infect Dis J 2004;23:985–9.
[59] Forsyth KD, Campins-Marti M, Caro J, et al. New pertussis vaccination strategies beyond infancy: recommendations by the global pertussis initiative. Clin Infect Dis 2004;39:1802–9.
[60] Scuffham P, McIntyre P. Pertussis vaccination strategies for neonates—an exploratory cost-effectiveness analysis. Vaccine 2004;22:2953–64.
[61] Burd EM. Human papillomavirus and cervical cancer. Clin Microbiol Rev 2003;16:1–17.
[62] Harro CD, Pang YY, Roden RB, et al. Safety and immunogenicity trial in adult volunteers of a human papillomavirus 16 L1 virus-like particle vaccine. J Natl Cancer Inst 2001;93:284–92.
[63] Koutsky LA, Ault KA, Wheeler CM, et al. A controlled trial of a human papillomavirus type 16 vaccine. N Engl J Med 2002;347:1645–51.
[64] Harper DM, Franco EL, Wheeler C, et al. Efficacy of a bivalent L1 virus-like particle vaccine in prevention of infection with human papillomavirus types 16 and 18 in young women: a randomised controlled trial. Lancet 2004;364:1757–65.
[65] Zanardi LR, Haber P, Mootrey GT, Niu MT, Wharton M. Intussusception among recipients of rotavirus vaccine: reports to the Vaccine Adverse Event Reporting System. Pediatrics 2001;107:E97.
[66] Murphy TV, Gargiullo PM, Massoudi MS, et al. Intussusception among infants given an oral rotavirus vaccine. N Engl J Med 2001;344:564–72.
[67] Iwamoto M, Saari TN, McMahon SR, et al. A survey of pediatricians on the reintroduction of a rotavirus vaccine. Pediatrics 2003;112(1 Pt 1):e6–10. Available at: www.pediatrics.aappublications.org/cgi/reprint/112/1/e6?maxtoshow=&HITS=10&hits=10&RESULTFORMAT=&author1=Iwamoto&searchid=1107975380001_13871&stored_search=&FIRSTINDEX=0&sortspec=relevance&journalcode=pediatrics. Accessed February 2005.
[68] Seward JF, Watson BM, Peterson CL, et al. Varicella disease after introduction of varicella vaccine in the United States, 1995–2000. JAMA 2002;287:606–11.
[69] Seward JF, Zhang JX, Maupin TJ, Mascola L, Jumaan AO. Contagiousness of varicella in vaccinated cases: a household contact study. JAMA 2004;292:704–8.
[70] Thomas SL, Wheeler JG, Hall AJ. Contacts with varicella or with children and protection against herpes zoster in adults: a case-control study. Lancet 2002;360:678–82.
[71] Thompson WW, Shay DK, Weintraub E, et al. Influenza-associated hospitalizations in the United States. JAMA 2004;292:1333–40.

[72] Kobasa D, Takada A, Shinya K, et al. Enhanced virulence of influenza A viruses with the haemagglutinin of the 1918 pandemic virus. Nature 2004;431:703–7.

[73] Quach C, Piche-Walker L, Platt R, et al. Risk factors associated with severe influenza infections in childhood: implication for vaccine strategy. Pediatrics 2003;112:197–201.

[74] Neuzil KM, Zhu Y, Griffin MR, et al. Burden of interpandemic influenza in children younger than 5 years: a 25-year prospective prospective study. J Infect Dis 2002;185:147–52.

[75] Izurieta HS, Thompson WW, Kramarz P, et al. Influenza and the rates of hospitalization for respiratory disease among infants and young children. N Engl J Med 2000;342:232–9.

[76] Centers for Disease Control and Prevention. Prevention and control of influenza: recommendations of the Advisory Committee on Immunization Practices (ACIP). MMWR Morb Mortal Wkly Rep 2004;53(No. RR-6).

[77] Centers for Disease Control and Prevention. Update: influenza-associated deaths reported among children aged < 18 years—United States, 2003–04 influenza season. MMWR Morb Mortal Wkly Rep 2004;52:1286–8.

[78] Liu MA, Ulmer JB, O'Hagan D. Vaccine technologies. In: US Department of Health and Human Services, editor. The Jordan Report, 20th Anniversary Accelerated Development of Vaccines (2002). Bethesda (MD): The Institute; 2002. p. 32–7

[79] Vogel FR, Alving CR. Progress in immunologic adjuvant development: 1982–2002. In: US Department of Health and Human Services, editor. The Jordan Report, 20th Anniversary Accelerated Development of Vaccines (2002). Bethesda (MD): The Institute; 2002. p. 39–43

[80] Institute of Medicine. Financing vaccines in the 21st century: assuring access and availability. Washington, DC: National Academy of Sciences; 2003. Available at: www.iom.edu/vaccine priorities. Accessed February 2005.

[81] Li KS, Guan Y, Wang J, Smith GJ, et al. Genesis of a highly pathogenic and potentially pandemic H5N1 influenza virus in eastern Asia. Nature 2004;430:209–13.

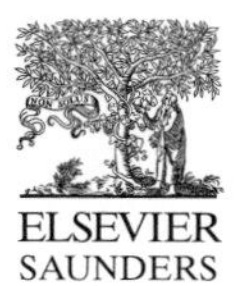

PEDIATRIC CLINICS
OF NORTH AMERICA

Pediatr Clin N Am 52 (2005) 695–710

Reducing the Impact of Viral Respiratory Infections in Children

H. Cody Meissner, MD

Division of Pediatric Infectious Disease, Tufts–New England Medical Center, Tufts University School of Medicine, 750 Washington Street, #321, Boston, MA 02111, USA

Recent years have witnessed a surge in understanding of viral upper and lower respiratory tract disease in children. Respiratory viruses include the following:

1. Respiratory syncytial virus (RSV)
2. Influenza viruses
3. Human metapneumovirus
4. Parainfluenza viruses
5. Coronaviruses (including SARS-CoV)
6. Adenoviruses
7. Rhinoviruses

The epidemiology of established viral pathogens (parainfluenza viruses, adenoviruses, rhinoviruses) continues to be clarified. New pathogens have been identified (human metapneumoviruses and the coronavirus that causes severe acute respiratory syndrome [SARS] [SARS-CoV]). The relentless emergence of antigenic variation among influenza viruses continues, but progress is being made in prevention and control of disease in children through active immunoprophylaxis (trivalent inactivated vaccine, live attenuated vaccine) and new antiviral agents (neuraminidase inhibitors). RSV causes two to three times more pediatric hospitalizations than influenza viruses, parainfluenza viruses, and human metapneumoviruses. Important advances in control of RSV infections among high-risk patients have been achieved using passive immunoprophylaxis despite slow progress in vaccine development. This article reviews current

E-mail address: cmeissner@tufts-nemc.org

0031-3955/05/$ – see front matter
doi:10.1016/j.pcl.2005.02.010

understanding of the major causes of viral respiratory tract disease with an emphasis on prevention and control.

Respiratory syncytial virus

In 1956, Morris et al [1] published a report of a virus that caused upper respiratory infections in chimpanzees. The pathogen was named *chimpanzee coryza agent* because it was initially isolated from chimps with coryza. A similar virus soon was isolated from a child with pneumonia, and the name was changed to *RSV,* reflecting the tendency of RSV-infected cells in vitro to fuse and form syncytia. RSV is a nonsegmented, negative strand RNA virus that encodes for 10 viral proteins. Two subgroups of RSV (A and B) each with multiple genotypes may circulate during annual outbreaks, although it has not been possible to associate more severe disease with one subgroup or another on a consistent basis [2,3].

RSV is the leading cause of hospitalization among infants and young children with respiratory tract disease. The outcome of RSV infection varies from mild upper respiratory tract infection, which occurs in approximately 75% of infected infants, to severe life-threatening disease in a small percentage of patients [4]. Each year in the United States, RSV accounts for 50% to 90% of the approximately 120,000 hospitalizations attributable to bronchiolitis and 20% to 50% of pediatric hospitalizations attributable to pneumonia [5]. During the 17-year period between 1980 and 1996, hospitalization rates for bronchiolitis in infants younger than 12 months old increased by more than twofold, whereas hospitalization rates for other respiratory diseases (pneumonia, asthma) showed little change [5]. Approximately 500 RSV-associated deaths occur each year in the United States, and most occur in non–high-risk patients [6]. Outbreaks of nosocomial RSV disease on pediatric wards continue to be a serious problem when effective infection control policies are not followed [7]. Serologic surveys show that by 2 years of age, more than 90% of children have been infected by RSV at least once. Reinfection throughout life is common, indicating that immunity to RSV after natural infection is inadequate. Whether RSV infection early in life predisposes to subsequent reactive airway disease is an important but unresolved question [8].

RSV lower respiratory tract disease (bronchiolitis, pneumonia) occurs primarily in infants younger than 1 year old. Premature infants and infants with chronic lung disease of prematurity constitute high-risk groups with rates of RSV hospitalization that are approximately five times the hospitalization rate in full-term, healthy infants [9]. Several factors place preterm infants at risk for severe RSV disease, including a relative lack of maternal antibodies, an immature immune response, and underdeveloped lungs with small bronchioles and reduced pulmonary reserve [10]. Transfer of maternal antibodies occurs mainly after the 28th week of pregnancy, so infants born before this time are likely to have lower antibody concentrations. In addition, maternal antibody concentrations to RSV show seasonal variation, and infants born in the early fall or soon after the start of the respiratory virus season are more likely to be born to mothers with low serum antibody concentrations [11]. A low concentration of antibody to RSV correlates with susceptibility to severe RSV in infants [12].

Congenital heart disease in the United States occurs in 4 to 8 infants per 1000 live births. Morbidity and mortality resulting from RSV infection are increased in infants younger than 24 months old with hemodynamically significant congenital heart disease, including infants with large left-to-right shunts, pulmonary hypertension greater than half the systemic pressure, cyanotic heart disease, and complex heart disease such as single ventricular anatomy [13]. Other groups of patients, such as pre-engraftment bone marrow transplant recipients, solid organ transplant recipients, and lymphopenic children receiving chemotherapy, have high hospitalization rates secondary to RSV [14]. The average hospital stay and intensity of care for children in high-risk groups may be several times that of previously healthy infants.

In the Northern Hemisphere and particularly in the United States, RSV circulates predominantly between November and March [9]. In the United States, the inevitability of the RSV season is predictable, but the severity of the season, the time of onset, the peak of activity, and the end of the season cannot be predicted precisely. There can be substantial variation in timing of community outbreaks of RSV disease from year to year in the same community and between communities in the same year even in the same region. These variations occur, however, within the overall pattern of RSV outbreaks, usually beginning in November or December, peaking in January or February, and ending by the end of March or by April [15]. Communities in the southern states tend to experience the earliest onset of RSV activity, and midwestern states tend to experience the latest onset. The duration of the season for western and northeastern regions typically is between that noted in the South and the Midwest [15].

Despite the importance of RSV as a pathogen, options for prevention and treatment of disease are limited. Aerosolized ribavirin was licensed in 1986 for treatment of children hospitalized with severe RSV lower respiratory tract infection. Because of high cost and conflicting data regarding efficacy, however, this drug is not widely used. A vaccine remains the most practical means of reducing the burden of disease attributable to RSV, but it has proved difficult to develop an effective vaccine for young infants that produces protective immunity but does not enhance natural infection [16]. In contrast, remarkable progress has been achieved in showing the efficacy, ease of administration, and safety of passive immunoprophylaxis against RSV. In slightly more than 10 years, the field of passive immunoprophylaxis has evolved from clinical trials with standard intravenous immunoglobulin to the use of a RSV-hyperimmune, polyclonal intravenous globulin (RespiGam) to an intramuscular, humanized murine monoclonal antibody (palivizumab) directed against a conserved epitope on the fusion glycoprotein [4,17].

The US Food and Drug Administration licensed palivizumab in 1998 for monthly intramuscular administration for prevention of RSV lower respiratory tract infections in high-risk infants and children. Results from two blinded, randomized, placebo-controlled trials with palivizumab involving 2789 infants and children with prematurity, chronic lung disease, or congenital heart disease showed a reduction in RSV hospitalization rates of 39% to 78% in different groups [13,18]. Results from postlicensure, observational studies suggest that monthly immunoprophylaxis with palivizumab may reduce rates of RSV-induced hospitalization to an even greater extent than rates reported in clinical trials [19].

Despite the fact that the highest rate of RSV hospitalization occurs in high-risk infants, most infants hospitalized with severe RSV disease are previously healthy infants who were born at term. Studies confirm that prematurity, chronic lung disease of prematurity, congenital heart disease, and young age at the beginning of the RSV season constitute the major risk factors for RSV hospitalization [20]. Household crowding seems to be another important risk factor for severe viral lower respiratory illness including that caused by RSV. As the number of household members increases, the risk of exposure to infectious respiratory secretions also increases. Numerous other risk factors have been associated with severe RSV disease, including gender (males > females), low socioeconomic status, daycare attendance, exposure to passive smoke, lack of breastfeeding, limited maternal education, and malnutrition. These factors have an inconsistent association with hospitalization across studies, however, and at most account for only a modest increase in risk [10,21]. The American Academy of Pediatrics has published guidelines for selection of high-risk infants who are most likely to benefit from monthly prophylaxis with palivizumab [22].

A crucial aspect of RSV prevention in high-risk infants is education of parents and other caregivers about the importance of decreasing infants' exposure to RSV. High-risk infants should be excluded from situations where exposure to infected individuals cannot be controlled, such as daycare centers. Emphasis on hand hygiene is important in all settings, including the home, and exposure to passive smoke should be avoided.

Influenza viruses

Influenza viruses are negative sense RNA viruses containing eight segments of RNA, which encode for 10 viral proteins. The segmented genome is one of the key features explaining the ability of influenza viruses to undergo antigenic change and cause annual outbreaks of disease. Influenza viruses are classified as one of three types (A, B, C) based on antigenic differences in the nucleocapsid protein. Type A strains infect humans and animals and are associated with the most severe disease, causing epidemics and pandemics on a worldwide basis. Influenza A viruses are categorized further into subtypes based on two surface glycoproteins, hemagglutinin and neuraminidase. Type B strains tend to cause less severe illness than type A, do not circulate in animals, and are not categorized into subtypes. Type C strains cause mild disease and have little public health impact.

The two major surface glycoproteins of the influenza virion are important in understanding epidemiology, pathogenesis, and treatment. The hemagglutinin glycoprotein enables viral attachment to respiratory epithelial cells that support influenza virus replication. The neuraminidase glycoprotein possesses enzymatic activity that cleaves sialic acid residues that is essential for efficient release of progeny virions as they escape from an infected cell. Antibodies directed against hemagglutinin and neuraminidase proteins confer immunity against a specific strain of influenza.

Annual outbreaks of influenza occur because types A and B undergo constant antigenic change classified as either antigenic shift or antigenic drift. *Antigenic drift* refers to mutations (nucleotide substitutions or deletions) in the hemagglutinin or neuraminidase genes. Selective pressure favors the emergence of antigenically altered strains as an increasing number of individuals in the community develop antibody against the circulating strain. New antigenic stains emerge, circulate, and are replaced by the next emerging strain against which the population has limited immunity. Depending on the extent of antigenic variation from strain to strain, the new circulating virus may cause more or less severe outbreaks of disease.

Antigenic shift refers to a different mechanism by which a new strain of influenza suddenly emerges. Type A viruses with genes encoding for different subtypes of hemagglutinin and neuraminidase reside in a diverse range of host species, including birds, horses, swine, and humans, although birds are considered to be the natural reservoir. To date, 15 immunologically distinct subtypes of hemagglutinin and 9 distinct subtypes of neuraminidase have been described. If a new gene encoding for either neuraminidase or hemagglutinin is acquired, a new strain may begin to circulate. Antigenic shift occurs less frequently than antigenic drift. Antigenic shift has not been described in influenza type B viruses.

In temperate climates, disease resulting from influenza activity peaks between late December and early March. Data from the Centers for Disease Control and Prevention (CDC) indicate that during 28 years, the month of peak activity due to influenza occurred in November in 4% of the years, December in 14%, January in 21%, February in 43%, March in 10%, April in 4%, and May in 4%. [23] On a yearly basis, influenza is responsible for approximately 36,000 deaths in the United States. Most deaths occur in the elderly, although there are few data on pediatric deaths. Approximately 200,000 excess hospitalizations occur each year because of complications of influenza.

Studies have determined that children age 6 to 23 months are at increased risk for influenza-related hospitalization [24,25]. This figure has been difficult to determine because of overlap of the RSV and influenza seasons. It now seems that in children 0 to 4 years old, hospitalization rates because of influenza in high-risk children are approximately 5 per 1000 and approximately 1 per 1000 for children without underlying disease. These rates are similar to hospitalization rates in adults 65 years old and older and for whom annual immunization is strongly recommended [23].

During an influenza outbreak, the highest attack rates occur in school-age children and may exceed 30%, whereas the attack rates among adults average 10% to 20% in interpandemic years [23]. Families with school-age children are twice as likely to experience influenza than families with older children, reflecting the importance of young children in transmission of influenza in a community. Influenza is highly contagious, and secondary spread to adults in the same household is common. Patients may be infectious for 24 hours before the onset of symptoms and continue to shed virus in nasal secretions for about 5 days after onset of symptoms. Young children may shed virus for longer periods. Annual outpatient visits because of complications of influenza vary from 6 to 29 per 100 children depending on the virulence of the circulating strain and the relatedness between the vaccine and the circulating strains. Complications from influenza infections are estimated to account for a 10% to 30% increase in antibiotic courses in infected children. In 2004, because of the high risk of influenza infection in young children, the Advisory Committee on Immunization Practices to the CDC and the American Academy of Pediatrics changed the recommendation for routine annual influenza vaccination to include infants 6 to 23 months old [23].

Transmission of influenza virus results from airborne spread of respiratory secretions generated by coughing, sneezing, or talking. Inhalation of small airborne particles accounts for most infections. Viral transmission also can occur by direct contact with contaminated secretions. Influenza has a short incubation period of 18 to 72 hours, with the shorter period occurring after exposure to a larger innoculum. Influenza infection typically begins with sudden onset of fever, followed by myalgia, malaise, headache, nonproductive cough, rhinitis, and sore throat (Table 1). Individuals with underlying medical conditions are at increased risk of pneumonia, which may be due to viral extension to the lungs or bacterial superinfection. Less severe complications of influenza include otitis media and sinusitis.

Primary influenza viral pneumonia is manifest by rapid onset of cough and dyspnea. It is associated with a high morbidity rate. In contrast, secondary bac-

Table 1
Influenza versus cold symptoms

Signs and symptoms	Influenza	Cold
Onset	Sudden	Gradual
Fever	>101 °F lasting >3 d	Rare
Cough	Can become severe	Less common
Headache	Prominent	Rare
Myalgia	Severe	Slight
Fatigue	Fatigue lasting >1 wk	Mild
Extreme exhaustion	Early and prominent	Rare
Chest discomfort	Common	Mild
Stuffy nose	Sometimes	Common
Sneezing	Sometimes	Common
Sore throat	Sometimes	Common

terial pneumonia caused by pneumococcus, group A beta-hemolytic streptococcus, or *Staphylococcus aureus* generally follows a period of improvement with recrudescence of fever associated with symptoms of pneumonia. Other pulmonary complications in children include croup and bronchiolitis. Children with a history of asthma may experience an acute exacerbation. Myositis, particularly in the gastrocnemius and soleus muscles, is a recognized complication of influenza. In severe cases, myoglobinuria with progression to renal failure may occur. Myocarditis and pericarditis also have been described. CNS complications include Guillain-Barré syndrome, transverse myelitis, postinfectious encephalitis, and encephalopathy [27].

The most important means of control of influenza is active immunization with either the killed inactivated trivalent influenza vaccine (TIV) or the live attenuated influenza vaccine (LAIV) [23,26]. When vaccine and epidemic strains are well matched, the vaccine confers protection in 70% to 90% of vaccinees. The optimal time for vaccination is between the beginning of October and the end of November. Vaccine should be offered throughout the influenza season as long as vaccine is available and until virus is no longer circulating (Box 1). Protective antibodies develop within 2 weeks after vaccination. The immunogenicity of a single dose of vaccine in young children is limited, especially if they have not been vaccinated previously or infected by influenza virus. Two doses of intramuscular vaccine should be administered at least 1 month apart to children younger than 9 years old (Table 2). The duration of immunity is likely to be less

Box 1. Target groups for influenza vaccination

1. Chronic pulmonary disorders, including asthma
2. Hemodynamically significant heart disease
3. Regular medical follow-up or hospitalization in the past year for any of the following:
   Metabolic disease, including diabetes mellitus
   Renal dysfunction
   Hemoglobinopathy
   Immunosuppression due to medical therapy or HIV infection
4. Persons 6 months old to 18 years old receiving long-term aspirin therapy
5. Women who will be pregnant during the influenza season
6. Infants 6 to 23 months old
7. Persons ≥65 years old
8. Persons ≥50 years old when vaccine supplies are adequate
9. Close contacts of high-risk persons, including household and other close contacts of infants <6 months old
10. Health care personnel
11. Anyone who wishes to reduce the risk of influenza infection

Table 2
Influenza vaccine schedule

Age group	Dose (mL)	No. doses
6–35 mo	0.25	1 or 2
3–8 y	0.50	1 or 2
≥9 y	0.50	1

than 12 months, so yearly vaccination is necessary to boost the immune response and to provide immunity to new antigenic strains. Hospitalization rates secondary to influenza in infants younger than 6 months old may be greater than 10 per 1000 [25]. Influenza vaccine is not recommended for this age group, however, because it has not been evaluated in such young children. It is important to vaccinate the contacts of these young, at-risk infants. The most frequent side effect of vaccination is soreness at the vaccination site, which occurs in 10% to 64% of vaccinees. Fever, malaise, and myalgia occur most often in young children who have had no previous exposure to influenza virus antigens.

A topical live attenuated, temperature-sensitive, cold-adapted, trivalent influenza vaccine administered by nasal spray was licensed by the Food and Drug Administration in 2003 (Table 3). Temperature-sensitive strains preferentially replicate at the lower temperature of the nasal cavity and less efficiently at core body temperature. Intranasal administration of vaccine results in a subclinical infection that induces immunity by simulating a natural infection of the upper airways. This vaccine was approved as an alternative to TIV for healthy persons 5 to 49 years old. It is likely that approval will be extended beyond these age limits. The advantages of LAIV are avoidance of intramuscular injection and possibly greater protection against mutated strains than that found with TIV [23,28]. LAIV should not be used to immunize persons who have close contact with severely immunocompromised patients who require isolation [23].

Antiviral drugs for treatment or prophylaxis are not a substitute for vaccination. Four influenza antiviral drugs are presently licensed in the United States: amantadine, rimantadine, zanamivir, and oseltamivir. Three drug are approved for treatment of influenza in children younger than 13 years old (Table 4). When therapy is initiated within the first 2 days of illness, all four medications are similarly effective in reducing the duration of symptoms by about 1 day [23,26]. Antiviral therapy with oseltamivir or zanamivir has been shown to decrease influenza-associated otitis media and antibiotic use in children. Amantadine,

Table 3
Comparison of live attenuated influenza vaccine versus killed inactivated trivalent influenza vaccine

Factor	LAIV	TIV
Route	Intranasal spray	Intramuscular injection
Type of vaccine	Live virus	Killed virus
Number of strains in vaccine	2 type A and 1 type B	2 type A and 1 type B
Vaccine strains updated	Annually	Annually
Approved age and risk groups	Healthy persons; age 5–49 y	Persons ≥6 mo old

Table 4
Antiviral drugs for influenza

	Amantadine	Rimantadine	Zanamivir	Oseltamivir
Virus	A	A	A and B	A and B
Administration	Oral	Oral	Inhalation	Oral
Treatment indications	$\geq$1 y	$\geq$13 y	$\geq$7 y	$\geq$1 y
Prophylaxis indications	$\geq$1 y	$\geq$1 y	Not licensed	$\geq$13 y
Adverse effects	CNS, GI	GI	Bronchospasm	Nausea, vomiting

rimantadine, and oseltamivir are the three antiviral medications approved for chemoprophylaxis of influenza in children [23,26,29].

Any person 1 year old or older experiencing a potentially life-threatening infection should be treated with antiviral medication. Any person 1 year old or older who is at risk of serious complications of influenza should be treated with antiviral medication, ideally within 48 hours of onset of symptoms. Treatment of persons who do not have conditions placing them at greater risk of serious complications also may benefit from antiviral therapy begun within 48 hours of onset of symptoms. For treatment of illness resulting from influenza A or if the type is unknown, oseltamivir or zanamivir is recommended to reduce the risk of development of amantadine-resistant isolates, which could be transmitted to contacts [26,30,31].

Persons who live or work in an institution caring for people at high risk of serious complications should receive prophylaxis during an institutional outbreak. Prophylaxis also may be considered for persons at high risk who cannot be vaccinated, vaccinated high-risk persons who are exposed within 2 weeks of immunization (before time for an adequate antibody response), immunosuppressed persons who may not respond to the vaccine, and health care workers who are not able to obtain vaccine [26,32,33]. For prophylaxis against influenza A, amantadine or rimantadine is encouraged because of greater availability and lower cost relative to the neuraminidase inhibitors.

Influenza pandemics refer to the sudden emergence and rapid spread throughout the world of a new strain of influenza virus that causes extensive social disruption and severe disease with increased mortality relative to typical annual epidemics. Three influenza pandemics occurred in the last century (Table 5). The occurrence of the next pandemic seems to be inevitable. Estimates from the CDC project that 200 million people may be infected during the next pandemic. Between 300,000 and 800,000 persons in the United States may re-

Table 5
Influenza pandemics in twentieth century

Years	Influenza	Virus
1918–19	Spanish	Type A (H1N1)
1957–58	Asian	Type A (H2N2)
1968–69	Hong Kong	Type A (H3N2)

quire hospitalization, resulting in 88,000 to 300,000 deaths. Because pandemic strains typically appear in the United States less than 6 months after detection elsewhere in the world, vaccine may be unavailable or in limited supply. Health care workers are at increased risk of early exposure and may become ill before much of the general population, compromising the delivery of health care.

Type A influenza virus is capable of infecting numerous different animal species, including birds, pigs, horses, whales, and humans. Birds are considered to be the natural host of influenza viruses because all known subtypes of influenza A have been isolated from birds. Wild birds generally do not develop symptoms when infected by influenza virus. In contrast, domesticated birds, such as chickens or turkeys, often become sick or die when infected. Influenza virus survives in the intestine and is spread in the saliva, nasal secretions, and feces of infected birds, although fecal-oral spread of virus among susceptible birds is the most common route of transmission. Transmission of avian influenza directly from birds to humans generally does not occur. The first reported instance of human infection by avian influenza A (H5N1) occurred in Hong Kong in 1997. During this outbreak, 18 people were infected, and 6 died. Killing 1.5 million chickens in Hong Kong removed the reservoir of virus and helped control the outbreak. In early 2004, widespread outbreaks of avian influenza H5N1 occurred in Cambodia, China, Indonesia, Japan, Laos, South Korea, Thailand, and Vietnam. More than 100 million birds died or were killed to control the outbreak. In summer 2004, a second wave of disease due to H5N1 was reported among poultry in China, Indonesia, Thailand, and Vietnam. If H5N1 strains acquire the ability for efficient human-to-human transmission, this strain could cause the next pandemic. The CDC recommends testing for H5N1 strains in patients with radiographically confirmed pneumonia or severe respiratory illness for whom a diagnosis has not been established and who have a history of travel within 10 days of onset of symptoms to a country with documented H5N1 avian influenza in poultry.

Human metapneumoviruses

Human metapneumoviruses were identified as a cause of respiratory tract disease in 2001 [34]. The spectrum of disease and the epidemiology of this RNA virus resemble that of RSV. Findings to date suggest this virus may cause hospitalization in young children at a rate that is second only to RSV [35–37].

Human metapneumoviruses cause upper and lower respiratory tract disease with symptoms including the common cold, bronchiolitis, pneumonia, croup, and exacerbation of reactive airway disease. Results from the New Vaccine Surveillance study found that approximately 4% of 668 hospitalizations of children were associated with human metapneumovirus, and that requirements for supplemental oxygen and mechanical ventilation were similar to the requirements in RSV-infected children [35]. Although the most serious lower respiratory tract infections occur in children in the first year of life, symptomatic reinfection by human metapneumovirus seems to be common. Risk factors for severe human metapneumovirus disease are similar to the risk factors associated with severe RSV illness. Most cases of lower tract disease occur before 12 months of age, although the median age of human metapneumovirus–infected children in one study of hospitalized patients was greater than the age of RSV-infected children (3 months versus 11.5 months) [35]. Similar to RSV, the incidence of human metapneumovirus infection is greatest during the winter and early spring months, although human metapneumovirus activity seems to peak later in the season than the peak in RSV activity. No vaccine is available. Disease prevention in certain high-risk populations with passively administered antibody may be an option to vaccine development.

Parainfluenza viruses

Parainfluenza viruses that infect humans are divided into four categories, types 1 to 4, based on genetic and antigenic characteristics [38]. Parainfluenza viruses 1 through 3 are important causes of upper and lower respiratory infection in infants and young children, whereas parainfluenza virus 4 is isolated infrequently and seldom associated with severe disease. Although most parainfluenza virus infections in healthy children are restricted to the upper respiratory tract, parainfluenza viruses 1 through 3 are isolated from 9% to 30% of children hospitalized with viral lower respiratory disease. As with RSV, primary infection is more likely to be associated with severe disease in children, whereas recurrent infections typically result in mild illness, especially in adults. Among immunocompromised patients, such as bone marrow transplant patients or solid organ transplant patients, pneumonia is associated with high mortality rates.

Epidemiologic studies suggest that parainfluenza viruses 1 and 2 cause disease in the fall months of alternate years [39,40]. Parainfluenza virus 3 tends to be endemic through the year, with a peak in activity in the spring and early summer months. Most symptomatic infections resulting from parainfluenza viruses occur between 6 months and 3 years of age, although parainfluenza virus 3 is an important cause of bronchiolitis in the first 6 months of life. Upper respiratory tract symptoms secondary to parainfluenza viruses 1 through 3 tend to be similar and consist of coryza, cough, conjunctivitis, hoarseness, and fever. Manifestations of lower respiratory tract disease secondary to parainfluenza virus include croup, bronchiolitis, and pneumonia.

Efforts at disease control through vaccination are progressing slowly. Inactivated or subunit vaccines have met with limited success [16]. Experience with live attenuated vaccines is more promising [41]. A report describes the initial results from a clinical trial with a bivalent RSV/parainfluenza virus 3 intranasal vaccine and supports the feasibility of such a vaccine [42]. Subjects responded with an immune response to both components of the vaccine (no significant interference), and the vaccine strains seemed to be genetically stable (no evidence of back mutation to a virulent phenotype). Questions to be resolved include shedding and transmissibility of the vaccine strain and development of symptoms in some subjects suggesting insufficient attenuation.

Coronaviruses

Coronaviruses have been classified into four groups based on antigenic and genetic characteristics. Coronaviruses have been recognized for several decades as a cause of respiratory and enteric disease in humans and animals. Human coronaviruses OC43 and 229E cause a common cold syndrome with symptoms similar to those of rhinovirus infection. Common symptoms include malaise, headache, nasal discharge, sore throat, and cough lasting 6 to 7 days. Fever is frequently absent. Asymptomatic infection is common, whereas lower tract disease in infants and children is uncommon. In temperate climates, coronavirus infection is more common in winter and spring than in summer and fall. Because there are multiple strains of coronaviruses, and because reinfection is common, a vaccine is unlikely to be developed.

In November 2002, the first reports of an atypical pneumonia were issued from Guangdong province, mainland China. In less than 1 year, more than 8000 patients (mostly adults) from 26 countries were diagnosed with SARS. Within months, the etiologic agent of SARS was determined to be a coronavirus (SARS-CoV). This virus is now known to circulate in animals, particularly Himalayan palm civets [43,44]. Seroepidemiologic data suggest that SARS-CoV did not infect humans previously. SARS provided a dramatic example of the sudden appearance of a new human respiratory virus arising from an animal source.

The incubation period of SARS is approximately 2 to 10 days. The use of appropriate infection control policies and public health measures showed that epidemics could be prevented. Most transmission of SARS-CoV occurred in health care settings, accounting for the high attack rate seen in medical personnel. SARS-CoV is spread when infectious respiratory droplets come in contact with mucous membranes of susceptible persons. SARS-CoV seems to be more stable than other respiratory pathogens, such as RSV. Profuse watery diarrhea that contains virus is a common feature of infection, and fecal-oral transmission may be another route of transmission [43].

Transmission of disease from adults to children seems to be rare. Infection in children younger than 12 years old is associated with milder disease and a lower fatality rate than infection in adults [45]. Disease in teenagers resembles disease in adults. SARS in patients older than 65, particularly in patients with chronic illnesses, such as diabetes mellitus or heart disease, may produce mortality rates that exceed 50%.

No specific treatment regimen has been shown to prevent disease progression. Supportive care includes supplemental oxygen and mechanical ventilation.

Adenoviruses

Adenoviruses are nonenveloped DNA viruses first observed in human adenoid tissue in 1953. Forty-nine serotypes have been identified. Adenoviruses cause a range of respiratory symptoms, including coryza, pharyngitis, tonsillitis, bronchitis, pneumonia, and conjunctivitis. Infection predisposes to otitis media and sinusitis. Although these viruses can produce sporadic outbreaks of disease, adenoviruses are not associated with the seasonality that characterizes other respiratory viruses. In contrast to some other respiratory viruses that show tropism for only the respiratory tract, adenovirus infection is not restricted to the respiratory tract and has the ability to cause multiorgan involvement, particularly including the gastrointestinal tract, heart, and CNS.

Most adenovirus respiratory infections are self-limited and resolve without long-term complications. There are no licensed antiviral agents for treatment of adenovirus infections. A live oral adenovirus vaccine consisting of serotypes 4 and 7 for use in military recruits was available for many years but was not studied in civilians. This vaccine is no longer available [46].

Rhinoviruses

Rhinoviruses are the principal cause of the common cold. Serotype immunity persists after infection, but there are more than 100 serotypes, and there is no cross-protection. Transmission of rhinovirus infection is common among school-age children, who transmit infection to family members. The peak incidence of colds secondary to rhinovirus in the United States occurs in the fall, when approximately 80% of colds are associated with positive cultures or reverse-transcriptase polymerase chain reaction assays for rhinoviruses. Symptoms in older children and adults consist of runny nose, nasal congestion, sore throat, and malaise, with a median duration of 11 days [47].

There are no licensed antiviral agents for treatment of rhinoviral infections, although pleconaril and interferon alfa have been studied. Because of the numerous serotypes, vaccination against rhinovirus infection is not practical.

Summary

Respiratory infections caused by RNA viruses continue to challenge clinicians' ability to prevent and control outbreaks of disease. In the years ahead, entirely new viral respiratory diseases will continue to emerge, previously unrecognized viruses will be identified using new techniques, and known viruses will continue to mutate. To address the growing public health threat posed by respiratory viruses, surveillance will be essential for establishing public health policy and for directing federal and industry-sponsored research efforts. Perhaps the greatest capacity for widespread disease and social disruption will come from new strains of influenza viruses that acquire the capacity to move between species, from birds to humans, owing to natural evolution or to an act of bioterrorism with an intentionally altered strain. Determination of population-based incidence rates is a first step on the road to development of new vaccines and novel antiviral agents. The CDC has established the New Vaccine Surveillance Network to assess the disease burden attributable to certain viral illnesses against which new vaccines are likely to become available [48,49]. Data provided from ongoing surveillance of respiratory hospitalization in children younger than 5 years old will be useful in assessing the effectiveness of new vaccines and therapies.

References

[1] Morris JA, Blount RE, Savage RE. Recovery of cytopathic agent from chimpanzees with coryza. Proc Soc Exp Biol Med 1956;92:544–50.

[2] Hall CB, Walsh EE, Schanbel KC. Occurrence of groups A and B of RSV over 15 years: associated epidemiologic and clinical characteristics in hospitalized and ambulatory children. J Infect Dis 1990;162:1283–90.

[3] Martinello RA, Chen MD, Weibel C, Kahn JS. Correlation between RSV genotype and severity of illness. J Infect Dis 2002;186:839–42.

[4] Meissner HC, Long SS. Revised indications for the use of palivizumab and respiratory syncytial virus immune globulin intravenous for the prevention of respiratory syncytial virus infection. Pediatrics 2003;112:1447–52.

[5] Shay DK, Holman RC, Newman RD, Liu LL, Stoput JW, Anderson LJ. Bronchiolitis associated hospitalization among United States children 1980–1996. JAMA 1999;282:1440–6.

[6] Shay DK, Holman RC, Roosevelt GE, Clarke MJ, Anderson LJ. Bronchiolitis associated mortality and estimates of respiratory syncytial virus associated deaths among United States children 1979–97. J Infect Dis 2001;183:16–22.

[7] McCarney KK, Gorelick MH, Manning ML, Hodinka RI, Bell LM. Nosocomial respiratory syncytial virus infections: the cost effectiveness and cost benefit of infection control. Pediatrics 2000;106:520–6.

[8] Martinez FD. Respiratory syncytial virus bronchiolitis and the pathogenesis of childhood asthma. Pediatr Infect Dis J 2003;22:S76–82.

[9] Meissner HC, Anderson LJ, Pickering LK. Annual variation in respiratory syncytial virus season and decisions regarding immunoprophylaxis with palivizumab. Pediatrics 2004;114:1082–4.

[10] Meissner HC. The unresolved issue of risk factors for hospitalization of infants with respiratory syncytial virus infection born after 33–35 weeks gestation. Pediatr Infect Dis J 2004;23:821–3.

[11] LeSaux N, Gaboury I, MacDonald N. Maternal respiratory syncytial virus antibody titers: season and children matter. Pediatr Infect Dis J 2003;22:563–4.

[12] Glezen WP, Paredes A, Allison JE, Taber LH, Frank AL. Risk of respiratory syncytial virus infection for infants from low-income families in relationship to age, sex, ethnic group and maternal antibody level. J Pediatr 1981;98:708–15.

[13] Feltes TF, Cabalka AK, Meissner HC, et al, and Cardiac Synagis study group. Palivizumab prophylaxis reduces hospitalization due to respiratory syncytial virus in young children with hemodynamically significant congenital heart disease. J Pediatr 2003;143:532–40.

[14] Meissner HC. Selected populations at increased risk from respiratory syncytial virus infection. Pediatr Infect Dis J 2003;22:S40–5.

[15] Mullins JA, Lamonte AC, Bresee JS, Anderson LJ. Substantial variability in community respiratory syncytial virus season timing. Pediatr Infect Dis J 2003;22:857–62.

[16] Durbin AP, Karron RA. Progress in the development of RSV and parainfluenza virus vaccines. Clin Infect Dis 2003;37:1668–77.

[17] Johnson S, Oliver C, Prince GA, et al. Development of humanized monoclonal antibody (MEDI-493) with potent in vitro and in vivo activity against respiratory syncytial virus. J Infect Dis 1997;176:1215–24.

[18] The IMpact-RSV study group. Palivizumab, a humanized respiratory syncytial virus monoclonal antibody, reduces hospitalization from respiratory syncytial virus infection in high-risk infants. Pediatrics 1998;102:531–7.

[19] Romero JR. Palivizumab prophylaxis of respiratory syncytial virus disease from 1998 to 2002: results from four years of palivizumab usage. Pediatr Infect Dis J 2003;22:S46–54.

[20] Meissner HC, Welliver RC, Chartrand SA, et al. Immunoprophylaxis with palivizumab, a humanized RSV monoclonal antibody, for prevention of respiratory syncytial virus infection in high risk infants: a consensus opinion. Pediatr Infect Dis J 1999;18:223–31.

[21] Simoes EAF. Environmental and demographic risk factors for respiratory syncytial virus lower respiratory tract disease. J Pediatr 2003;143:S118–26.

[22] American Academy of Pediatrics. Revised indications of the use of palivizumab and respiratory syncytial virus immune globulin intravenous for the prevention of respiratory syncytial virus infections. Pediatrics 2003;112:1442–6.

[23] Centers for Disease Control and Prevention. Prevention and control of influenza. MMWR Morb Mortal Wkly Rep 2003;52(RR-8):1–36.

[24] Izurieta HS, Thompson WW, Kramarz P, et al. Influenza and the rates of hospitalizations for respiratory disease among infants and young children. N Engl J Med 2000;342:232–9.

[25] Neuzil KM, Mellen BG, Wright PE, Mitchel EF, Griffin MR. The effect of influenza on hospitalizations, outpatient visits and courses of antibiotic in children. N Engl J Med 2000;342: 225–31.

[26] Rennels MB, Meissner HC. Reduction of the influenza burden in children. Pediatrics 2002; 110:e80–98.

[27] Weitkamp J, Spring MD, Brogan T, et al. Influenza A virus-associated acute necrotizing encephalopathy in the United States. Pediatr Infect Dis J 2004;23:259–63.

[28] Belshe RB, Gruber WC, Mendelman PM, et al. Efficacy of vaccination with live attenuated cold-adapted, trivalent, intranasal influenza virus vaccine against a variant (A/Sydney) not contained in the vaccine. J Pediatr 2000;136:168–75.

[29] Centers for Disease Control and Prevention. Neuraminidase inhibitors for treatment of influenza A and B infections. MMWR Morb Mortal Wkly Rep 1999;48(RR-14):1–9.

[30] Hedrick JA, Barzilai A, Behre U, et al. Zanamivir for treatment of symptomatic influenza A and B infection in children five to twelve years of age: a randomized controlled trial. Pediatr Infect Dis J 2000;19:410–7.

[31] Whitely RJ, Hayden FG, Reisinger KS, et al. Oral oseltamivir treatment of influenza in children. Pediatr Infect Dis J 2001;20:127–33.

[32] Welliver R, Monto AS, Carewicz O, et al. Effectiveness of oseltamivir in preventing influenza in household contacts. JAMA 2001;285:748–54.

[33] Hayden FG, Gubareva LV, Monto AS, et al. Inhaled zanamivir for the prevention of influenza in families. N Engl J Med 2000;343:1282–9.

[34] van den Hoogen BG, deJong JC, Groen J, et al. A newly discovered human pneumovirus isolated from young children with respiratory tract disease. Nat Med 2001;7:719–24.

[35] Mullins JA, Erdman DD, Weinberg GA, et al. Human metapneumovirus infection among children hospitalized with acute respiratory illness. Emerg Infect Dis 2004;10:700–5.

[36] Williams JV, Harris PA, Tollefson SJ, et al. Human metapneumovirus and lower respiratory tract disease in otherwise healthy infants and children. N Engl J Med 2004;350:443–50.

[37] van den Hoogen BG, Osterhaus ME, Pouchier RAM. Clinical impact and diagnosis of human metapneumovirus infection. Pediatr Infect Dis J 2004;23:S25–32.

[38] Henrickson KJ. Parainfluenza viruses. Clin Microbiol Rev 2003;16:242–64.

[39] Knott AM, Long CE, Hall CB. Parainfluenza viral infections in pediatric outpatients: seasonal patterns and clinical characteristics. Pediatr Infect Dis J 1994;13:269–73.

[40] Reed G, Jewett PH, Thompson J, Tollefson S, Wright PF. Epidemiology and clinical impact of parainfluenza virus infections in otherwise healthy infants and young children < 5 years old. J Infect Dis 1997;175:807–13.

[41] Karron RA, Belshe RB, Wright PF, et al. A live human parainfluenza type 3 virus vaccine is attenuated and immunogenic in young infants. Pediatr Infect Dis J 2003;22:394–405.

[42] Belshe BB, Newman FK, Anderson EL, et al. Evaluation of combined live, attenuated respiratory syncytial virus and parainfluenza 3 virus vaccines in infants and young children. J Infect Dis 2004;190:2096–103.

[43] Ksiazek TG, Erdman D, Goldsmith CS, et al. A novel coronavirus associated with severe acute respiratory syndrome. N Engl J Med 2003;348:1953–66.

[44] Peris JSM, Yeun KY, Osterhaus ADME, Stohr K. The acute respiratory syndrome. N Engl J Med 2003;349:2431–41.

[45] Leung C, Kwan Y, Ko P, et al. Severe acute respiratory syndrome in children. Pediatrics 2004; 113:e535–43.

[46] Katz SL. A tale of two vaccines. Clin Infect Dis 2000;31:671–2.

[47] Arruda E, Pitkaranta A, Witek TJ, Doyle CA, Hayden FG. Frequency and natural history of rhinovirus infections in adults during autumn. J Clin Microbiol 1997;35:2864–8.

[48] Griffin MR, Walker FJ, Iwane MK, Weinberg GA, Staat MA, Erdman DD, and the New Vaccine Surveillance Network Study Group. Epidemiology of respiratory infections in young children: insights from the New Vaccine Surveillance Network. Pediatr Infect Dis J 2004;23:S193–201.

[49] Iwane MK, Edwards KM, Szilagyi PG, et al. Population-based surveillance for hospitalizations associated with RSV, influenza virus, and parainfluenza viruses among young children. Pediatrics 2004;113:1758–64.

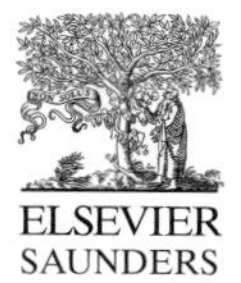

ELSEVIER
SAUNDERS

Pediatr Clin N Am 52 (2005) 711–728

PEDIATRIC CLINICS
OF NORTH AMERICA

Otitis Media: Re-Evaluation of Diagnosis and Treatment in the Era of Antimicrobial Resistance, Pneumococcal Conjugate Vaccine, and Evolving Morbidity

Stephen I. Pelton, MD[a,b,*]

[a] *Departments of Pediatrics and Epidemiology, Boston University Schools of Medicine and Public Health, Boston, MA 02118, USA*
[b] *Division of Pediatric Infectious Diseases, Boston Medical Center, Boston, MA 02118, USA*

The changing susceptibility of bacterial otopathogens is only one aspect of the evolving concepts regarding pathogenesis, immunoprophylaxis, pharmacodynamics, and sequelae of acute otitis media (AOM) that mandates new insights for achieving a successful outcome. 2004 guidelines by the American Academy of Pediatrics (AAP) for the treatment of AOM provide one perspective that proposes a rethinking of the routine use of antimicrobial therapy with the hope of preventing further increases in bacterial resistance among otopathogens. The goals of this article are to incorporate the advances in diagnosis, treatment, prevention, and management of sequelae into strategies that optimize the outcome of AOM and limit further emergence of resistant otopathogens.

Etiology: changing microbiology in the era of pneumococcal conjugate vaccine

Initial episodes

A phase III clinical trial of seven-valent pneumococcal conjugate vaccine (PVC7) conducted in Finland showed a 55% reduction in episodes of AOM

* Maxwell Finland Laboratory for Infectious Diseases, 774 Albany Street, Boston, MA 02118.
E-mail address: spelton@bu.edu

doi:10.1016/j.pcl.2005.02.013

secondary to vaccine serotypes (4, 6B, 9V, 14, 18C, 19F, and 23F) and an overall reduction of 34% in pneumococcal otitis media [1]. Comparison of the otopathogens recovered by tympanocentesis from immunized children compared with controls showed a shift in the proportion of disease resulting from *S. pneumoniae,* nontypable *H. influenzae,* and *Moraxella catarrhalis* (Table 1). Episodes of AOM resulting from vaccine serotypes of *S. pneumoniae* declined, but disease resulting from nonvaccine serotypes increased. Nontypable *H. influenzae* also accounted for a greater number and proportion of disease in immunized children. These changes were observed even though only a portion of children in the community received PCV7. The changes have the potential to be more pronounced where the use of PCV7 is universal in children younger than 2 years old. Several studies conducted in the United States support this hypothesis. One study observed that the proportion of nonvaccine serogroups of *S. pneumoniae* recovered by tympanocentesis from children with otitis media increased from 14.8% (13 of 88) to 36.5% (23 of 63) between 1999 and 2001 [2]. Almost 50% (7 of 15) of the isolates of *S. pneumoniae* recovered from children who had received at least two doses of PCV7 were nonvaccine serogroup isolates compared with only about 20% (26 of 125) of the isolates from children who did not receive vaccine. These data are consistent with other reports showing a decline in nasopharyngeal carriage of vaccine serotypes of *S. pneumoniae* in young infants and toddlers and an increase in carriage of nonvaccine serotypes [3,4]. Further evidence of change in the microbiology of AOM resulting from universal immunization with PCV7 was reported in two articles. A comparison of the microbiology of AOM in infants with either persistent or recurrent AOM undergoing tympanocentesis from periods before and after licensure of PCV7 [5,6] showed an increase in disease secondary to nontypable *H. influenzae* and a decline in pneumococcal episodes. This change is especially relevant because most of the isolates of nontypable *H. influenzae* produced β-lactamase [5,6].

What are the implications of this transition from disease primarily resulting from vaccine serotypes of *S. pneumoniae* to nonvaccine serotypes of *S. pneu-*

Table 1
Microbiology of acute otitis media in children immunized with PCV7 or control vaccine

	No. episodes	
Microbiology of acute otitis media	PCV 7 No. (%)	Control No. (%)
Pneumococci (all)	271 (28)	414 (35)
Vaccine serotype		
Streptococcus pneumoniae	107	250
Cross-reactive serotypes	41	84
Nonvaccine serotypes	125	95
Haemophilus influenzae	315 (33)	287 (26.5)
Moraxella catarrhalis	379 (39)	381 (35)

Data from Eskola J, Kilpi T, Palmu A, et al. Efficacy of a pneumococcal conjugateres vaccine against acute otitis media. N Engl J Med 2001;344:403–9.

moniae and an increase in the proportion of disease resulting from nontypable *H. influenzae*? Because most nonvaccine serotypes of *S. pneumoniae* are more susceptible to β-lactam and macrolide antibiotics, it is postulated that the shift in *S. pneumoniae* otopathogens would result in infection more responsive to traditional antimicrobial agents. Consistent with this hypothesis, a 24% decline in persistent symptomatic AOM and treatment failures has been observed in one study conducted after the introduction of PCV7 [6]. Other investigators have observed a decline in episodes of chronic otorrhea in aboriginal children immunized with PCV7 compared with historic controls, suggesting a less severe course of disease, perhaps as a result of a shift in otopathogens toward nonvaccine serotypes of *S. pneumoniae* and nontypable *H. influenzae*. It also is crucial to anticipate that the antimicrobial susceptibility of nonvaccine serotypes of *S. pneumoniae* will not remain low. Porat et al [7] reported recovering nonvaccine *S. pneumoniae* serotypes from the middle ear of children with AOM that were not susceptible to penicillin. Finkelstein (personal communication, 2004) also observed an increase in nonvaccine, penicillin-nonsusceptible isolates of *S. pneumoniae* in the nasopharynx of Massachusetts children after introduction of PCV7.

Treatment failure and early recurrences

The antimicrobial susceptibility of bacteria responsible for treatment failures is influenced by the antibiotic used to treat the previous infection and the timing of the recurrence. Early recurrences are more likely due to the original pathogen compared with recurrences occurring later. In one study, 16 of 39 (41%) recurrences occurring within 7 days of completing therapy were due to the original pathogen, whereas only 1 of 10 (10%) occurring between days 22 and 28 after completing therapy were due to the same bacteria [8]. Recurrent episodes of AOM are often due to multidrug-resistant otopathogens that persist in the nasopharynx after antibiotic therapy [9]. β-Lactamase–producing nontypable *H. influenzae* has become the most common otopathogen recovered from children failing therapy, especially when high-dose amoxicillin or amoxicillin-clavulanate was prescribed initially. Such treatment does not eradicate or prevent colonization with these β-lactamase–producing nontypable *H. influenzae*.

Clinical manifestations and diagnosis of acute otitis media

Distinguishing acute otitis media from otitis media with effusion

Until recently, little attention was given to distinguishing AOM from otitis media with effusion (OME). In part, this situation resulted from studies of OME that recovered bacterial otopathogens from a small proportion of middle ear samples from children undergoing myringotomy and tympanostomy tube insertion. In retrospect, the absence of inflammatory cells and the lack of a substantial response to antimicriobial therapy strongly suggests the presence of bacteria within the gluelike substance observed at the time of surgery was coincidental. The failure to distinguish AOM and OME contributed to widespread use of antibiotics in children with middle ear disease, reaching 2.5 prescriptions per year in children younger than 3 years old in 1996 [10]. The AAP guidelines published in 2003 suggested principles for improving the diagnosis of AOM (Fig. 1). The presence of middle ear effusion is a crucial criterion. This effusion can be confirmed by the existence of an air-fluid level, air bubbles behind the tympanic membrane, or reduced mobility when pneumo-otoscopy or a type B tympanogram is performed. In addition to middle ear effusion, diagnosis of AOM requires the recent onset of signs and symptoms of acute inflammation, such as earache, ear tugging, or a bulging tympanic membrane. The more specific the ear findings (eg, earache and ear tugging), the more likely the presence of bacterial otopathogens in the middle ear. In one study, approximately 85% of children with earache, ear tugging, or bulging or extreme redness of the tympanic membrane had positive bacterial cultures from fluid obtained from the middle ear cleft. In contrast, among children with nonspecific symptoms, such as fever and irritability, bacterial pathogens were found at tympanocentesis in about 50% [11]. The implication is that the less likely a child is to have bacterial otitis media, the less likely he or she would benefit from antimicrobial therapy. Greater than 96% of children with nonbacterial AOM are

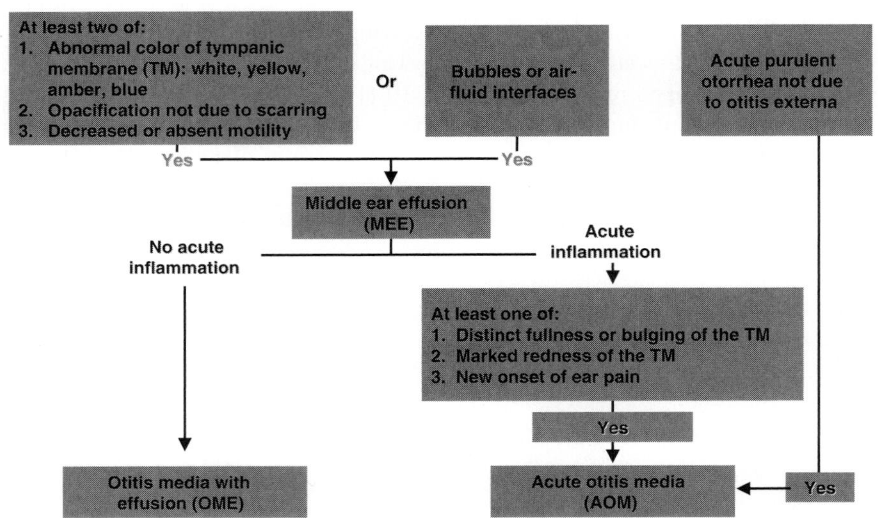

Fig. 1. Diagnostic criteria: acute otitis media and otitis media with effusion. (*Adapted from* Hoberman A, Marchant CD, Kaplan SL, et al. Treatment of acute otitis media: consensus recommendations. Clin Pediatr 2002;141:373–90; with permission.)

cured or improved within 10 days with only supportive therapy (Dagan, personal communication, 2004).

The implications of inaccurate diagnosis cannot be overstated, although the magnitude of the problem has not been studied extensively. Some informative data have been published, however. Blomgren et al [12] observed a 50% decline in episodes of otitis media in otitis-prone children in Finland when a senior resident performed all of the otoscopic examinations during a 6-month period compared with the number of episodes in the same population diagnosed by primary clinicians in the prior 6 months. Pichichero and Poole [13] found pediatricians frequently misclassified videotapes of pneumo-otoscopic middle ear examinations representing AOM, OME, and normal tympanic membranes. Inaccurate diagnosis has implications for the individual child and the community. For the child, unnecessary exposure results in increased risk of adverse side effects; for the community, it provides a selective advantage for otopathogens with reduced antibiotic susceptibility.

Correlating clinical manifestations with specific bacterial otopathogens

Several studies have attempted to correlate presenting signs and symptoms of AOM with the otopathogen recovered at tympanocentesis [14–16]. Dagan [17] used a scoring system based on fever, irritability, ear tugging, and bulging and redness of the tympanic membrane to assess the association between severity and specific bacterial etiology. Rodriguez and Schwartz [15] used fever, pain, and severity of tympanic membrane changes. Palmu et al [16] analyzed a spectrum of signs and symptoms. In general, disease resulting from *S. pneumoniae* was associated more often with severe symptoms and signs; however, the low positive predictive value limited the clinical utility of this association. The most useful clinical indicator of the presence of a specific pathogen was the association between signs of conjunctivitis and infection caused by nontypable *H. influenzae*. This observation had been described previously by Boder [18] and is referred to as the *otitis-conjunctivitis syndrome*.

Outcome of acute otitis media

AOM is most often a complication of viral upper respiratory tract infection resulting in inflammatory exudates within the middle ear cavity. More than 70% of culture-positive episodes have a purulent exudate within the middle ear, with the remainder either mucoid or serous [16]. Fever greater than 38°C is present in approximately one third of episodes; earache or ear pulling, in more than half; and restlessness, restless sleep, or excessive crying, in nearly three quarters [16]. Suppurative complications of AOM are now rare in the United States, although more recent data suggest an increase in the occurrence of mastoiditis in association with multidrug-resistant *S. pneumoniae* [19–21]. A retrospective 10-year survey in Finland (1990–2000) identified only 33 children with suppurative complications of AOM; 32 were intratemporal, and 1 was intracranial [22]. Children younger than 2 years old had approximately fourfold greater risk (3.6 per 100,000 per year) compared with children 2 to 14 years old. It is presumed that the low rate of suppurative complications observed reflects the benefits of immunization with *Haemophilus* conjugate vaccines, the decline in virulence in group A streptococcal infections over the last 50 years, and the introduction of effective antimicrobial therapy for AOM. The most frequent complications of AOM currently are persistent middle ear fluid and perforation of the tympanic membrane. Kacmarynski et al [23] reviewed complications in children with recurrent otitis or persistent effusion younger than 10 years old before tympanostomy tube insertion between June 1999 and December 2000. Among otherwise healthy children, 24.5% were found to have persistent perforation; 78.8%, moderate hearing loss greater than 20 db; 21.1%, speech or language delay; 0.7%, balance "difficulties"; and 0.7%, chronic tinnitus. Resolution of acute signs and symptoms of AOM and management of persistent middle ear fluid and its complications have become the outcomes of concern in the management of children with AOM.

Resolution of acute signs and symptoms

In 1991, Kaleida et al [24] reported that antibiotics were more effective in the therapy of AOM than mechanical drainage (myringotomy). Antibiotics, antibiotics plus myringotomy, and myringotomy alone were compared in children older that 2 years of age with severe disease (high fever with significant otalgia). The treatment failure rate in the myringotomy-alone group (23%) was more than five times greater than the failure rates in children assigned to either antibiotic treatment group (Table 2). The differences in outcome were less dramatic, however, in children who had only minimal symptoms (low or no fever and mild otalgia). The clinical failure rates in the antibiotic-treated and placebo groups

Table 2
Initial treatment failure in severe and nonsevere acute otitis media: amoxicillin* versus placebo/myringotomy alone

	Initial treatment failure		
Classification	Amoxicillin (%)	Placebo (%)	Relative risk
Nonsevere			
Age <2 y	6.5	9.8	
Age ≥2 y	0.5	5.5	
All	3.9	7.7	2
Severe			
Age ≥2 y	3.6	23.5	6.5

* With or without myringotomy in the severe category.
From Kaleida PH, Casselbrant ML, Rockette HE, et al. Amoxicillin or myringotomy or both for acute otitis media: results of a randomized clinical trial. Pediatrics 1991;87:466–74.

were 3.9% and 7.7% (see Table 2). Two recent studies questioned the value of antibiotic therapy for children with AOM. In one study, immediate antibiotic therapy was compared with delayed antibiotic therapy or supportive therapy only [25]. A greater proportion of children randomized to early antibiotic therapy were symptom-free at each time point during follow-up. The investigators concluded that a benefit was apparent in the early treatment group only after the first 24 hours and did not warrant routine early therapy for AOM. In another study that compared treatment with amoxicillin with placebo, the median duration of fever in the active treatment group was reduced by 1 day (2 versus 3 days), and analgesic consumption was higher in the placebo group during the first 10 days [26]. The investigators also concluded that such differences did not warrant routine treatment of AOM with antimicrobial therapy [26]. Limitations of both of these studies were the use of numerous study sites and lack of rigid criteria for the diagnosis of AOM. Many of the children in these studies are likely not to have had AOM, diluting any potential benefit of antimicrobial therapy. In a study using objective criteria for diagnosing AOM and a limited number of investigators, children with mild disease (defined as symptom scores in the lower 50th percentile on a symptom severity assessment) were assigned to immediate therapy with an antibiotic or "watchful waiting" [27]. In the 126 children younger than 2 years old, "watchful waiting" was associated with a twofold increase in treatment failure or relapse. No differences in outcome were observed by day 30 among the children with mild AOM who were older than 2.

Compared with no antimicrobial therapy, there is evidence that immediate antibiotic therapy for children with AOM results in a more rapid resolution of symptomatic disease and a reduced rate of treatment failure or relapse. The benefits are most notable in children younger than 2 and children with severe symptoms. The AAP guidelines for AOM are consistent with these studies. The AAP acknowledges that younger children and children with more severe symptoms are most likely to benefit from antimicrobial therapy. The AAP suggests that "watchful waiting" should be considered only for children with minimal symptoms and children older than 2 [28].

Correlation between microbiologic and clinical end points

Effective antimicrobial therapy eradicates otopathogens from the middle ear space more rapidly than placebo or ineffective therapy [29,30]. Based on rigorously conducted double tympanocentesis studies, it has been observed repeatedly that the middle ear is sterilized within 3 to 5 days of initiation of appropriate antibiotic therapy. Dagan et al [31] reported that more than 95% of otopathogens are eradicated when high-dose amoxicillin-clavulanate or an experimental quinolone is prescribed. In contrast, less than 50% of isolates of nontypable *H. influenzae* are eradicated if an antimicrobial with insufficient *Haemophilus* activity is administered, and less than 20% of isolates of *S. pneumoniae* are eliminated when a macrolide is used in the therapy of AOM caused by multidrug-resistant *S. pneumoniae* [31–34]. The correlation between microbiologic and clinical outcome is incomplete, however, resulting in controversy as to which end points should be regarded as paramount [28]. Several studies have attempted to correlate the relationship between microbiologic eradication and symptomatic relief. The relative risk of persistent symptoms at the end of therapy (clinical failure) has been observed to be 5-fold to 14-fold greater among children when there is failure to eradicate bacterial otopathogens from the middle ear by day 4 to 6 of antibiotic treatment (Table 3) [31,32,35]. Dagan et al [31] reported that children with AOM in whom otopathogens persisted in the middle ear on days 4 to 6 had higher symptom scores (eg, fever, irritability, bulging tympanic membrane) compared with children in whom the middle ear contents were sterile. These studies support the concept that there would be more rapid clinical improvement if children were treated with antibiotics that result in early sterilization of middle ear fluid.

Role of watchful waiting

The decline in suppurative complications of AOM and decrease in the number of children with chronic otitis media has been attributed to the routine use of antibiotics for these infections in the United States over the past 50 years. Controversy over the benefits of routine antibiotic therapy has emerged, however, in light of the emergence of resistance among otopathogens. Meta-analyses of placebo-controlled clinical trials of antimicrobial therapy for AOM have suggested that many children need to be treated with antibiotics to realize a small benefit in outcome [36,37]. In the Netherlands, symptomatic therapy (antipyretics and analgesia) without the use of antibiotics is recommended for nontoxic children older than 6 months of age with AOM. Based on this practice, investigators in the Netherlands have concluded that although early symptom resolution is more frequent with amoxicillin therapy, the benefit is not sufficient to recommend routine antibiotic use in every child with AOM [26]. The AAP guidelines for the treatment of AOM include a "watchful waiting" option for nontoxic children older than 2 with AOM.

Table 3
Outcome of acute otitis media in children with and without sterilization of middle ear exudate on day 4–6

Study	Microbiologic outcome day 4–6	Clinical failure at end of treatment (%)	Relative risk of failure in culture-positive children
Carlin et al [33]	Culture +	38	5.4
	Culture −	7	
Dagan et al [32]	Culture +	37	12.3
	Culture −	3	
Piglansky et al [30]	Culture +	21	>14
	Culture −	0	

Therapy of acute otitis media

Selection of initial therapy

Acute otitis media usually is treated empirically because the specific otopathogen rarely is determined by tympanocentesis in clinical practice (Table 4). Cultures of material obtained from the nasopharynx may reflect the etiology of AOM because bacterial pathogens usually gain entry into the middle ear after ascent from the nasopharynx. Because the nasopharynx typically contains multiple otopathogens, however, the specificity of these cultures is limited. The specific etiology of AOM cannot be predicted reliably on the basis of clinical findings; however, clinicians can determine if the child is at high risk for disease resulting from an antibiotic-resistant otopathogen. Studies repeatedly have identified recent antibiotic exposure, young age, attendance at daycare, and residence in a community with high rates of antimicrobial resistance as risk features for infection with multidrug-resistant *S. pneumoniae* [38,39]. In this context, the term *multidrug resistance* refers to the observation that isolates of *S. pneumoniae* resistant to β-lactam antibiotics have a high likelihood of resistance to multiple classes of antimicrobials, including macrolides and trimethoprim-sulfamethoxazole [40]. In the absence of risk features, it is most likely that susceptible otopathogens will be present, and amoxicillin would achieve a successful outcome.

The AAP guidelines also suggest that severity of infection be considered in the selection of specific antimicrobial therapy. This concept evolves from evidence that more severe episodes of AOM are more likely to take a longer time for resolution or to fail therapy, justifying a different approach in the selection of therapy [24,40]. The classification of AOM by severity does not reflect a concern that such episodes are more likely to be caused by antibiotic-resistant pathogens.

Table 4
Antibiotic management of children with initial or uncomplicated episode of acute otitis media

Temperature ≥39°C, severe earache, or both	For treatment of initial episodes with antibacterial agents	
	Recommended	Alternative for penicillin allergy
No	Amoxicillin 80–90 mg/kg/d	Nontype I Cefdinir Cefuroxime Cefpodoxime Type I Azithromycin Clarithromycin
Yes	Amoxicillin-clavulanate 90/6.4 mg/kg/d	Nontype I Ceftriaxone (3 d)

Modified from Lieberthal AS, Ganiates TG, Cox EO, et al. Clinical practice guidelines: diagnosis and treatment of acute otitis media. Pediatrics 2004.

Rather, the goal of broader spectrum therapy in patients with severe infection is to increase the likelihood of effective sterilization of the middle ear with more rapid resolution of clinical signs and symptoms.

The AAP guidelines recommend amoxicillin, 90 mg/kg/d administered twice daily, as the antibiotic of choice for initial therapy in most children with AOM [28]. The major determinant of effectiveness for β-lactam antibiotics is the amount of time drug concentration in the middle ear exceeds the minimal inhibitory concentration (MIC) for a given pathogen [41]. In general, effective bacterial killing occurs when the serum concentration exceeds the MIC for 40% to 50% of the dosing interval [41]. Among β-lactam antibiotics, only oral "high-dose" amoxicillin and intramuscular ceftriaxone achieve middle ear concentrations high enough to exceed the MIC of all *S. pneumoniae* that are intermediately sensitive to penicillin and many, but not all, highly resistant strains and strains of nontypable *H. influenzae* that do not produce β-lactamases. Cefuroxime axetil, cefprozil, and cefpodoxime represent alternatives to high-dose amoxicillin; however, each agent achieves sufficient middle ear concentration to be effective against only approximately 50% of *S. pneumoniae* isolates that are intermediately susceptible to penicillin. Also, cefprozil has limited activity against nontypable *H. influenzae* [42]. Macrolides have limited efficacy in the therapy of AOM at current doses. Successful eradication of otopathogens requires sufficient extracellular middle ear concentrations with current dosing regimen. Extracellular middle ear fluid concentrations of macrolides are below the MIC for almost all nontypable *H. influenzae* and *S. pneumoniae* isolates that show either efflux or ribosomal mechanisms of resistance. Macrolides are able to sterilize the middle ear only when isolates of *S. pneumoniae* that are fully susceptible are present.

Amoxicillin-clavulanate is an alternative for initial therapy of children with "severe" disease, such as children with temperatures greater than 102°F and substantial otalgia. Amoxicillin is ineffective against β-lactamase–producing isolates of nontypable *H. influenzae*. Because amoxicillin-clavulanate resists destruction by the β-lactamase, it effectively eradicates middle ear infection caused by all nontypable *H. influenzae* isolates [32,43]. Although the AAP guidelines recommend the consideration of amoxicillin-clavulanate as initial therapy only for children with severe disease, the increasing prevalence of AOM resulting from nontypable *H. influenzae* associated with universal PCV7 immunization may warrant broader use of amoxicillin-clavulanate as first-line therapy in the future. Ongoing evaluation of the rate of treatment failure after therapy with amoxicillin is required to assess the relative merits of amoxicillin versus amoxicillin-clavulanate as initial therapy.

Initial therapy for a child with type I allergy to penicillin (urticaria, laryngeal spasm, wheezing, or anaphylaxis) is currently challenging. The choice of alternative classes of antimicrobials is limited by a substantial prevalence of resistance. Macrolides, including azithromycin and clarithromycin, show in vitro activity against most pneumococcal isolates; however, 25% to 40% of *S. pneumoniae* have MICs that are too high for these agents to be effective [44]. Resistance to trimethoprim-sulfamethoxazole among *S. pneumoniae* and nontypable

H. influenzae also is substantial in most communities [3]. The AAP guidelines acknowledge the potential limitations of these agents, but recommend their use as the best alternative. For a child with "severe" disease, a combination of agents, such as clindamycin (for *S. pneumoniae*) and sulfasoxazole (for nontypable *H. influenzae*), may be effective. In contrast to other macrolides, clindamycin is effective against isolates of *S. pneumoniae* with the efflux mechanism of resistance and maintains activity against approximately 90% of *S. pneumoniae* isolates in the United States.

Analgesia also should be used for children with AOM. A few studies suggest ibuprofen or acetaminophen is effective [45]. Topical agents (eg, Auralgan Otic) also may offer temporary symptomatic relief [46]. For children with severe pain, myringotomy is an effective method to attain relief.

Antimicrobial therapy in a child who fails to respond to initial therapy or with early recurrence

Two studies have evaluated the microbiology of AOM in children failing initial management (Table 5) [5,6]. Infection in this setting is enriched for otopathogens with reduced susceptibility to antimicrobial agents. β-lactamase–producing nontypable *H. influenzae* is the predominant pathogen, especially in children initially treated with amoxicillin, cefdinir, or cefpodoxime. Penicillin-resistant *S. pneumoniae* is found in a small proportion of cases. Dagan et al [43,47] showed that high-dose amoxicillin-clavulanate and multidose regimens of ceftriaxone sterilize the middle ear in greater than 95% of children when either of these pathogens is present. The AAP guidelines are consistent with these observations.

Options are limited for the treatment of a child with type I allergy to penicillin and persistent severe signs and symptoms or early recurrence of AOM. Performing a tympanocentesis to provide symptomatic relief and define the specific

Table 5
Antibiotic management of children with acute otitis media who fail initial treatment

Temperature ≥39°C, severe earache, or both	Clinically defined treatment failure at 48–72 hours after initial management with antibacterial agents	
	Recommended	Alternative for penicillin allergy
No	Amoxicillin-clavulanate 90/6.4 mg/kg/d	Nontype I Ceftriaxone 3 d Type I Clindamycin plus sulfonamide
Yes	Ceftriaxone 3 d	Tympanocentesis Clindamycin plus sulfonamide

Modified from Lieberthal AS, Ganiates TG, Cox EO, et al. Clinical practice guidelines: diagnosis and treatment of acute otitis media. Pediatrics 2004;113:1451–65.

etiology is one option. The use of combination therapy with clindamycin and sulfonamide may be effective but is limited by the need for multiple doses of each agent daily. Off-label use of a quinolone is another potential option. Studies of gatifloxacin show in vitro activity against virtually all isolates of nontypable *H. influenzae* and more than 98% of *S. pneumoniae* and rapid sterilization and clinical resolution of middle ear infection resulting from either of these pathogens [33].

Acute otitis media in a child with tympanostomy tubes

Acute otorrhea is the most common complication after tube insertion. *S. pneumoniae* and nontypable *H. influenzae* are the most common pathogens associated with acute otorrhea through a tympanostomy tube. *Staphylococcus aureus* and *Pseudomonas aeruginosa* are occasional pathogens under these circumstances. An increasing proportion of the *S. aureus* isolates, even isolates acquired in the community, are resistant to methicillin. Amoxicillin is generally effective for the therapy of acute otorrhea through a tympanostomy tube. Compared with placebo, amoxicillin results in rapid clearing of bacterial pathogens and a shortened duration of otorrhea [48]. An alternative to oral antimicrobial therapy is topical otic suspensions, either ofloxacin or ciprofloxacin. Both agents have shown efficacy, provide a broader spectrum of activity that includes *Pseudomonas* and quinolone-susceptible *Staphylococcus,* and exert little selective pressure on nasopharyngeal flora [49,50]. Topical vancomycin (25 mg/mL) drops seem to be effective when methicillin-resistant *S. aureus* is the putative etiologic agent [51].

Therapy for otitis media with effusion

The management of OME continues to be debated. More recent studies, including a meta-analysis, fail to show significant language delay or cognitive impairment in otherwise healthy children with persistent middle ear effusion, and spontaneous resolution occurs in most cases [52–54]. The management of OME with tympanostomy tube placement may not be benign. Consequences of tube placement may include recurrent otorrhea, persistent perforation, development of granulation tissue, chronic otitis media, and cholesteatoma [55]. Repeated insertions of tympanostomy tubes also have been associated with mild hearing loss, including a sensorineural component [56]. Guidelines on management of OME jointly published by the AAP and American Academy of Otolaryngology [55] stress the need to identify children at risk for speech, language, and cognitive impairment early in the course of disease. The guidelines assert that certain sensory, physical, cognitive, or behavioral features may increase the risk of developmental difficulties (Box 1) [56], and their presence should warrant earlier intervention. The guidelines recommend early hearing testing and language assessment and tympanostomy tube insertion in these situations. For otherwise

Box 1. Comorbid conditions that increase the risk for developmental difficulties in children with otitis media with effusion

1. Permanent hearing loss separate from OME
2. Suspected speech language delay or disorder
3. Autism spectrum disorders
4. Uncorrectable visual disorders or blindness
5. Cleft palate
6. Congenital syndromes associated with cognitive, speech, or language delays
7. Documented developmental delay of unknown etiology

healthy children, watchful waiting for 6 months, with hearing evaluation at 3 months, is suggested.

The primary intervention for OME is surgical; antihistamines and decongestants are ineffective, and therapy with antimicrobials or corticosteroids does not result in lasting benefit [55]. Tympanostomy tube insertion for otherwise healthy children is recommended when persistent hearing loss of 40 db or greater is documented, or symptomatic disease is present (balance difficulties or sleep disturbance associated with intermittent ear pain, fullness, or popping). Tympanostomy tube insertion results in improved hearing, a decrease in days spent with effusion, and decline in recurrent episodes of AOM. Adenoidectomy often is performed as an adjunct to tympanostomy tube placement in children older than 2 years of age undergoing tube reinsertion after spontaneous extrusion [55]. Adenoidectomy seems to reduce the need for subsequent tube insertions. Tonsillectomy alone and myringotomy alone are not effective interventions for OME.

Prevention of acute otitis media

The goals of prevention are a reduction in the burden of middle ear disease during the vulnerable period of speech and language development. Epidemiologic studies identify onset of disease early in the first year of life, male gender, and family history as risk features for frequently recurrent infections [56,57]. Although it is not possible to alter these factors, there are several environmental risks that increase the likelihood of respiratory infection and subsequent otitis media, and these factors can be altered. Most more recent studies identify daycare attendance as a major risk. Hypothetically, changing the daycare environment might reduce the frequency of AOM; however, definitive studies addressing this hypothesis have not been conducted. Breastfeeding for the first 6 months of life seems to delay the age of onset of AOM. Other risk factors for AOM that could be modulated, with the hope of reducing the frequency of recurrent infections, include use of pacifiers and exposure to passive tobacco smoke and indoor wood burning stoves. Antibiotic prophylaxis can be effective in reducing the frequency of AOM in otitis-prone children. Because chronic antibiotic use may result in the emergence of drug-resistant otopathogens, however, there has been a dramatic reduction in the use of this intervention [58,59]. Presently, antibiotic prophylaxis should be considered only for a severely afflicted child with multiple episodes of AOM occurring over a brief time. Prevention of recurrent episodes over a limited time is not curative, and most often recurrent episodes recur when prophylaxis is discontinued.

The use of influenza vaccine has been shown to reduce the frequency of AOM during the respiratory virus season [60,61]. The role of preceding influenza infection in the total burden of AOM is relatively small, however, and a substantial reduction in disease burden is not observed in immunized children [62]. Two studies clearly show a reduction in the number of pneumococcal episodes of AOM in children immunized with pneumococcal conjugate vaccines and a reduction in the frequency of all episodes of AOM. In these studies, the overall benefit of vaccination for reduction of recurrent AOM in an individual child is small, however [30,63]. It has been hypothesized that a more substantial reduction would be observed with immunization of a larger proportion of children than achieved in the clinical trials. Data to examine this hypothesis are still being collected. Immunization of an otitis-prone child with pneumococcal conjugate vaccine has not been proved to result in fewer overall episodes [64].

Summary

Successful therapy for AOM results in the rapid resolution of signs and symptoms of acute inflammation and reduction in fever. More rapid resolution accompanies the prompt use of antibiotics active against the infecting pathogen. Although controversial, some experts suggest that the magnitude of the benefit of prompt antibiotic therapy, low risk of suppurative complications, and emergence of otopathogens with reduced susceptibility to antimicrobial therapy justify a watchful waiting approach for children older than 2 with AOM, with antimicrobial therapy being reserved for children without spontaneous resolution. An alternative approach for reducing unnecessary antibiotic use is a continued refining of diagnostic criteria that distinguish AOM from OME.

Amoxicillin is the drug of choice for the initial therapy of uncomplicated AOM. An increase in the proportion of disease resulting from nontypable *H. influenzae,* as a result of universal immunization of infants and toddlers with PCV7, requires careful monitoring. If this trend continues, and if the rate of treatment failure increases, amoxicillin-clavulanate may become the agent recommended for initial therapy. For children failing initial therapy with amoxicillin, β-lactamase–producing nontypable *H. influenzae* has become an important etiology, and antimicrobial therapy should have a spectrum of activity that includes this otopathogen.

Currently, there are limited strategies that are likely to lessen substantially the burden of AOM early in life. The efficacy of vaccination with PCV7 has not been determined fully because clinical trials that immunized only a small fraction of the population do not provide the herd benefit that would be observed when vaccine supply is sufficiently replete to support universal immunization. The frequency of infections caused by vaccine serotypes would be reduced. In addition, it is likely that there would continue to be an increasing proportion of nonvaccine serotypes of pneumococcus and other pathogens causing AOM. This shift toward less virulent otopathogens can be expected to have a favorable impact on the course of a typical episode of AOM.

References

[1] Eskola J, Kilpi T, Palmu A, et al. Efficacy of a pneumococcal conjugate vaccine against acute otitis media. N Engl J Med 2001;344:403–9.

[2] McEllistrem MC, Adams J, Mason EO, Wald ER. Epidemiology of acute otitis media caused by *Streptococcus pneumoniae* before and after licensure of the 7-valent pneumococcal protein conjugate vaccine. J Infect Dis 2003;188:1679–84.

[3] Pelton SI, Loughlin A, Marchant CD. Seven valent pneumococcal vaccine immunization in two Boston communities: changes in serotypes distribution and antimicrobial susceptibility among *Streptococcus pneumoniae* isolates. Pediatr Infect Dis J 2004;23:1015–22.

[4] Ghaffar F, Barton T, Lozano J, et al. Effect of 7-valent pneumococcal conjugate vaccine on nasopharyngeal colonization by *Streptococcus pneumoniae* in the first two years of life. Clin Infect Dis 2004;39(7):930–8.

[5] Block SL, Hecrick J, Harrison CJ, et al. Community-wide vaccination with the heptavalent pneumococcal conjugate significantly alters the microbiology of acute otitis media. Pediatr Infect Dis J 2004;23:829–33.

[6] Casey JR, Pickickero ME. Change in frequency and pathogens causing acute otitis media in 1995–2003. Pediatr Infect Dis J 2004;23:824–8.

[7] Porat N, Barkai G, Jacobs MR, Trefler R, Dagan R. Four antibiotic-resistant *Streptococcus pneumoniae* clones unrelated to the pneumococcal conjugate vaccine serotypes, including 2 new serotypes, causing acute otitis media in southern Israel. J Infect Dis 2004;189:385–92.

[8] Leibovitz E, Greenberg D, Piglansky L, et al. Recurrent acute otitis media occurring within one month from completion of antibiotic therapy: relationship to the original pathogen. Pediatr Infect Dis J 2003;22:209–15.

[9] Leibovitz E, Libson S, Greenberg D, Porat N, Leiberman A, Dagan R. The presence of *Streptococcus pneumoniae* (Pnc) in nasopharynx (NP) after successful treatment of acute otitis media (AOM) predicts its etiologic role in the next AOM episode. Abstract No. G-1855–2003. Presented at 44th ICAAC. Washington, DC, October 30, 2004.

[10] Finkelstein JA, Stille C, Nordin J, et al. Reduction in antibiotic use among US children 1999–2000. Pediatrics 2003;112:620–7.

[11] Pelton SI. Otoscopy for the diagnosis of otitis media. Pediatr Infect Dis J 1998;17:540–3.

[12] Blomgren K, Pohjavuori S, Poussa T, Hatakka K, Korpela R, Pitkaranta A. Effect of accurate diagnostic criteria on incidence of acute otitis media in otitis-prone children. Scand J Infect Dis 2004;36:6–9.

[13] Pichichero ME, Poole MD. Assessing diagnostic accuracy and tympanocentesis skill in the management of otitis media. Arch Pediatr Adolesc Med 2001;155:P1137–42.

[14] Leibovitz E, Satran R, Piglansky L, et al. Can acute otitis media caused by *Haemophilus influenzae* be distinguished from that caused by *Streptococcus pneumoniae*? Pediatr Infect Dis J 2003;22:509–14.

[15] Rodriguez WJ, Schwartz RH. *Streptococcus pneumoniae* causes otitis media with higher fever and more redness of tympanic membranes than *Haemophilus influenzae* or *Moraxella catarrhalis*. Pediatr Infect Dis J 1999;18:942–4.
[16] Palmu AA, Herva E, Savolainen H, Karma P, Makela PH, Kilpi TM. Association of clinical signs and symptoms with bacterial findings in acute otitis media. Clin Infect Dis 2004;38:234–42.
[17] Dagan R, Leibovitz E, Greenberg D, et al. Early eradication of pathogens from middle ear fluid during antibiotic treatment of acute otitis media is associated with improved clinical outcome. Pediatr Infect Dis J 1998;17:776–82.
[18] Bodor EF. Conjunctivitis-otitis syndrome. Pediatrics 1982;69:695–8.
[19] Dhooge IJM, Albers FWJ, Van Cauwenberge PB. Intratemporal and intracranial complications of acute suppurative otitis media in children: renewed interest. Int J Pediatr Otorhinolaryngol 1999;49:S109–14.
[20] Bahadori RS, Schwartz RH, Ziai M. Acute mastoiditis in children: an increase in frequency Northern Virginia. Pediatr Infect Dis J 2000;19:212–5.
[21] Ghaffar FA, Wördemann M, McCracken Jr H. Acute mastoiditis in children: a seventeen-year experience in Dallas, Texas. Pediatr Infect Dis J 2001;20:376–80.
[22] Leskinen K, Jero J. Complication of acute otitis media in children in southern Finland. Int J Pediatr Otorhinolaryngol 2004;68:317–24.
[23] Kacmarynski DS, Levine SC, Pearson SE, Maisel RH. Complications of otitis media before placement of tympanostomy tubes in children. Arch Otolaryngol Head Neck Surg 2004;103: 289–92.
[24] Kaleida PH, Casselbrant ML, Rockette HE, et al. Amoxicillin or myringotomy or both for acute otitis media: results of a randomized clinical trial. Pediatrics 1991;87:466–74.
[25] Little P, Gould C, Williamson I, Moore M, Warner G, Dunleavey J. Pragmatic randomized controlled trial of two prescribing strategies for childhood acute otitis media. BMJ 2001;322: 336–42.
[26] Damoiseaux RAMJ, van Balen FAM, Hoes AW, et al. Primary care based randomized double blind trial of amoxicillin versus placebo for acute otitis media in children aged under 2 years. BMJ 2000;320:350–4.
[27] McCormick DP, Chonmaitree T, Pittman C, et al. Non-severe acute otitis media: a clinical trial comparing outcomes of watchful waiting versus immediate antibiotic treatment. Presented at the Pediatric Academic Society, San Francisco, 2004.
[28] Lieberthal AS, Ganiates TG, Cox EO, et al. Clinical practice guidelines: diagnosis and treatment of acute otitis media. Pediatrics 2004;113:1451–65.
[29] Schaad UB. Correlation between bacteriologic eradication and clinical cure in acute otitis media. Pediatr Infect Dis J 2004;23:281–2.
[30] Dagan R. Correlation between bacteriologic eradication and clinical cure in acute otitis media: in reply. Pediatr Infect Dis J 2004;23:281–2.
[31] Dagan R, Leibovitz E, Greenberg D, Yagupsky P, Fliss DM, Leiberman A. Early eradication of pathogens from middle ear fluid during antibacterial agent treatment of acute otitis media is associated with improved clinical outcome. Pediatr Infect Dis J 1998;17:776–82.
[32] Piglansky L, Leibovitz E, Raiz S, et al. Bacteriologic and clinical efficacy of high dose amoxicillin for therapy of acute otitis media in children. Pediatr Infect J 2003;22:405–12.
[33] Leibovitz E, Piglanksky L, Raiz S, et al. Bacteriological and clinical efficacy of oral gatifloxacinin the treatment of recurrent/non-responsive acute otitis media: an open label, single center, non-comparative, double tympanocentesis study. Pediatr Infect Dis J 2003;22:1–7.
[34] Carlin SA, Marchant CD, Shurin PA, Johnson CE, Super DM. Host factors and early therapeutic response in acute otitis media. J Pediatr 1991;118:178–83.
[35] Leiberman A, Leibovitz E, Piglansky L, et al. Bacteriologic and clinical efficacy of TMP/SMX for the treatment of AOM. Pediatr Infect Dis J 2001;20:260–4.
[36] Rosenfeld RM, Vertrees JE, Carr J, et al. Clinical efficacy of antibacterial drugs for acute otitis media: meta-analysis of 5400 children from thirty-three randomized trials. J Pediatr 1994;124: 355–67.

[37] Rosenfeld RM, Kay D. Natural history of untreated otitis media. In: Rosenfeld RM, Bluestone CD, editors. Evidence-based otitis media. Hamilton, Ontario: Decker; 2003. p. 180–98.
[38] Dowell SF, Butler JC, Giebink SG, et al. The Drug-resistant *Streptococcus pneumoniae* Therapeutic Working Group. Acute otitis media: management and surveillance in an era of pneumococcal resistance—a report from the Drug-resistant Streptococcus pneumoniae Therapeutic Working Group. Pediatr Infect Dis J 1999;18:1–9.
[39] Dowell SF, Marcy SM, Phillips WR, Gerber MA, Schwartz B. Otitis media—principles of judicious use of antimicrobial agents. Pediatrics 1998;101:165–71.
[40] Little P, Gould C, Moore M, Warner G, Dunleavey J, Williamson I. Predictors of poor outcome and benefits from antibacterial agents in children with acute otitis media: pragmatic randomized trial. BMJ 2002;325:22.
[41] Craig W. Pharmacokinetic/pharmacodynamic parameters: rationale for antibacterial dosing of mice and men. Clin Infect Dis 1998;26:1–12.
[42] Jacobs MR. Increasing antibiotic resistance among otitis media pathogens and their susceptibility to oral agents based on pharmacodynamic parameters. Pediatr Infect Dis J 2000;19:S47–55.
[43] Dagan R, Hoberman A, Johnson C, et al. Bacteriologic and clinical efficacy of high dose amoxicillin/clavulanate in children with acute otitis media. Pediatr Infect Dis J 2001;20:829–37.
[44] Dagan R, Leibovitz E, Fliss DM, et al. Bacteriologic efficacies of oral azithromycin and oral cefaclor in treatment of acute otitis media in infants and young children. Antimicrob Agents Chemother 2000;44:43–50.
[45] Bertin L, Pons G, d'Athis P, et al. A randomized, double-blind, multicenter controlled trial of ibuprofen versus acetaminophen and placebo for symptoms of acute otitis media in children. Fundam Clin Pharmacol 1996;10:387–92.
[46] Hoberman A, Paradise JL, Reynolds EA, Urkin J. Efficacy of auralgan for treating ear pain in children with acute otitis media. Arch Pediatr Adolesc Med 1997;151:675–8.
[47] Leibovitz E, Piglansky L, Raiz S, Press J, Leiberman A, Dagan R. Bacteriologic and clinical efficacy of one day vs. three day intramuscular ceftriaxone for treatment of nonresponsive acute otitis media in children. Pediatr Infect Dis J 2000;19:1040–5.
[48] Ruohola A, Heikkinen T, Meurman O, Puhakka T, Lindblad N, Ruuskanen O. Antibiotic treatment of acute otorrhea through tympanostomy tube: randomized double-blind placebo-controlled study with daily follow- up. Pediatrics 2003;111:1061–7.
[49] Roland PS, Dohar JE, Lanier BJ, et al. Topical ciproflaxacin/dexamethosone otic suspension is superior to ofloxacin otic solution in the treatment of granulation tissue in children with acute otitis media with otorrhea through tympanostomy tubes. Otolaryngol Head Neck Surg 2004; 130:736–41.
[50] Dohar JE, Garner ET, Nielsen RW, et al. Topical ofloxacin treatment of otorrhea in children with tympanostomy tubes. Arch Otolaryngol Head Neck Surg 1999;125:537–45.
[51] Hwang JH, Tsai HY, Liu TC. Community-acquired methicillin-resistant *Staphylococcus aureus* infections in discharging ears. Acta Otolyaryngol 2002;122:827–30.
[52] Paradise JL, Feldman HM, Campbell TF, et al. Early versus delayed insertion of tympanostomy tubes for persistent otitis media: developmental outcomes at the age of three years in relation to prerandomization illness patterns and hearing levels. Pediatr Infect Dis J 2003;22:309–14.
[53] Roberts J, Hunter L, Gravel J, et al. Otitis media, hearing loss and language learning: controversies and current research. Dev Behav Pediatr 2004;25:110–22.
[54] Roberts JE, Rosenfeld RM, Zeisel SA. Otitis media and speech and language: a meta-analysis of prospective studies. Pediatrics 2004;113:e238–48.
[55] Rosenfeld RM, Culpepper L, Doyle KJ, et al. Clinical practice guideline: otitis media with effusion. Otolaryngol Head Neck Surg 2004;130:s95–118.
[56] Daly KA, Casselbrant ML, Hoffman HJ, et al. Epidemiology, natural history and risk factors. Ann Otol Rhinolaryngol 2002;111:19–25.
[57] Daly KA, Giebink GS. Clinical epidemiology of otitis media. Pediatr Infect Dis J 2000; 19(Suppl 5):S31–6.
[58] Casselbrant ML, Kaleida PH, Rockette HE, Paradise JL, Bluestone CD, Kurs-Lasky M. Efficacy

of antimicrobial prophylaxis and of tympanostomy tube insertion for prevention of recurrent acute otitis media: results of a randomized clinical trial. Pediatr Infect Dis J 1992;11:278–86.

[59] Williams RL, Chalmers TC, Stange KC, Chalmers FT, Bowlin SJ. Use of antibiotics in preventing recurrent acute otitis media and in treating otitis media with effusion: a meta-analytic attempt to resolve the brouhaha. JAMA 1993;270:1344–51.

[60] Clements DA, Langdon L, Bland C, et al. Influenza A vaccine decreases the incidence of otitis media in 6- to 30-month-old children in day care. Arch Pediatr Adolesc Med 1995;149:1113–7.

[61] Belshe RB, Gruber WC. Prevention of otitis media in children with live attenuated influenza vaccine given intranasally. Pediatr Infect Dis J 2000;19(Suppl 5):S66–71.

[62] Hoberman A, Greenberg DP, Paradise JL, et al. Efficacy of inactivated influenza vaccine in preventing acute otitis media in young children: a randomized controlled trial. JAMA 2003;290:1608–16.

[63] Fireman B, Black SB, Shinefield HR, Lee J, Lewis E, Ray P. Impact of the pneumococcal conjugate vaccine on otitis media. Pediatr Infect Dis J 2003;22:10–6.

[64] Veenhoiven R, Bogaert D, Uiterwaal C, et al. Effect of conjugate pneumococcal vaccine followed by polysaccharide pneumococcal vaccine on recurrent acute otitis media: a randomized study. Lancet 2003;361:2189–95.

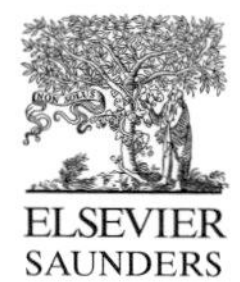

ELSEVIER
SAUNDERS

Pediatr Clin N Am 52 (2005) 729–747

PEDIATRIC CLINICS
OF NORTH AMERICA

Diagnosis and Treatment of Pharyngitis in Children

Michael A. Gerber, MD[a,b,*]

[a]Department of Pediatrics, University of Cincinnati College of Medicine, Cincinnati, OH 45229, USA
[b]Division of Infectious Diseases MC 5019, Cincinnati Children's Hospital Medical Center, 3333 Burnet Avenue, Cincinnati, OH 45229, USA

Pharyngitis is an inflammation of the mucous membranes and underlying structures of the throat. Acute pharyngitis is one of the most common illnesses for which children visit primary care physicians; pediatricians in the United States make the diagnosis of acute pharyngitis, acute tonsillitis, or streptococcal sore throat more than 7 million times annually [1]. Many viral and bacterial agents are capable of producing pharyngitis, either as a separate entity or as part of a more generalized illness (Table 1). Most cases of acute pharyngitis in children are caused by viruses and are benign and self-limited. Group A beta-hemolytic streptococcus (GAS) is the most important of the bacterial causes of acute pharyngitis. Strategies for the diagnosis and treatment of pharyngitis are directed at distinguishing children with viral pharyngitis, who would not benefit from antimicrobial therapy, from children with group A beta-hemolytic streptococcal pharyngitis, for whom antimicrobial therapy would be beneficial. Making this distinction is crucial in attempting to minimize the unnecessary use of antimicrobial agents in children.

Etiology

Viruses are the most common cause of acute pharyngitis in children. Respiratory viruses, such as influenza virus, parainfluenza virus, rhinovirus,

* Division of Infectious Diseases MC 5019, Cincinnati Children's Hospital Medical Center, 3333 Burnet Avenue, Cincinnati, OH 45229.

E-mail address: michael.gerber@cchmc.org

doi:10.1016/j.pcl.2005.02.004 **pediatric.theclinics.com**

Table 1
Etiology of acute pharyngitis

Etiologic agent	Associated disorders or clinical findings
Bacterial	
Streptococci	
Group A	Scarlet fever
Groups C and G	
Mixed anaerobes	Vincent's angina
Neisseria gonorrhoeae	
Corynebacterium diphtheriae	Diphtheria
Arcanobacterium haemolyticum	Scarlatiniform rash
Yersinia enterocolitica	Enterocolitis
Yersinia pestis	Plague
Francisella tularensis	Tularemia (oropharyngeal form)
Viral	
Rhinovirus	Common cold
Coronavirus	Common cold
Adenovirus	Pharyngoconjunctival fever; acute respiratory disease
Herpes simplex virus types 1 and 2	Gingivostomatitis
Parainfluenza virus	Common cold; croup
Coxsackievirus A	Herpangina; hand-foot-and-mouth disease
Epstein-Barr virus	Infectious mononucleosis
Cytomegalovirus	Cytomegalovirus mononucleosis
HIV	Primary HIV infection
Influenza A and B viruses	Influenza
Mycoplasmal: *Mycoplasma pneumoniae*	Acute respiratory disease; pneumonia
Chlamydial	
Chlamydia psittaci	Acute respiratory disease; pneumonia
Chlamydia pneumoniae	Pneumonia

Modified from Bisno AL, Gerber MA, Gwaltney JM, Kaplan EL, Schwartz RH. Practice guideline for the diagnosis and management of group A streptococcal pharyngitis. Clin Infect Dis 2002;35:113–25.

coronavirus, adenovirus, and respiratory syncytial virus, are frequent causes of acute pharyngitis. Other viral causes of acute pharyngitis include coxsackievirus, echovirus, and herpes simplex virus. Epstein-Barr virus is a frequent cause of acute pharyngitis that is often accompanied by other clinical findings of infectious mononucleosis (eg, splenomegaly, generalized lymphadenopathy). Systemic infections with other viral agents, including cytomegalovirus, rubella virus, and measles virus, may be associated with acute pharyngitis.

GAS is the most common bacterial cause of acute pharyngitis, accounting for 15% to 30% of cases of acute pharyngitis in children. Other bacteria also can cause acute pharyngitis, however, including groups C and G beta-hemolytic streptococci and *Corynebacterium diphtheriae*. *Arcanobacterium haemolyticum* is a rare cause of acute pharyngitis, particularly in teenagers, and *Neisseria gonorrhoeae* occasionally can cause acute pharyngitis in sexually active adolescents. Other bacteria, such as *Francisella tularensis* and *Yersinia enterocolitica,* and mixed infections with anaerobic bacteria (eg, Vincent's angina) are rare causes of acute pharyngitis. *Chlamydia pneumoniae* and *Mycoplasma pneumoniae* have been implicated as causes of acute pharyngitis, particularly in adults. Although other bacteria, such as *Staphylococcus aureus, Haemophilus influenzae,* and *Streptococcus pneumoniae,* are cultured frequently from the throats of children with acute pharyngitis, their etiologic role in this disease has not been established.

Epidemiology

Most cases of pharyngitis occur during the colder months of the year, when respiratory viruses (eg, rhinovirus, coronavirus, influenza virus, and adenovirus) are prevalent. Spread among family members in the home is a prominent feature of the epidemiology of most of these agents, with children being the major reservoir of infection. Group A beta-hemolytic streptococcal pharyngitis is primarily a disease of children age 5 to 15. In temperate climates, it usually occurs in the winter and early spring.

The incidence of gonococcal pharyngitis is highest among older adolescents and young adults. The usual route of infection is orogenital sexual contact with an infected sexual partner. Sexual abuse must be strongly considered if *N. gonorrhoeae* is isolated from the pharynx of a prepubertal child. Widespread immunization with diphtheria toxoid has made diphtheria a rare disease in the United States, with fewer than five cases reported annually in recent years.

Groups C and G beta-hemolytic streptococci can cause acute pharyngitis with clinical features similar to those of group A beta-hemolytic streptococcal pharyngitis. Group C streptococcus is a relatively common cause of acute pharyngitis among college students and adults evaluated in emergency departments [2,3]. Group C streptococcus also can cause epidemic food-borne pharyngitis; family and school outbreaks of group C streptococcal pharyngitis related to ingestion of contaminated food products, such as unpasteurized cow's milk, have been described [4]. Although there have been several well-documented food-borne outbreaks of group G streptococcal pharyngitis, the etiologic role of group G streptococcus in acute, endemic pharyngitis is unclear. A community-wide, respiratory outbreak of group G streptococcal pharyngitis in a pediatric population was described in which group G streptococcus was isolated from 56 of 222 (25%) consecutive children with acute pharyngitis seen in a private pediatric office [5]. Results of DNA fingerprinting of the group G streptococcus isolates suggested that 75% of them were the same strain.

The role of groups C and G streptococci in acute pharyngitis may be underestimated for several reasons. Anaerobic incubation increases the yield of these organisms, but many laboratories do not use anaerobic incubation routinely for throat cultures. In addition, because many groups C and G streptococci are bacitracin resistant, and laboratories may report only bacitracin-sensitive streptococci (consistent with GAS), many groups C and G streptococci would be missed. Finally, many clinicians no longer perform throat cultures, but instead rely solely on rapid antigen detection tests (RADTs), and groups C and G streptococci would not be identified by a RADT for GAS [6].

Clinical manifestations

Acute group A beta-hemolytic streptococcal pharyngitis has certain clinical characteristics and epidemiologic patterns (Table 2). Patients with group A beta-hemolytic streptococcal pharyngitis commonly present with sore throat (generally of sudden onset), severe pain on swallowing, and fever. Headache, nausea, vomiting, and abdominal pain also may be present. On examination, patients typically have tonsillopharyngeal erythema with or without exudates and tender, enlarged anterior cervical lymph nodes. Other findings include a beefy, red, swollen uvula; petechiae on the palate; excoriated nares (especially in infants); and a scarlitiniform rash. None of these findings is specific for group A beta-hemolytic streptococcal pharyngitis. Many patients with streptococcal pharyngitis exhibit signs and symptoms that are milder than a "classic" case of this illness. Some of these patients have bona fide group A beta-hemolytic streptococcal pharyngitis, whereas others are merely colonized with GAS and have pharyngitis resulting from an intercurrent viral illness.

Scarlet fever is an upper respiratory tract infection associated with a characteristic rash, which is caused by an infection with pyrogenic exotoxin (erythrogenic toxin)–producing GAS in individuals who do not have antitoxin antibodies. Scarlet fever is encountered less commonly and is less virulent than in the past, but the incidence is cyclical, depending on the prevalence of toxin-producing strains and the immune status of the population. The modes of trans-

Table 2
Clinical and epidemiologic findings and diagnosis of group A streptococcal pharyngitis

Features suggesting group A streptococcus as etiologic agent
Sudden onset
Sore throat
Fever
Scarlet fever rash
Headache
Nausea, vomiting, and abdominal pain
Inflammation of pharynx and tonsils
Patchy discrete exudates
Tender, enlarged anterior cervical nodes
Patient age 5–15 y
Presentation in winter or early spring
History of exposure
Features suggesting viral etiology
Conjunctivitis
Coryza
Cough
Diarrhea
Characteristic exanthems
Characteristic enanthems

Modified from Bisno AL, Gerber MA, Gwaltney JM, Kaplan EL, Schwartz RH. Practice guideline for the diagnosis and management of group A streptococcal pharyngitis. Clin Infect Dis 2002;35:113–25.

mission, age distribution, and other epidemiologic features are otherwise similar to the features for group A beta-hemolytic streptococcal pharyngitis.

The rash of scarlet fever appears within 24 to 48 hours after the onset of symptoms, although it may appear with the first signs of illness. The rash often begins around the neck and spreads over the trunk and extremities. It is a diffuse, finely papular, erythematous eruption producing a bright red discoloration of the skin, which blanches on pressure. Involvement is often more intense along the creases of the elbows, axillae, and groin. The involved skin has a goose-pimple appearance and feels rough. The face is usually spared, although the cheeks may be erythematous with pallor around the mouth. After 3 to 4 days, the rash begins to fade and is followed by desquamation, first on the face, progressing downward, and often resembling that seen after a mild sunburn. Occasionally, sheetlike desquamation may occur around the free margins of the fingernails, palms, and soles. Examination of the pharynx of a patient with scarlet fever reveals essentially the same findings as with group A beta-hemolytic streptococcal pharyngitis. In addition, the tongue usually is coated, and the papillae are swollen. After desquamation, the reddened papillae are prominent, giving the tongue a strawberry appearance.

The absence of fever or the presence of clinical features such as conjunctivitis, cough, hoarseness, coryza, anterior stomatitis, discrete ulcerative lesions, viral exanthem, and diarrhea suggests a viral etiology rather than GAS. Acute pharyngitis caused by adenovirus typically is associated with fever, erythema of the pharynx, enlarged tonsils with exudate, and enlarged cervical lymph nodes. Adenoviral pharyngitis may be associated with conjunctivitis, and, when it is, it is referred to as pharyngoconjunctival fever. The pharyngitis of pharyngoconjunctival fever can persist for 7 days, the conjunctivitis can persist for 14 days, and both resolve spontaneously. Outbreaks of pharyngoconjunctival fever have been associated with transmission in swimming pools; widespread epidemics and sporadic cases also occur.

Enteroviruses (coxsackievirus, echovirus, and newer enteroviruses) can cause acute pharyngitis, especially during the summer and early fall. The pharynx may be erythematous, but tonsillar exudate and cervical adenopathy are unusual. Fever may be prominent. Resolution usually occurs within a few days. Herpangina is a specific syndrome caused by coxsackievirus A or B or echoviruses and is characterized by fever and painful, discrete, gray-white papulovesicular lesions on an erythematous base in the posterior oropharynx. These lesions become ulcerative and usually resolve within 7 days. Hand-foot-mouth disease is a specific syndrome caused by coxsackievirus A16. It is characterized by painful vesicles and ulcers throughout the oropharynx associated with vesicles on the palms, soles, and sometimes on the trunk or extremities. These lesions usually resolve within 7 days.

Primary oral herpes simplex virus infections usually occur in young children and typically produce acute gingivostomatitis associated with ulcerating vesicular lesions throughout the anterior mouth, including the lips, but sparing the posterior pharynx. The gingivostomatitis can last 2 weeks and often is associated with high fever. The pain may be intense, and the oral intake of fluids may be impaired, leading to dehydration. Herpes simplex virus also can produce a mild pharyngitis in adolescents and adults that may or may not be associated with typical ulcerating vesicular lesions.

Acute pharyngitis is a common finding in adolescents and young adults with infectious mononucleosis caused by Epstein-Barr virus. The pharyngitis of infectious mononucleosis can be severe with clinical findings virtually identical to those of group A beta-hemolytic streptococcal pharyngitis. Generalized lymphadenopathy and hepatosplenomegaly also may be present, however. Fever and pharyngitis typically last 1 to 3 weeks; the lymphadenopathy and hepatosplenomegaly resolve over 3 to 6 weeks. Laboratory findings include the presence of atypical lymphocytosis, heterphil antibody, and specific antibodies to Epstein-Barr virus antigens.

The acute pharyngitis caused by *A. haemolyticum* may closely resemble group A beta-hemolytic streptococcal pharyngitis, including the presence of a scarlitiniform rash in many patients. In rare cases, *A. haemolyticum* can produce a membranous pharyngitis that can be confused with diphtheria.

Pharyngeal diphtheria is characterized by a grayish brown pseudomembrane that may be limited to one or both tonsils or may extend widely to involve the nares, uvula, soft palate, pharynx, larynx, and tracheobronchial tree. Involvement of the tracheobronchial tree may lead to life-threatening respiratory obstruction. Soft tissue edema and prominent cervical and submental lymphadenopathy may create a bull-neck appearance.

Diagnosis

The decision to perform a microbiologic test on a patient presenting with acute pharyngitis should be based on the clinical and epidemiologic characteristics of the illness (see Table 2). A history of close contact with a well-documented case of group A beta-hemolytic streptococcal pharyngitis or a high prevalence of group A beta-hemolytic streptococcal infections in the community also may be helpful. Testing usually does not need to be performed on patients with acute pharyngitis whose clinical and epidemiologic features do not suggest GAS as the etiology. Selective use of diagnostic studies for GAS not only increases the proportion of positive test results, but also the percentage of patients with positive tests who are truly infected rather than merely GAS carriers.

Efforts have been made to incorporate clinical and epidemiologic features of acute pharyngitis into scoring systems that attempt to predict the probability that a particular illness is caused by GAS [7–9]. These clinical scoring systems are helpful in identifying patients at such low risk of infection with GAS that a throat culture or RADT is usually unnecessary. The signs and symptoms of group A beta-hemolytic streptococcal and non–group A beta-hemolytic streptococcal pharyngitis overlap too broadly, however, and the clinical diagnosis of group A beta-hemolytic streptococcal pharyngitis cannot be made with accuracy even by the most experienced physicians. Guidelines from the Infectious Diseases Society of America (IDSA) [10], American Academy of Pediatrics [11], and American Heart Association [12] indicate that microbiologic confirmation (with a throat culture or RADT) is required for the diagnosis of group A beta-hemolytic streptococcal pharyngitis.

New practice guidelines from the Centers for Disease Control and Prevention (CDC), American Academy of Family Physicians (AAFP), and American College of Physicians–American Society of Internal Medicine (ACP-ASIM) recommend the use of a clinical algorithm without microbiologic confirmation as an acceptable approach to the diagnosis of group A beta-hemolytic streptococcal pharyngitis in adults only [12,13]. Although the goal of this algorithm-based strategy was to reduce the inappropriate use of antibiotics in adults with pharyngitis, there was concern that their use would result in the administration of antimicrobial treatment to an unacceptably large number of adults with non–group A beta-hemolytic streptococcal pharyngitis [14].

The authors of the CDC/AAFP/ACP-ASIM guidelines suggested that prospective studies should be conducted to compare this particular strategy with other strategies in terms of relevant patient outcomes and cost. McIsaac et al [15] performed a retrospective analysis to assess the impact of six different guidelines (including the IDSA and CDC/AAFP/ACIP-ASIM guidelines) on identification and treatment of group A beta-hemolytic streptococcal pharyngitis in children and adults. Guidelines that recommend selective use of RADTs or throat cultures and treatment based only on positive test results significantly reduced the inappropriate use of antibiotics in adults. In contrast, the empirical strategy proposed in the CDC/AAFP/ACIP-ASIM guidelines resulted in the administration of unnecessary antibiotics to an unacceptably large number of adults. Before abandoning the concept of treatment only after laboratory confirmation of GAS in adults with pharyngitis (IDSA guideline), additional prospective studies need to be performed to compare empirical and laboratory-based strategies in terms of relevant patient outcomes and cost.

Throat cultures

Culture of a specimen obtained by throat swab on a sheep blood agar plate is the standard laboratory procedure for the microbiologic confirmation of the clinical diagnosis of acute group A beta-hemolytic streptococcal pharyngitis [16]. If performed correctly, a single throat swab has a sensitivity of 90% to 95% in detecting the presence of GAS in the pharynx [17].

Several variables may affect the accuracy of the throat culture results. One of the most important is the manner in which the swab is obtained [18,19]. Throat swab specimens should be obtained from the surface of both tonsils (or tonsillar fossae) and the posterior pharyngeal wall. Other areas of the pharynx and mouth are not acceptable sites and should not be touched during the culturing procedure. Even with an appropriately collected specimen, false-negative results may be obtained if the patient has received antibiotics before the throat swab is taken.

Anaerobic incubation and the use of selective culture media have been reported to increase the sensitivity of throat cultures [20,21]. The data regarding the impact of the atmosphere of incubation and the culture media conflict, however, and, in the absence of definite benefit, the increased cost and effort associated with anaerobic incubation and selective culture media are difficult to justify, particularly for physicians processing throat cultures in their own offices [22–24].

Duration of incubation is another variable that can affect the yield of throat cultures. When plated, cultures should be incubated at 35°C to 37°C for 18 to 24 hours before reading. An additional overnight incubation at room temperature would identify a considerable number of positive throat cultures, however, that would not otherwise have been identified. Armengol et al [25] found that more than 40% of the positive confirmatory throat cultures obtained on patients with pharyngitis and negative RADTs were negative after 24 hours of incubation, but positive after 48 hours. Although initial therapeutic decisions may be made on the basis of an overnight culture, it is advisable to examine plates that are negative at 24 hours again at 48 hours.

The clinical significance of the number of colonies of GAS present on the throat culture plate is controversial. Patients with bona fide acute group A beta-hemolytic streptococcal pharyngitis are likely to have more colonies of GAS on their culture plates than patients who are GAS carriers. There is too much overlap in the colony count, however, between patients acutely infected with GAS and GAS carriers to permit differentiation on the basis of degree of positivity [24].

Probably the most widely used test for differentiation of GAS from other beta-hemolytic streptococci in physicians' offices is the bacitracin disk test. This test provides a presumptive identification based on the observation that greater than 95% of GAS show a zone of inhibition around a disk containing 0.04 units of bacitracin, whereas 83% to 97% of non-GAS are not inhibited by bacitracin [24].

An alternative and highly specific method for the differentiation of GAS from other beta-hemolytic streptococci is the detection of the group-specific cell wall carbohydrate antigen directly on isolated bacterial colonies. Commercial kits employing group-specific antisera are available for this purpose. Such tests are appropriate for use by clinical microbiology laboratories, but most physicians performing throat cultures would find it difficult to justify the additional expense for the minimal improvement in accuracy that serogrouping of beta-hemolytic streptococci would provide over the bacitracin disk test [24].

Rapid antigen detection tests

The major disadvantage of culturing a specimen obtained by throat swab on blood agar plates is the delay in obtaining culture results. RADTs have been developed for the identification of GAS directly from throat swabs. Although RADTs are more expensive than blood agar plate cultures, the advantage they offer over the traditional procedure is the speed with which they can provide results. Rapid identification and treatment of patients with group A beta-hemolytic streptococcal pharyngitis can reduce the risk of the spread of GAS, allow the patient to return to school or work sooner, and speed clinical improvement [17,26]. In addition, in certain environments (eg, emergency departments), the use of RADTs has been shown to increase significantly the number of patients appropriately treated for group A beta-hemolytic streptococcal pharyngitis compared with the use of throat cultures [27].

Most currently available RADTs have specificities of 95% or greater compared with blood agar plate cultures [28]. False-positive test results are unusual, and therapeutic decisions can be made with confidence on the basis of a positive RADT result. The sensitivity of most RADTs is 80% to 90% [28]. Although it has been suggested that many false-negative RADT results occur in patients who are GAS carriers, it has been shown that a large proportion of patients with false-negative RADT results are truly infected with GAS [29].

The first RADTs used latex agglutination methodology, were relatively insensitive, and had unclear end points [28]. Subsequent tests based on enzyme immunoassay techniques had a more sharply defined end point and increased sensitivity. More recently, RADTs using optical immunoassay and chemiluminescent DNA probes have been developed [28]. These tests may be more sensitive than other RADTs and perhaps even as sensitive as blood agar plate cultures [28]. Because of conflicting and limited data about the optical immunoassay [28] and other commercially available RADTs, however, advisory groups recommend that physicians electing to use any RADT in children and adolescents without culture backup of negative results should do so only after showing in their own practice that the RADT is as sensitive as throat culture [10,11].

Currently, two of the most important issues regarding the use of RADTs for the diagnosis of group A beta-hemolytic streptococcal pharyngitis are the relative sensitivities of the different tests and whether any RADTs are sensitive enough to mitigate against the need to perform throat cultures in patients with negative test results. Most studies that have evaluated the sensitivities of RADTs have compared the performance of a single type of RADT with a standard culture. Because of considerable variability in study designs and culture techniques, it is difficult to compare the sensitivity of a RADT as determined in one study with the sensitivity of another RADT as determined in a different study [28]. The relative sensitivities of different RADTs can be determined only by direct comparisons. There have been to date only four direct comparisons of different RADTs reported in the English literature (one of which was a letter to the editor) [30–33]. The relative sensitivities of different RADTs have not been established.

Few studies have investigated the performance of the RADTs currently being used in clinical practice [25,31–35]. Armengol et al [25] attempted to validate the sensitivity of the specific RADT being used in their practice before abandoning confirmatory throat cultures for negative RADT results [10,11]. In this study performed over three winter seasons and using the on-site physician office laboratory at the pediatric group practice, they found that the RADT had a sensitivity of approximately 85% compared with a single blood agar plate culture. The investigators concluded that the sensitivity of this particular RADT was too low for them to consider abandoning the confirmatory throat culture in their practice. In contrast, Mayes and Pichichero [36] reviewed the experience with RADTs in a different pediatric group practice between January 1996 and June 1999. During this period, 11,427 RADTs were performed, and 8385 (73.4%) were negative. A confirmatory blood agar plate culture was performed for 8234 (98.2%) of these 8385 negative tests. Of these, 200 (2.4%) were determined to have been negative RADT results with a positive throat culture. A cost analysis showed that elimination of confirmatory throat cultures for negative RADT results could produce substantial saving to a practice and to patients. The investigators concluded that culture confirmation of negative RADT results may not be necessary in all circumstances [36].

Neither the blood agar plate culture nor the RADT can differentiate accurately individuals with bona fide group A beta-hemolytic streptococcal pharyngitis from asymptomatic GAS carriers with intercurrent viral pharyngitis. They do facilitate, however, the withholding of antibiotics from most patients with sore throats, whose cultures or RADTs are negative, and this is extremely important. There are an estimated 6.7 million visits to primary care providers by adults who complain of sore throat each year in the United States, and antibiotics are prescribed at 73% of these visits [14]. Although more recent trends suggest a decline in the use of antibiotics in children and adolescents with pharyngitis, in 1999–2000, 68.6% of children and adolescents who were seen by their primary care provider for pharyngitis received a prescription for antibiotics [37].

Antistreptococcal antibody titers reflect past and not present immunologic events and are of no value in the diagnosis of acute group A beta-hemolytic streptococcal pharyngitis. They are valuable for confirmation of prior group A beta-hemolytic streptococcal infections in patients suspected of having acute rheumatic fever or poststreptococcal acute glomerulonephritis. Antistreptococcal antibody titers also are helpful in prospective epidemiologic studies in trying to differentiate patients with acute group A beta-hemolytic streptococcal infections from patients who are GAS carriers.

Repeat diagnostic testing

Most asymptomatic patients who have confirmed positive throat cultures after completing a course of appropriate antimicrobial therapy are GAS carriers [38]. Follow-up throat cultures (or RADTs) are not routinely indicated for asymptomatic patients who have completed a course of antibiotic therapy for GAS. There are specific situations, however, when follow-up throat cultures (or RADTs) on asymptomatic individuals should be performed. Patients with a history of rheumatic fever should have routine follow-up testing. Such testing also should be considered in patients who develop acute pharyngitis during outbreaks of either acute rheumatic fever or poststreptococcal acute glomerulonephritis and during outbreaks of group A beta-hemolytic streptococcal pharyngitis in closed or semiclosed communities [38].

Treatment

Antimicrobial therapy is indicated for individuals with symptomatic pharyngitis after the presence of GAS in the throat has been confirmed by either throat culture or RADT. In situations in which the clinical and epidemiologic evidence results in a high index of suspicion, antimicrobial therapy can be initiated while awaiting laboratory confirmation, provided that such therapy is discontinued if the diagnosis of group A beta-hemolytic streptococcal pharyngitis is not confirmed by a laboratory test. Early initiation of antimicrobial therapy for group A beta-hemolytic streptococcal pharyngitis results in a shortening of the clinical course of the illness [26]. Group A beta-hemolytic streptococcal pharyngitis is usually a self-limited disease, however, and most signs and symptoms resolve spontaneously within 3 or 4 days of onset even without antimicrobial therapy [39]. In addition, the initiation of antimicrobial therapy can be delayed for 9 days after the onset of symptoms and still prevent the occurrence of acute rheumatic fever [40]. There can be flexibility in initiating antimicrobial therapy during the evaluation of an individual patient with presumed group A beta-hemolytic streptococcal pharyngitis.

Numerous antimicrobial agents have been shown to be effective in the treatment of group A beta-hemolytic streptococcal pharyngitis, including penicillin and its congeners (eg, ampicillin and amoxicillin) and numerous cephalosporins, macrolides, and clindamycin. When selecting an antimicrobial for the treatment of group A beta-hemolytic streptococcal pharyngitis, it is important to consider efficacy, safety, antimicrobial spectrum (narrow versus broad), dosing schedules, compliance, and cost. Based on such considerations, several advisory bodies recommend penicillin as the treatment of choice for this infection [9–11]. Although the problem of increasing antimicrobial resistance among bacteria is one of the most important current infectious disease issues, GAS has never developed resistance to any of the penicillins or cephalosporins or shown any increase in penicillin minimal inhibitory concentrations over at least 5 decades [41]. Amoxicillin often is used in place of oral penicillin V in young children; the efficacy appears equal. This choice is related primarily to acceptance of the taste of amoxicillin suspension. Orally administered erythromycin is indicated for patients allergic to penicillin. Other macrolides, such as clarithromycin or azithromycin, also are effective. First-generation cephalosporins also are acceptable in penicillin-allergic patients who do not manifest immediate-type hypersensitivity to β-lactam antibiotics.

Casey and Pichichero [42] presented a meta-analysis of 35 clinical trials performed between 1970 and 1999 in which a cephalosporin was compared with penicillin for the treatment of group A beta-hemolytic streptococcal pharyngitis.

Based on this analysis, they concluded that cephalosporins should be added "as a treatment of choice for [group A beta-hemolytic streptococcal] tonsillo-pharyngitis...." This report has several major flaws, however, that make it impossible to accept the validity of this conclusion [43].

Although the use of cephalosporins for group A beta-hemolytic streptococcal pharyngitis could reduce the number of patients (most merely chronic carriers) who continue to harbor the organism in their throats after completing therapy, the economic and ecologic costs involved would make this a Pyrrhic victory for those who advocate the use a cephalosporin as the drug of choice for streptococcal pharyngitis. Penicillin has stood, the test of time satisfactorily for 5 decades, and there are compelling reasons (eg, its narrow antimicrobial spectrum, inexpensive cost, and impressive safety profile) to continue to recommend it as the drug of choice.

Most oral antibiotics must be administered for 10 days to achieve maximal pharyngeal eradication rates of GAS. It has been reported that several antimicrobial agents, including clarithromycin, cefuroxime, cefixime, ceftibuten, cefdinir, cefpodoxime, and azithromycin, are effective in eradication of GAS from the pharynx when administered for 5 or fewer days [10,44]. Many of the studies of short-course therapy have serious methodologic flaws, however, that raise questions about the validity of their conclusions. In addition, the spectra of these antibiotics are much broader than that of penicillin, and even when they are administered for short courses, they are more expensive [44]. Additional studies are needed before these short-course regimens can be recommended [10,11].

Attempts to treat group A beta-hemolytic streptococcal pharyngitis with a single daily dose of penicillin have been unsuccessful [45]. In recent years, investigators have shown that several antimicrobial agents, including azithromycin, cefadroxil, cefixime, ceftibuten, cefpodoxime, cefprozil, and cefdinir, are effective in eradicating pharyngeal streptococci when given as a single daily dose [10,44]. These agents are expensive, however, and have broad spectra of activity compared with penicillin. Preliminary investigations have shown that once-daily amoxicillin therapy is effective in the treatment of group A beta-hemolytic streptococcal pharyngitis [46,47]. If confirmed by additional investigations, once-daily amoxicillin therapy, because of its low cost and relatively narrow spectrum, could become an alternative regimen for the treatment of group A beta-hemolytic streptococcal pharyngitis.

Antimicrobial therapy for group A beta-hemolytic streptococcal pharyngitis may be given orally or parenterally. Table 3 gives recommendations for several antimicrobials proved to be effective for the treatment of group A beta-hemolytic streptococcal pharyngitis [10]. Intramuscular benzathine penicillin G is preferred in patients who are unlikely to complete a full 10-day course of oral therapy.

Antimicrobial resistance has not been a significant issue in the treatment of group A beta-hemolytic streptococcal pharyngitis in the United States [48]. There has never been a clinical isolate of GAS documented to be resistant to penicillin anywhere in the world. Although there have been geographic areas with relatively high levels of resistance to macrolide antibiotics [49,50], the rate

Table 3
Antimicrobial therapy for group A streptococcal pharyngitis

Route of administration, antimicrobial agent	Dosage	Duration
Oral		
Penicillin*	Children: 250 mg bid or tid	10 d
	Adolescents and adults: 250 mg tid or qid	10 d
	Adolescents and adults: 500 mg bid	10 d
Intramuscular		
Benzathine penicillin G	1.2×10^6 U (for patients $\geq$27 kg)	1 dose
	6×10^5 U (for patients <27 kg)	1 dose
Mixtures of benzathine and procaine penicillin G	Varies with formulation[†]	1 dose
Oral, for patients allergic to penicillin		
Erythromycin	Varies with formulation	10 d
First-generation cephalosporins[‡]	Varies with agent	10 d

* Amoxicillin is often used in place of oral penicillin V in young children because of the acceptance of the taste of the suspension, not because of any microbiologic advantage.

[†] Dose should be determined on basis of benzathine component.

[‡] These agents should not be used to treat patients with immediate-type hypersensitivity to β-lactam antibiotics.

Modified from Bisno AL, Gerber MA, Gwaltney JM, Kaplan EL, Schwartz RH. Practice guideline for the diagnosis and management of group A streptococcal pharyngitis. Clin Infect Dis 2002;35:113–25.

of macrolide resistance among isolates of GAS in the United States generally has remained low at less than 5%. In an investigation of antibiotic resistance patterns of 245 pharyngeal isolates and 56 invasive isolates of GAS obtained between 1994 and 1997 from 24 states and the District of Columbia, only 8 (2.6%) of the 301 isolates were determined to be macrolide resistant [41]. Higher resistance rates occasionally have been reported, however. Nine percent of pharyngeal and 32% of invasive GAS strains collected in San Francisco during 1994–1995 were reported to be macrolide resistant [51]. Martin et al [52], during a longitudinal investigation of group A beta-hemolytic streptococcal disease in a single elementary school in Pittsburgh, Pennsylvania, found that 48% of the isolates of GAS collected between October 2000 and May 2001 were resistant to erythromycin. None were resistant to clindamycin. Molecular typing indicated that this outbreak was due to a single strain of GAS. In addition, of 100 randomly selected isolates of GAS obtained from the community between April and June 2001, 38 (38%) were resistant to erythromycin [52].

Tanz et al [53] reported the results of a prospective, multicenter, community-based surveillance of pharyngeal isolates of GAS recovered from children 3 to 18 years old during three successive respiratory seasons between 2000 and 2003. During this 3-year period, the macrolide resistance rate among pharyngeal GAS in the United States was less than 5%, and it was stable. Clindamycin resistance was found in 1.04% of isolates over the 3-year study period and did not vary by study year. There was no evidence of wide dissemination of specific macrolide-resistance clones, increasing clindamycin resistance, or increasing erythromycin minimal inhibitory concentrations over the 3-year study period. There was, however, considerable geographic variability in macrolide resistance rates in each study year and year-to-year variability at individual study sites [53].

Although these results are reassuring, clinicians need to be aware of local resistance rates. In the future, if there are significant increases in rates of macrolide resistance among GAS strains, it may be necessary to reconsider recommendations for treatment of group A beta-hemolytic streptococcal pharyngitis in penicillin-allergic patients.

The primary reason to identify either group C or group G streptococcus as the cause of acute pharyngitis is to initiate antimicrobial therapy that may mitigate the clinical course of the infection. There is currently no convincing evidence, however, from controlled studies of clinical response to antimicrobial therapy in patients with acute pharyngitis and either group C or group G streptococcus isolated from their pharynx. If one elects to treat either group C or group G streptococcal pharyngitis, the treatment should be similar to that for group A beta-hemolytic streptococcal pharyngitis with penicillin as the antimicrobial agent of choice [6].

Complications

Group A beta-hemolytic streptococcal pharyngitis can be associated with suppurative and nonsuppurative complications. Suppurative complications result from the spread of GAS to adjacent structures and include peritonsillar abscess, retropharyngeal abscess, cervical lymphadenitis, sinusitis, otitis media, and mastoiditis. Before antimicrobial agents were available, suppurative complications of group A beta-hemolytic streptococcal pharyngitis were common; however, antimicrobial therapy has reduced greatly the frequency of such complications.

Acute rheumatic fever, acute poststreptococcal glomerulonephritis, and poststreptococcal reactive arthritis are recognized nonsuppurative sequelae of group A beta-hemolytic streptococcal pharyngitis. Acute rheumatic fever occurs after an episode of group A beta-hemolytic streptococcal pharyngitis (usually after a 2- to 4-week latent period) and not after group A beta-hemolytic streptococcal infections of the skin. Appropriate antimicrobial therapy begun within 9 days of the onset of pharyngitis can prevent this complication. In contrast to acute rheumatic fever, acute poststreptococcal glomerulonephritis can occur after a group A beta-hemolytic streptococcal infection of either the pharynx or skin and does not seem to be prevented by antimicrobial therapy of the antecedent group A beta-hemolytic streptococcal infection. The latent period for glomerulonephritis is about 3 weeks after a skin infection and 10 days after an upper respiratory tract infection. Poststreptococcal reactive arthritis is similar to other postinfectious arthritides. The relationship of this entity to acute rheumatic fever is still unclear.

Acute glomerulonephritis has been reported as an extremely unusual complication of group C streptococcal pharyngitis, but a causal relationship between group G streptococcal pharyngitis and acute glomerulonephritis has not been established. Acute rheumatic fever has not been described as a complication of either group C or group G streptococcal pharyngitis [6].

Treatment failures, chronic, carriage and recurrences

Antimicrobial treatment failures with group A beta-hemolytic streptococcal pharyngitis traditionally have been classified as either clinical or bacteriologic failures. The significance of clinical treatment failures (usually defined as persistent or recurrent signs or symptoms suggesting group A beta-hemolytic streptococcal pharyngitis) is difficult to determine, however, because group A beta-hemolytic streptococcal pharyngitis is a self-limited illness even without antimicrobial therapy [39]. In addition, without the repeat isolation of the infecting strain of GAS (ie, true bacteriologic treatment failure), it is particularly difficult to determine the clinical significance of persistent or recurrent signs or symptoms suggesting group A beta-hemolytic streptococcal pharyngitis.

Bacteriologic treatment failures can be classified as either *true* or *apparent* failures. *True* bacteriologic failure refers to the inability to eradicate the specific strain of GAS causing an acute episode of pharyngitis with a complete course of appropriate antimicrobial therapy. *Apparent* bacteriologic treatment failure reflects a variety of circumstances.

Most *apparent* bacteriologic treatment failures are patients who are GAS carriers (ie, patients with GAS in the upper respiratory tract, but without illness or immunologic response). GAS carriers are unlikely to spread GAS to their close contacts and are at low, if any risk, for developing suppurative or nonsuppurative complications [54]. During the winter and spring in temperate climates, 20% of asymptomatic school-age children are GAS carriers [54]. *Apparent* bacteriologic failure also can occur when newly acquired GAS isolates are mistaken for the original infecting strain of GAS, when the infecting strain of GAS is eradicated but then rapidly reacquired, or when compliance with antimicrobial therapy is poor.

Although the specific reasons for true bacteriologic treatment failures have not been determined, several explanations have been proposed. It has been suggested that GAS may have become more resistant to penicillin; however, there is no evidence to support this hypothesis [48], and no penicillin-resistant strains of GAS have been identified. It also has been suggested that some strains of GAS have developed penicillin tolerance (ie, a discordance between the concentration of penicillin required to inhibit and to kill the organisms); however, the role of penicillin tolerance in true bacteriologic treatment failures has never been established [55,56]. It also has been suggested that other species of bacteria present in the normal pharyngeal flora contribute to true bacteriologic failures either by enhancing the colonization and growth of GAS in the upper respiratory tract or by producing β-lactamases that inactivate penicillin. The precise role, if any, of these other organisms has not been determined yet, however [48].

Routine throat cultures (or RADTs) for asymptomatic individuals after completion of antibiotic therapy for group A beta-hemolytic streptococcal pharyngitis are generally not indicated. The interpretation of a positive throat culture (RADT) after a course of treatment may be difficult even if the patient remains symptomatic because it is not possible to distinguish persistent carriage from persistent or recurrent infection. Under these circumstances, many clinicians elect to administer a second course of antimicrobials.

When the physician suspects "ping pong" spread to be associated with multiple repeated episodes of group A beta-hemolytic streptococcal infections in a family, simultaneous cultures of all family contacts and treatment of persons whose cultures are positive may be helpful. There is no credible evidence that family pets are reservoirs for GAS, and they do not contribute to familial spread.

A patient with repeated episodes of acute pharyngitis associated with a positive throat culture (or RADT) is a common and difficult problem for the practicing physician. The fundamental question that must be addressed is whether this patient is experiencing repeated episodes of bona fide group A beta-hemolytic streptococcal pharyngitis or is a GAS carrier experiencing repeated episodes of viral pharyngitis. The latter situation is considerably more common than the former. Such a patient is likely to be a GAS carrier if (1) the clinical and epidemiologic findings suggest a viral etiology, (2) there is little clinical response to appropriate antimicrobial therapy, (3) throat cultures (or RADTs) are also positive between episodes of pharyngitis, and (4) there is no serologic response to GAS extracellular antigen (eg, antistreptolysin O, anti-DNase B).

In contrast, a patient with repeated episodes of acute pharyngitis associated with positive throat cultures (or RADTs) for GAS is likely to be experiencing repeated episodes of bona fide group A beta-hemolytic streptococcal pharyngitis if (1) the clinical and epidermiologic findings suggest group A beta-hemolytic streptococcal pharyngitis as the etiology, (2) there is a demonstrable clinical response to appropriate antimicrobial therapy, (3) throat cultures (or RADTs) are negative between episodes of pharyngitis, and (4) there is a serologic response to GAS extracellular antigens. When it has been determined that the patient is experiencing repeated episodes of bona fide group A beta-hemolytic streptococcal pharyngitis, some have suggested prophylactic oral penicillin V. The efficacy of this regimen has never been proved, however, and antimicrobial prophylaxis is not recommended except to prevent recurrences of rheumatic fever in patients who have experienced a previous episode of rheumatic fever. Tonsillectomy may be considered in a rare patient whose symptomatic episodes do not diminish in frequency over time and in whom no alternative explanation for the recurrent group A beta-hemolytic streptococcal pharyngitis is evident. Tonsillectomy has been shown to be beneficial for a relatively small group of these patients, however, and any benefit can be expected to be relatively short-lived [57–59].

References

[1] Woodwell D. Office visits to pediatric specialists: 1989. Advance Data from Vital and Health Statistics. No. 208. Hyatttsville (MD): National Center for Health Statistics; 1992.

[2] Meier FA, Centor RM, Graham Jr I, et al. Clinical and microbiological evidence for endemic pharyngitis among adults due to group C streptococci. Arch Intern Med 1990;150:825–9.

[3] Turner JC, Hayden FG, Lobo MC, et al. Epidemiologic evidence for Lancefield group C beta-hemolytic streptococci as a cause of exudative pharyngitis in college students. J Clin Microbiol 1997;35:1–4.

[4] Arditi M, Shulman ST, Davis AT, et al. Group C beta-hemolytic streptococcal infections in children: nine pediatric cases and review. Rev Infect Dis 1989;11:34–45.

[5] Gerber MA, Randolp MF, Martin NJ, et al. Community wide outbreak of group G streptococcal pharyngitis. Pediatrics 1991;87:598–606.

[6] Kaplan EL, Gerber MA. Group A, group C, and group G beta-hemolytic streptooccal infections. In: Feigin R, Cherry J, Demmler G, Kaplan S, editors. Textbook of pediatric infectious diseases. 5th edition. Philadelphia: WB Saunders; 2004. p. 1142–56.

[7] Centor RM, Witherspoon JM, Dalton HP, Brody CE, Link K. The diagnosis of strep throat in adults in the emergency room. Med Decis Making 1981;1:239–46.

[8] Wald ER, Green MD, Schwartz B, Barbadora K. A streptococcal score card revisited. Pediatr Emerg Care 1998;14:109–11.

[9] Attia MW, Zaoutis T, Klein JD, Meier FA. Performance of a predictive model for streptococcal pharyngitis in children. Arch Pediatr Adolesc Med 2001;155:687–91.

[10] Bisno AL, Gerber MA, Gwaltney JM, Kaplan EL, Schwartz RH. Practice guidelines for the diagnosis and management of group A streptococcal pharyngitis. Clin Infect Dis 2002;35: 113–25.

[11] American Academy of Pediatrics Committee on Infectious Diseases. Red Book: report of the Committee on Infectious Diseases. 26th edition. Elk Grove Village (IL): American Academy of Pediatrics; 2003.

[12] Snow V, Mottur-Pilson C, Cooper RJ, Hoffman JR. Principles of appropriate antibiotic use of acute pharyngitis in adults. Ann Intern Med 2001;134:506–8.

[13] Cooper JR, Hoffman JR, Bartlett JG, et al. Principles of appropriate antibiotic use for acute pharyngitis in adults: background. Ann Intern Med 2001;134:509–17.

[14] Bisno AL, Peter GS, Kaplan EL. Diagnosis of strep throat in adults: are clinical criteria really good enough? Clin Infect Dis 2002;35:126–9.

[15] McIsaac WJ, Kellner JD, Aufricht P, Vanjaka A, Low DE. Empirical validation of guidelines for the management of pharyngitis in children and adults. JAMA 2004;291:1587–95.

[16] Breese BB, Disney FA. The accuracy of diagnosis of beta-streptococcal infections on clinical grounds. J Pediatr 1954;44:670–3.

[17] Gerber MA. Comparison of throat cultures and rapid strep tests for diagnosis of streptococcal pharyngitis. Pediatr Infect Dis J 1989;8:820–4.

[18] Brien JH, Bass JW. Streptococcal pharyngitis: optimal site for throat culture. J Pediatr 1985; 106:781–3.

[19] Gunn BA, Mesrobian R, Keiser JF, Bass J. Cultures of *Streptococcus pyogenes* from the oropharynx. Lab Med 1985;16:369–71.

[20] Schwartz RH, Gerber MA, McCoy P. Effect of atmosphere of incubation on the isolation of group A streptococci from throat cultures. J Lab Clin Med 1985;106:88–92.

[21] Lauer BA, Reller LB, Mirrett S. Effect of atmosphere and duration of incubation on primary isolation of group A streptococci from throat cultures. J Clin Microbiol 1983;17:338–40.

[22] Schwartz RH, Gerber MA, McCoy P. Effect of atmosphere of incubation on the isolation of group A streptococci from throat cultures. J Lab Clin Med 1985;106:88–92.

[23] Roddey Jr OF, Clegg HW, Martin ES, Swetenburg RL, Koonce EW. Comparison of throat culture methods for the recovery of group A streptococci in a pediatric office setting. JAMA 1995;274:1863–5.

[24] Gerber MA. Diagnosis of pharyngitis: methodology of throat cultures. In: Shulman ST, editor. Pharyngitis: management in an era of declining rheumatic fever. New York: Praeger; 1984. p. 61–72.
[25] Armengol CE, Schlager TA, Hendley JO. Sensitivity of a rapid antigen detection test for group A streptococci in a private pediatric office setting: answersing the Red Book's request for validation. Pediatrics 2004;113:924–6.
[26] Randolph MF, Gerber MA, DeMeo KK, Wright L. Effect of antibiotic therapy on the clinical course of streptococcal pharyngitis. J Pediatr 1985;106:870–5.
[27] Lieu TA, Fleisher GR, Schwartz JS. Clinical evaluation of a latex agglutination test for streptococcal pharyngitis: performance and impact on treatment rates. Pediatr Infect Dis J 1988;7: 847–54.
[28] Gerber MA, Shulman ST. Rapid diagnosis of pharyngitis caused by group A streptococci. Clin Microbiol Rev 2004;17:571–80.
[29] Gerber MA, Randolph MF, Chanatry J, Wright LL, DeMeo KK, Anderson LR. Antigen detection test for streptococcal pharyngitis: evaluation of sensitivity with respect to true infections. J Pediatr 1986;108:654–8.
[30] Roe M, Kishiyama C, Davidson K, Schaefer L, Todd J. Comparison of BioStar Strep A OIA optical immunoassay, Abbott Test Pack Plus Strep A, and culture with selective media for diagnosis of group A streptococcal pharyngitis. J Clin Microbiol 1995;33:1551–3.
[31] Roosevelt GE, Kaulkarni MS, Shulman ST. Critical evaluation of a CLIA-waived streptococcal antigen detection test in the emergency department. Ann Emerg Med 2001;37:377–81.
[32] Gieseker KE, MacKenzie T, Roe MH, Todd JK. Comparison of two rapid *Streptococcus pyogenes* diagnostic tests with a rigorous culture standard. Pediatr Infect Dis J 2002;21:922–6.
[33] Schwartz RH. Evaluation of rapid streptococcal detection tests. Pediatr Infect Dis J 1997; 16:1099–100.
[34] Nerbrand C, Jasir A, Schalen C. Are current rapid detection tests for group A streptococci sensitive enough? Scand J Infect Dis 2002;34:797–9.
[35] Gieseker KE, Roe MH, MacKenzie T, Todd JK. Evaluating the American Academy of Pediatrics diagnostic standard for *Streptococcus pyogenes* pharyngitis: backup culture versus repeat rapid antigen testing. Pediatics 2003;111:e666–70.
[36] Mayes T, Pichichero ME. Are follow-up throat cultures necessary when rapid antigen detection tests are negative for group A streptococci? Clin Pediatr 2001;40:191–5.
[37] McCaig LF, Besser RE, Hughes JM. Trends in antimicrobial prescribing rates for children and adolescents. JAMA 2002;287:3096–102.
[38] Gerber MA. Treatment failures and carriers: perception or problems? Pediatr Infect Dis J 1994;13:576–9.
[39] Brink WR, Rammelkamp Jr CH, Denny FW, Wannamaker LW. Effect of penicillin and aureomycin on the natural course of streptococcal tonsillitis and pharyngitis. Am J Med 1951; 10:300–8.
[40] Catanzaro FJ, Stetson CA, Morris AJ, et al. The role of streptococcus in the pathogenesis of rheumatic fever. Am J Med 1954;17:749–56.
[41] Kaplan EL, Johnson DR, Del Rosario MC, Horn DL. Susceptibility of group A beta-hemolytic streptococci to thirteen antibiotics: examination of 301 strains isolated in the United States between 1994 and 1997. Pediatr Infect Dis J 1999;18:1069–72.
[42] Casey JR, Pichichero ME. Meta-analysis of cephalosporin versus penicillin treatment of group A streptococcal tonsillopharyngitis in children. Pediatrics 2004;113:866–82.
[43] Shulman ST, Gerber MA. So what's wrong with penicillin for strep throat? Pediatrics 2004; 113:1816–8.
[44] Gerber MA, Tanz RR. New approaches to the treatment of group A streptococcal pharyngitis. Curr Opin Pediatr 2001;13:51–5.
[45] Gerber MA, Randolph MF, DeMeo K, Feder Jr HM, Kaplan EL. Failure of once-daily penicillin V therapy for streptococcal pharyngitis. Am J Dis Child 1989;143:153–5.
[46] Shvartzman P, Tabenkin H, Rosentzwaig A, Dolginov F. Treatment of streptococcal pharyngitis with amoxycillin once a day. BMJ 1993;306:1170–2.

[47] Feder HMJ, Gerber MA, Randolph MF, Stelmach PS, Kaplan EL. Once-daily therapy for streptococcal pharyngitis with amoxicillin. Pediatrics 1999;103:47–51.

[48] Gerber MA. Antibiotic resistance: relationship to persistence of group A streptococci in the upper respiratory tract. Pediatrics 1996;97:971–5.

[49] Cornaglia G, Ligozzi M, Mazzariol A, et al. Resistance of *Streptococcus pyogenes* to erythromycin and related antibiotics in Italy. Clin Infect Dis 1998;27(Suppl 1):S87–92.

[50] Seppala H, Klaukka T, Vuopio-Varkila J, et al. The effect of changes in the consumption of macrolide antibiotics on erythromycin resistance in group A streptococci in Finland. N Engl J Med 1997;337:441–6.

[51] York MK, Gibbs L, Perdreau-Remington R, Brooks GF. Characterization of antimicrobial resistance in *Streptococcus pyogenes* isolates from the San Francisco Bay area of Northern California. J Clin Microbiol 1999;37:1727–31.

[52] Martin JM, Green M, Barbadora KA, Wald ER. Erthromycin-resistant group A streptococci in school children in Pittsburgh. N Engl J Med 2002;346:1200–6.

[53] Tanz RR, Shulman ST, Shortridge VD, et al. Community-based surveillance in the United States of macrolide-resistant pediatric pharyngeal group A streptococci during 3 respiratory disease seasons. Clin Infect Dis 2004;39:1794–801.

[54] Kaplan EL. The group A streptococcal carrier state: an enigma. J Pediatri 1980;97:337–45.

[55] Smith TD, Huskins C, Kim KS, et al. Efficacy of beta-lactamase-resistant penicillin and influence of penicillin tolerance in eradicating streptococci from the pharynx after failure of penicillin therapy for group A streptococcal pharyngitis. J Pediatr 1987;110:777–82.

[56] Kim KS, Kaplan EL. Association of penicillin tolerance with failure to eradicate group A streptococci from patients with pharyngitis. J Pediatr 1985;107:681–4.

[57] Paradise JL, Blueston CD, Bachman RZ, et al. Efficacy of tonsillectomy for recurrent throat infection in severely affected children. N Engl J Med 1984;310:674–83.

[58] Paradise JL, Bluestone CD, Colborn DK, Bernard BS, Rockette HS, Kurs-Lasky M. Tonsillectomy and adenoidectomy for recurrent throat infection in moderately affected children. Pediatrics 2002;110:7–15.

[59] Discolo CM, Darrow DH, Koltai PJ. Infection indications for tonsillectomy. Pediatr Clin North Am 2003;50:455–8.

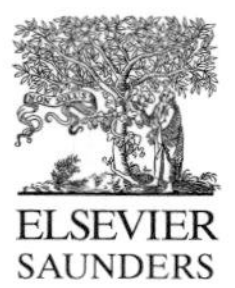

ELSEVIER
SAUNDERS

PEDIATRIC CLINICS
OF NORTH AMERICA

Pediatr Clin N Am 52 (2005) 749–777

Important Bacterial Gastrointestinal Pathogens in Children: A Pathogenesis Perspective

Manuel R. Amieva, MD, PhD*

Department of Pediatrics, Division of Infectious Diseases, and Department of Microbiology & Immunology, Stanford University School of Medicine, Stanford, CA, 94305-5208, USA

By necessity, pediatricians quickly become well versed in the management of common gastrointestinal illnesses in children, especially the diarrheal syndromes associated with acute gastroenteritis. Most infectious gastrointestinal syndromes resolve without complications if dehydration is avoided, and illnesses usually are managed without clear knowledge of the enteropathogen involved or its pathogenesis. Nevertheless, understanding the natural history and basic pathogenesis of most common enteropathogens adds another dimension to the clinical management of these syndromes. In each case of gastrointestinal infection, pediatricians should consider the following questions: What is the likelihood that the specific infectious agent will lead to more serious invasive disease? Is antibiotic therapy indicated? Should antimotility drugs be prescribed? Will the infection result in chronic gastrointestinal symptoms? What is the risk of post-infectious sequelae? How was the infection acquired?

The gastrointestinal tract is home to 10 times more bacteria than cells in the entire human body. It is the site of sophisticated interactions between microbial pathogens, commensals, host epithelial cells, and the immune system, a kind of jungle of biologic interactions, evolution, and natural history, whose balance is crucial for childhood growth and development.

This article focuses on the five most common bacterial enteropathogens of the developed world—*Helicobacter pylori, Escherichia coli, Shigella, Salmonella,*

* Department of Pediatrics, Division of Infectious Diseases, Stanford University Medical Center, G312, Stanford, CA, 94305-5208.

E-mail address: amieva@stanford.edu

doi:10.1016/j.pcl.2005.03.002 *pediatric.theclinics.com*

and *Campylobacter*—from the perspective of how they cause disease and how they relate to each other. Basic and recurring themes of bacterial pathogenesis, including mechanisms of entry, methods of adherence, sites of cellular injury, role of toxins, and how pathogens acquire particular virulence traits (and antimicrobial resistance), are discussed.

Because of space constraints, several bacterial enteropathogens that are important in pediatric practice have been omitted: *Vibrio cholerae* causes severe watery diarrhea in the developing world. *Yersinia enterocolitica* can cause enterocolitis and abdominal pain mimicking appendicitis, and its pathogenesis is similar to enteric fever caused by *Salmonella*. *Listeria monocytogenes* asymptomatically colonizes the gastrointestinal tract, occasionally causes gastroenteritis, but can cause bacteremia and meningitis in neonates. Toxin-mediated disease by *Clostridium difficile* is a common iatrogenic problem, secondary to antibiotic therapy.

Helicobacter pylori

H. pylori are gram-negative, microaerophilic, spiral-shaped bacilli with polar flagella. They efficiently colonize the harshest environment of the human body, the stomach. They were identified and cultured in the laboratory for the first time in 1988 [1], after being observed in histologic sections of biopsy specimens from people with gastritis and peptic ulcer disease. Since then, *H. pylori* also have been causally associated with gastritis and ulcers in children [2,3] and linked to the development of gastric adenocarcinoma and lymphoma of the stomach after long periods of chronic infection [4]. Despite their recent discovery, it is known that *H. pylori* have infected and co-evolved with humans for thousands of years, spreading within families [5,6]. Studies of the genetic makeup of *H. pylori* strains isolated from around the world indicate that they were derived from ancestral populations that diverged as human populations emigrated out of Africa, Central Asia, and East Asia [7]. Since the 1980s, a tremendous amount has been learned about the biology of *H. pylori,* its adaptations for survival in the stomach, and its association with disease. Nevertheless, relatively little is known about its effects on children.

Epidemiology and pathophysiology

H. pylori is the most common bacterial infection of humans; more than half of the human population is chronically infected. Transmission is probably oral-oral [8], and it is likely that children are the major vector of transmission and most susceptible to infection [9,10]. In areas of high prevalence, most children are infected by age 10 years [11], with some countries reaching 100% infection rate [12]. There are no proven environmental reservoirs of *H. pylori,* and the only known site of colonization is the human stomach. Because *H. pylori* best survive at neutral pH [13,14], colonization is limited to a narrow region overlying the stomach mucosal surface that is covered by protective mucus. To survive the rapid clearance of stomach contents, *H. pylori* have evolved rapid motility with their flagellar appendages and the ability to detect and move toward the epithelial surface [15]. They constantly swim "against the current" to stay near the epithelial surface and away from the stomach lumen [16]. As an additional buffering mechanism, *H. pylori* produce large amounts of urease enzyme, which catalyzes the breakdown of urea into ammonia and carbon dioxide. Ammonia is alkaline, creating a local environment capable of neutralizing nearby acidic pH [17]. This phenomenon is the basis of a diagnostic test, the urea breath test, in which a small amount of carbon-13 isotope–labeled urea is swallowed. *H. pylori* urease in the stomach releases carbon-13-labeled carbon dioxide, which can be detected in the breath [18].

Although most of the colonizing *H. pylori* are actively swimming in the mucus layer, some are found tightly adhering to the cell surface of mucus-producing epithelial cells on the surface and at the neck of the gastric glands [19]. Attachment to the cell surface is not only a way to avoid being removed with stomach contents, but also it facilitates the pathogen's delivery of toxic products directly to the epithelium [20]. The more pathogenic strains of *H. pylori* contain a molecular needle, a type 4 secretion system, through which they inject the bacterial protein CagA into the host cell after attachment [21–23]. CagA seems to act as a signaling molecule that affects cell behavior [24–27] and the attachment site on the cell surface [28,29]. *H. pylori* use CagA to adhere directly over the cell-cell junctions and perturb their function, perhaps as a way of acquiring nutrients that leak out from the interstitial space of the host (Fig. 1) [28,30–34]. A small percentage of bacteria are found inside mucosal epithelial cells, perhaps representing a reservoir of bacteria difficult to eradicate with antibiotics [35–38]. *H. pylori* also make at least one cytotoxin, VacA. This toxin disrupts endocytic trafficking of host cells, promotes cell death through apoptosis, suppresses the local immune system, and potentiates the development of ulcers [39]. These and multiple other adaptations allow *H. pylori* to colonize the stomach chronically and grow successfully, reaching concentrations of 100 million bacteria per mL of stomach mucus [40].

Clinical manifestations and complications

The clinical spectrum of *H. pylori* disease in children is not well characterized. It seems, however, that most infected children are asymptomatic, with few developing clinical disease during childhood [41–47]. Infection persists in most people for life, and 10% to 20% of infected individuals develop serious sequelae, such as peptic ulcer disease and gastric cancer. Because about half of the world's population is infected, *H. pylori* accounts for substantial mortality and morbidity from peptic ulcers and gastric cancer. Almost all asymptomatically infected children develop gross and histologic changes in the stomach resulting from chronic inflammation of the stomach mucosa (nodular gastritis) [48].

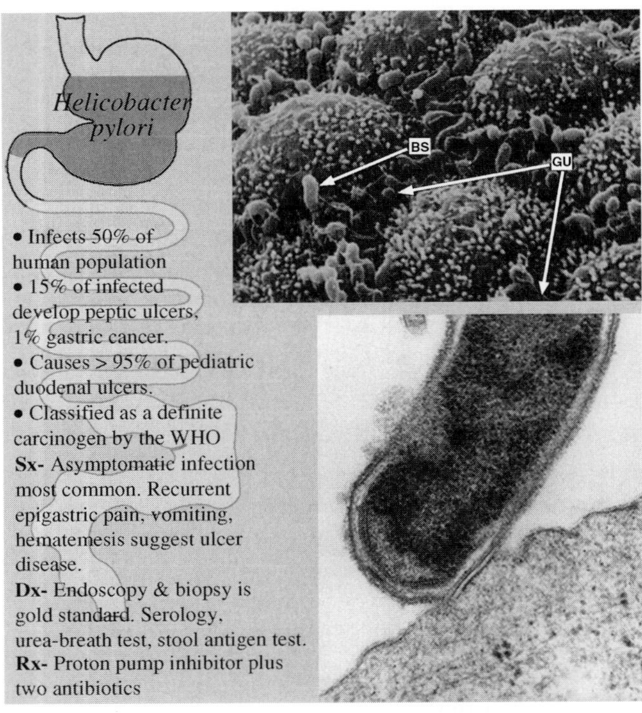

Fig. 1. *H. pylori* infects the stomach mucosa. Scanning electron micrograph (*top*) shows the bacteria adhering to the gastric epithelial cell surface of a prepyloric biopsy from a patient with duodenal ulceration. Numerous bacteria adhere to the junctions between mucus-producing cells. Transmission electron micrograph (*bottom*) shows close attachment of *H. pylori* and the cell surface in cell culture. *H. pylori* use specialized adhesion to the host cells to inject the bacterial protein CagA into the cytoplasm. Dx, diagnosis; Rx, treatment; Sx, symptoms. (*Scanning electron micrograph from* Steer HW. Surface morphology of the gastroduodenal mucosa in duodenal ulceration. Gut 1984;25:1203; with permission. Transmission electron micrograph courtesy of M. Amieva.)

Peptic ulcer disease is rare in children. Several studies have shown that duodenal ulcers in children almost always are associated with *H. pylori* infection [48,49]. Symptoms suggesting ulcer disease include recurrent abdominal pain, epigastric and food-related pain, recurrent vomiting, hematemesis, guaiac-positive stools, weight loss, and nocturnal abdominal pain. Because most infections are asymptomatic, and the infection is so prevalent, it has been difficult to ascertain whether *H. pylori* infection is a cause of dyspepsia or chronic abdominal pain in the absence of ulcer disease [50–53].

Numerous other pediatric illnesses have been associated with *H. pylori,* although the strength of these associations is limited [54]. All would benefit from further research, but these associations exemplify the notion that infectious agents, especially agents that cause chronic infections, may lead to noninfectious sequelae, such as autoimmune disorders. *H. pylori* infection has been proposed as a potential cause of chronic immune thrombocytopenic purpura. Antibiotic treatment results in resolution of chronic immune thrombocytopenic purpura in some cases [55–61]. Iron deficiency anemia also has been associated with *H. pylori* infection, independent of blood loss [62–66]. *H. pylori* infection also may contribute to short stature and poor growth independent of socioeconomic status [67–71]. *H. pylori* infection may affect the likelihood and outcome of other childhood gastrointestinal illnesses. Severe cholera [72], shigellosis [73], and typhoid fever [74] all have been reported to have increased prevalence in children with *H. pylori*.

Diagnosis and treatment

Four main diagnostic tools are available to detect *H. pylori* infection in children. The gold standard is direct visualization and biopsy of the stomach by endoscopy, followed by histologic examination of the biopsy specimens and culture of the organism. This approach, although invasive, yields the most valuable information because it establishes the presence of infection, gastritis, and ulcers, and the *H. pylori* isolates can be tested for antibiotic sensitivity. Serology is used widely in adults but is unreliable in children younger than 10 years of age [75]. The urea breath test is sensitive in children older than 2 years, but requires specialized equipment. A newer approach is the detection of *H. pylori* antigens in the stool [76]. This test is proving to be as sensitive and specific as the urea breath test; is noninvasive; and, in contrast to serology, is useful to monitor eradication after treatment.

Current guidelines for treatment of *H. pylori* in children are based on several consensus meetings of pediatric gastroenterologists [77–79]. The reports emphasize that the main goals of therapy for *H. pylori* infection in children are to heal peptic ulcer disease and relieve symptoms. Current knowledge is insufficient to determine whether treatment of asymptomatic *H. pylori* infection would prevent complications of cancer and peptic ulcer disease later in life [4]. Infected individuals with a strong family history of gastric cancer may benefit, however, from treatment aimed at eradication of *H. pylori* [78].

Treatment regimens for children should include a proton-pump inhibitor plus two antibiotics for 7 to 14 days. Failure rates of 25% are common [80,81], but reinfection is thought to be rare after 5 years of age [82]. The antibiotics of choice include amoxicillin plus either a macrolide (eg, erythromycin or azithromycin) or metronidazole. Follow-up noninvasive tests, such as the urea breath test or the stool antigen test, should be performed 8 weeks after treatment to document clearance of the infection because ulcers almost always recur in the presence of relapsed *H. pylori* infection.

Escherichia coli

E. coli are gram-negative rods that usually live as commensals in the gastrointestinal tract. They represent the best example of how evolution of a microbe within human and animal hosts can lead to multiple clinical manifestations of disease. Although most of the billion *E. coli* living in the large intestine are innocuous commensals, their ability to show different phenotypic traits has turned many of them into serious pathogens and given many other organisms the ability to survive antibiotic treatment.

Pediatricians frequently deal with gastrointestinal *E. coli* that become opportunistic pathogens when they enter the urinary tract or the bloodstream because they are a common cause of urinary tract infection, neonatal bacteremia, and meningitis. These strains of *E. coli* usually live only in the gastrointestinal tract, but have evolved adhesive mechanisms that increase their ability to persist on bladder epithelium [83] or adhere to meningeal vasculature [84,85].

E. coli also have evolved into true gastrointestinal pathogens by acquiring DNA in the form of plasmids, phages (bacterial viruses), transposons, or pathogenicity islands (pieces of DNA acquired from other bacteria, integrated into the chromosome) that confer the ability to cause disease in various ways. Enterotoxigenic (ETEC), enteropathogenic (EPEC), enteroaggregative, enterohemorrhagic (EHEC), and enteroinvasive (EIEC) *E. coli* all are basically the same organism, differing only by the acquisition of specific pathogenic traits [86]. Clinically significant *E. coli* that cause gastrointestinal illness can be grouped as causing nonbloody diarrhea (ETEC, EPEC, and enteroaggregative) and bloody diarrhea (EHEC, EIEC).

Enterotoxigenic E. coli

ETEC cause noninvasive watery diarrhea and together with rotavirus are responsible for most diarrheal illnesses in children. In developing countries, ETEC have a profound impact on mortality and on childhood growth and development [87,88]. ETEC do not damage the epithelium or invade cells, but they have acquired plasmids that allow them to make specialized attachment factors (fimbrial adhesins) for epithelial surfaces (Fig. 2) [89]. They also possess toxins that activate cellular switches, stimulating secretion of ions and water into the gastrointestinal lumen.

Two major classes of toxins have been identified in ETEC (LT [heat labile] and ST [heat stable]) [90]. The LT toxins are identical to cholera toxin in their mechanism of action (classic A-B toxins). They have five external "B" subunits that bind to cell surface lipids decorated with specific short chains of sugars (GM_1 gangliosides). This binding allows for the translocation of the "A" subunit across the cell membrane and into the cell. When inside the cell, the A subunit begins a cascade of modifications of host cell signals that result in the dysregulation of sodium and chloride transport, ion secretion, and massive water loss.

The second group of ETEC toxins, the ST toxins, also cause fluid and electrolyte secretion, without cell damage. Instead of being large multimeric proteins similar to LT, they are composed of small oligopeptides of 18 to 20 amino acids, which are not easily denatured and are stable at high temperature. In

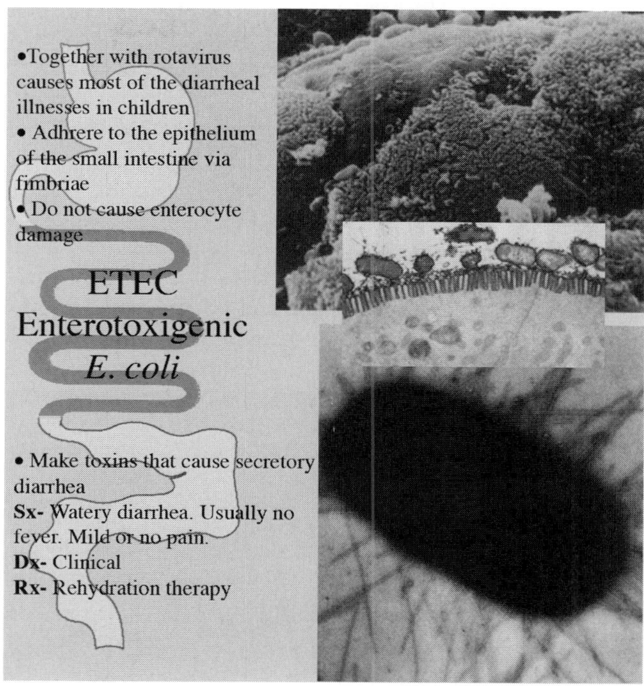

•Together with rotavirus causes most of the diarrheal illnesses in children
• Adhrere to the epithelium of the small intestine via fimbriae
• Do not cause enterocyte damage
ETEC
Enterotoxigenic
E. coli
• Make toxins that cause secretory diarrhea
Sx- Watery diarrhea. Usually no fever. Mild or no pain.
Dx- Clinical
Rx- Rehydration therapy

Fig. 2. Enterotoxigenic *E. coli* (ETEC) infect the small intestine. They adhere to enterocytes via type 1 fimbriae. Scanning electron micrograph (*top*) shows a human duodenal biopsy specimen that was cultured ex vivo in the presence of ETEC for 12 hours. Note the extensive bacterial colonization of the mucosal surface, also shown by transmission electron micrograph (*middle*). In the bottom transmission electron micrograph, an EPEC bacillus is negatively stained to show surface type 1 fimbriae. Dx, diagnosis; Rx, treatment; Sx, symptoms. (*Micrographs from* Knutton S, Lloyd DR, McNeish AS. Identification of a new fimbrial structure in enterotoxigenic *Escherichia coli* (ETEC) serotype O148:H28 which adheres to human intestinal mucosa: a potentially new human ETEC colonization factor. Infect Immun 1987;55:86; with permission.)

contrast to LT, they do not need to enter the cell for their effect because they function by activating a membrane receptor expressed on the apical surface of enterocytes called *guanylate cyclase type C* [91,92]. These peptide toxins mimic the function of endogenous gastrointestinal peptides, guanylin and uroguanylin, which are the natural ligands of guanylate cyclase type C and are involved in regulating salt homeostasis in the gastrointestinal tract and kidney.

The final common pathway for the LT and ST diarrheagenic toxins of ETEC (and cholera toxin) is activation of chloride secretion through the cystic fibrosis transmembrane conductance regulator (CFTR) [93]. Children that inherit mutations in both copies of the gene coding for CFTR develop cystic fibrosis. It has been postulated that the high prevalence of cystic fibrosis in some populations may have arisen as evolutionary selection of heterozygous carriers who could survive diarrheal illness better [94].

A corollary of this hypothesis is the idea that selective inhibitors of CFTR could function in the treatment of cholera and ETEC diarrhea. Attempts to develop these compounds are ongoing; success in animal models has been reported [95–98]. For now, the treatment of secretory diarrhea, regardless of etiology, is hydration and electrolyte management.

Enteropathogenic E. coli and other noninvasive E. coli

EPEC are an important cause of neonatal and infantile diarrhea in developing countries and a cause of diarrhea of long duration (>14 days) [99]. The precise

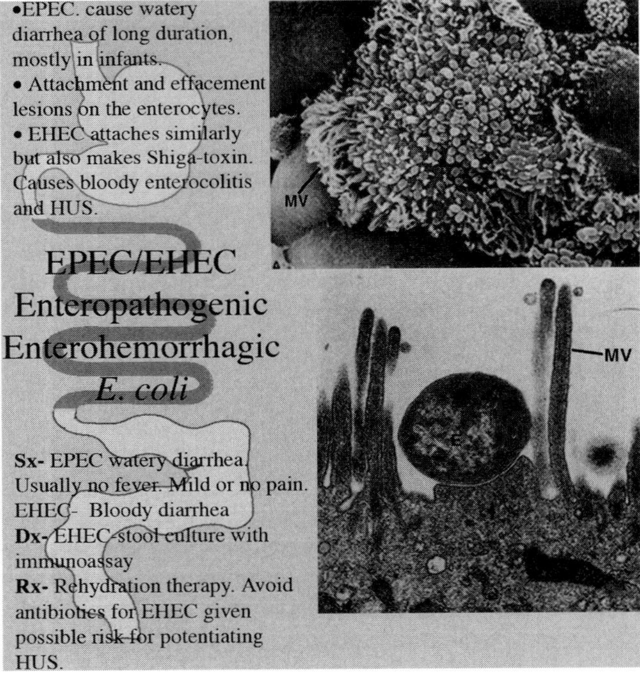

Fig. 3. Enteropathogenic *E. coli* (EPEC) and enterohemorrhagic *E. coli* (EHEC) are related to each other but cause different diseases. They both adhere to the surface of the enterocytes in the small intestine and modify the attachment site by injecting bacterial proteins into the host cell. Scanning electron micrograph (*top*) shows a human duodenal biopsy sample infected with EPEC for 6 hours. A dense microcolony is shown on the surface of enterocytes surrounded by normal cells. Transmission electron micrograph (*bottom*) shows a section through the attachment site of EPEC to cultured human intestinal mucosa. Note the intimate attachment at a cuplike projection of the enterocyte membrane. Microvilli (MV) are destroyed at the sites of attachment. EHEC (ie, *E coli* O157:H7) adheres to enterocytes in a similar manner, but also makes Shiga toxin and causes hemolytic uremic syndrome. Dx, diagnosis; Rx, treatment; Sx, symptoms. (*Micrographs from* Knutton S, Lloyd DR, McNeish AS. Adhesion of enteropathogenic *Escherichia coli* to human intestinal enterocytes and cultured human intestinal mucosa. Infect Immun 1987;55:69; with permission.)

mechanism by which EPEC cause diarrhea is not well understood, but bacteria have a characteristic way of attaching to the surface of enterocytes, effacing the microvilli, and growing as dense microcolonies directly on the membrane of infected cells (Fig. 3) [100]. EPEC is able to modify the cell surface to enhance its own adhesion [101] and does so by injecting bacterial effector proteins into the host cell through a molecular microsyringe (a type 3 secretion system), to control the organization of host molecules underneath the adherent bacteria [102,103]. By injecting other bacterial virulence factors into the cells, the junctions between enterocytes are disrupted [104]; this likely contributes to diarrhea by allowing fluid to leak out between the enterocytes.

Specialized adhesion with damage to the cell cytoskeleton is a recurrent pathogenic mechanism in *E. coli* that cause gastrointestinal disease. Numerous strains associated with diarrhea already have been identified that adhere in different ways to the cell surface. Enteroaggregative *E. coli* (also known as enteroadherent *E. coli*) are associated with persistent diarrhea in children [105–110] and secrete at least one toxin that disrupts the cell cytoskeleton [111,112].

Enterohemorrhagic E. coli (Shiga toxin–producing E. coli, O157:H7)

In the developed world, strains of *E. coli* derived from EPEC that have acquired the ability to produce Shiga toxin are emerging as a health threat that can cause serious disease. These strains of "killer *E. coli*" cause a hemorrhagic colitis that is complicated by hemolytic uremic syndrome (HUS) in 5% to 10% of infected children [113].

The source of these *E. coli* is not the human intestine, but cattle and sheep, and the emergence of this zoonotic disease in developed nations is related to mass production of bovine products, especially ground beef (ie, "hamburger disease"). EHEC is related most closely to EPEC strains and possesses some of the same cellular adhesion mechanisms, including the microsyringe, adhesion apparatus, and ability to modify the cytoskeleton underneath adherent bacteria (Fig. 3) [114]. In contrast to EPEC, however, EHEC also have acquired the ability to make cytotoxins related to those of *Shigella dysenteriae*.

It is thought that the Shiga toxins produced by EHEC are largely responsible for the development of HUS. The genes encoding these toxins were acquired by EPEC strains through infection with a bacteriophage. There are two major types of toxin, Stx1 and Stx2. Stx1 is identical to the toxin produced by *S. dysenteriae* type 1. Stx2 is structurally related and is more likely to lead to HUS [115,116].

Similar to cholera toxin, Shiga toxins are A-B toxins [117]. They consist of five B subunits that are arranged in a ring around an A subunit protein. The B subunits are involved in binding to a cell surface receptor, in this case a sugar decorated lipid termed *globotriosyl ceramide* (Gb3) [118]. The B subunits confer cell tropism and allow translocation of the A subunit into the cell. When inside, the A subunit intoxicates the cell by inactivating the protein synthesis machinery, eventually causing cell death. Intoxication also causes release of proinflammatory cytokines by the affected cells, which induces an inflammatory response that contributes to cellular damage [119–121]. Inflammation also increases the expression of the Gb3 receptor, making the inflamed tissue more susceptible to further damage by the toxins [122].

Clinical manifestations and complications

Infections with ETEC and EPEC, which are noninvasive, result in watery diarrhea. ETEC causes a clinical syndrome similar to cholera, with mild diarrhea in most cases, but which also can lead to severe dehydration. Most often the illness is self-limited and lasts less than 1 week. EPEC causes a similar syndrome, but diarrhea may be protracted, lasting 2 weeks or more [99]. The longer duration of symptoms probably is related to damage of the absorptive microvilli, causing malabsorption and food intolerance [123]. ETEC and EPEC are common causes of traveler's diarrhea. Other than acute dehydration, both also are associated with acute and long-term consequences of malnutrition in infants in developing nations [124].

Although EHEC use an attachment mechanism similar to EPEC, the clinical manifestations of EHEC infection are largely due to the destructive effects of Shiga toxin. Within 2 to 5 days of ingesting food contaminated with EHEC, some infected children develop hemorrhagic colitis with frank blood in the stool. The colitis may be painless or associated with abdominal pain. Symptoms usually subside spontaneously without sequelae, but some individuals develop HUS, which has become the leading cause of acute renal failure in children in the United States. HUS is characterized clinically by microangiopathic hemolytic anemia, thrombocytopenia, CNS findings, and acute renal failure.

The toxins affect enterocytes locally, but also injure the underlying microvasculature, and this is thought to cause the hemorrhagic gastroenteritis. Toxin also is transported in the circulation and concentrated in the kidney vasculature, where it leads to kidney damage [125]. CNS symptoms, such as lethargy and irritability, are common, and other complications, such as seizures, may accompany CNS vascular injury. Hypertension and electrolyte imbalances resulting from renal failure also contribute to CNS disease. More than half of patients with HUS require temporary renal dialysis [126,127]. Even with optimal therapy, the disease has a 5% to 10% mortality rate secondary to complications of renal failure [128,129].

Diagnosis and treatment

Definitive diagnosis of ETEC and EPEC diarrhea is not usually available because it requires distinguishing these strains from normal stool *E. coli*. As with other forms of noninvasive diarrhea, most cases of ETEC and EPEC infection should be treated by reestablishing optimal hydration and correcting electrolyte abnormalities. Continuation of breastfeeding and early restitution of feeding also are important in minimizing the impact on nutrition and growth. Although antibiotic therapy is useful in treating acute diarrhea from ETEC and protracted diarrhea from EPEC, defining an empirical antimicrobial treatment regimen is difficult. Antimicrobial susceptibilities vary widely in different *E. coli* strains, and ETEC and EPEC are often resistant to amoxicillin and clotrimazole [130,131]. Fluoroquinolones commonly are used in adults for traveler's diarrhea, but are not recommended for children. Clotrimazole and azithromycin may be useful in some cases of EPEC-induced or ETEC-induced diarrhea.

As with other pathogenic *E. coli,* identification of EHEC requires distinguishing it from commensal *E. coli* in the stool; this is done by screening for the ability of strains to ferment sorbitol, a characteristic of many (but not all) EHEC strains. Definitive diagnosis is based on enzyme immunoassays. More recently, polymerase chain reaction–based technologies have been developed that detect the presence of the Shiga toxin genes [132]. The ability of laboratories to identify EHEC quickly varies widely, and it is common for hospital laboratories to perform the initial screening tests, then refer suspicious specimens for final typing to reference and state laboratories. It is important for clinicians to understand this process in their local microbiology laboratories because positive identification of EHEC may not be timely.

The optimal treatment for children with EHEC aiming to prevent or ameliorate HUS is unknown. It is important to monitor children with bloody diarrhea for signs of hemolysis, thrombocytopenia, and renal failure. Intravenous hydration to reduce glomerular injury has been advocated [133]. Antimotility drugs probably worsen outcomes by increasing the concentrations of toxin [134,135]. The effect of antimicrobial therapy on the incidence of HUS has been controversial. Some studies show no relationship between antibiotic use and the development of HUS [134,136]. One study from Japan showed a reduction in risk with antibiotic treatment early in the disease [137]. Other studies have shown a higher risk of development of HUS after the use of antibiotics [138,139]. The reasons for these differences in outcome are still not well understood, but some insight has come from understanding the pathogenesis of the disease in animal models. Certain antibiotics, such as fluoroquinolones, cause DNA damage to the bacteria. When given in sublethal doses, these have been shown to induce the latent bacteriophages coding for Shiga toxin to increase production and release of the toxin and increase mortality [140]. Other antibiotics with different modes of action may not have the same effects. These results point to the danger in assuming that inflammatory gastroenteritis can be treated empirically with one antibiotic that covers all enteric pathogens. Until it is understand how best to prevent HUS, antimicrobial therapy for EHEC infections should be avoided. Promising therapies with biologically inert compounds that bind and neutralize the toxin in the intestine are under investigation [141,142], but they may not be useful if started after HUS has ensued [143], so methods for early detection of EHEC infection are important. Antibody-based therapies to neutralize the toxin in the bloodstream and kidneys also are being studied for the treatment of HUS [144]. To date, no published clinical trials have shown benefit of a particular therapeutic intervention in the prevention or treatment of HUS.

Shigella

Shigella are gram-negative nonmotile rods that are closely related to *E. coli*. In contrast to EHEC, which colonizes animals, humans are the only reservoir of *Shigella,* and transmission is fecal-oral. The inoculum needed to cause disease is small (10–100 organisms), increasing the risk of epidemic disease and transfer through vectors such as houseflies [145].

Epidemiology and pathogenesis

In addition to the toxin-producing properties of EHEC, *Shigella* have acquired the ability to invade the cells of the intestinal mucosa and spread within them. *Shigella,* similar to *Salmonella,* gain initial entry across the epithelial barrier by inducing their uptake into specialized immune-surveillance cells overlying Peyer's patches (M cells), but they have a predilection for the colonic epithelium [146]. The organisms then spread to adjacent enterocytes by invading them through their basolateral surface.

Invasion of the colonic epithelium is a pathogen-driven process in which *Shigella* bind to the cell surface and use a microsyringe (type 3 secretion system) to deliver bacterial effector proteins into host cells, which rearrange the cytoskeleton beneath adhered bacteria, inducing their uptake into a membrane bound vacuole [147]. When inside a cell, *Shigella* use other effector proteins to break out of the internalization vacuole [148], then harness the host cell cytoskeleton to move and spread within cells and from cell to cell without being exposed to the immune system [149]; this allows rapid spread within the mucosa.

Shigella also possess toxins. The best understood is Shiga toxin, which causes cell death by stopping protein synthesis and stimulates expression of proinflammatory cytokines, inducing a large amount of local inflammation.

Clinical manifestations and complications

The result of the invasive properties of *Shigella* is that a small bacterial inoculum spreads rapidly in the mucosa, causing ulcerations with substantial neutrophilic inflammation; the small-volume mucus and bloody diarrhea, lower abdominal pain, and tenesmus that are characteristic of *Shigella* dysentery. Generalized symptoms of malaise and fever may precede the diarrhea. In children, especially infants, *Shigella*-associated diarrhea also can be nonbloody, occur without fever or abdominal pain, and cause dehydration [150]. Different *Shigella* species predominate in developed (*S. sonnei*) versus developing (*S. dysenteriae, S. flexneri*) countries. *S. dysenteriae* is the only species that produces Shiga toxin, which increases the risk of complications such as HUS.

Diagnosis and treatment

Diagnosis of *Shigella* is made from stool culture. Treatment with antimicrobials should be considered for shigellosis because it can shorten the duration and severity of symptoms and reduce epidemic spread. The choice of antibiotics in children is limited because of increasing resistance of *Shigella* to ampicillin and clotrimazole (Septra, Bactrim) [151]. Oral and intravenously administered third-generation cephalosporins have proved useful in the treatment of shigellosis [152,153]. Azithromycin may be another useful choice for milder cases that do not require intravenous therapy because this antibiotic concentrates intracellularly and has been effective in several clinical studies [154–156].

Salmonella

Salmonella are members of the Enterobacteriaceae family and are closely related to *E. coli* and *Shigella*. They consist of a highly related group of gram-negative bacilli that has evolved the capacity to colonize the gastrointestinal tract of humans and many different animals, including mammals, birds, reptiles, and insects. Their classification has been confusing because more than 2000 different serovars have been identified [157,158]. Despite the great number of strains, DNA sequence analysis has revealed that *Salmonella* are so closely related that they belong to only two species, *S. enterica* and *S. bongori*. These are divided further into eight subspecies. Of the strains that cause disease in warm-blooded animals, 99% are members of *S. enterica* subspecies I. These highly related strains show great variety in their host preference and their ability to cause disease. The types of disease they cause range from asymptomatic carriage and mild gastroenteritis to bacteremia and enteric fever. Relatively small changes in genetic content can result in dramatic changes in host tropism and virulence.

For clinical purposes, the serovars most likely to cause bacteremia and enteric fever in humans are typhi and paratyphi. The rest (nontyphoidal *Salmonella*) are mostly responsible for noninvasive, self-limited gastroenteritis except in very young and immunocompromised patients. Diseases from nontyphoidal *Salmonella* are largely zoonoses because they colonize animals such as pets (turtles, snakes, birds, dogs, and cats), rodents, and farm animals.

Epidemiology and pathogenesis

In the United States, *S. enteriditis* is the most common cause of nontyphoidal salmonellosis. These bacteria colonize poultry, among other animals. Infection commonly is associated with contaminated eggs and broiler chickens [159]. The eggs usually are infected when egg-laying hens consume feed contaminated with mouse feces [160,161]. The bacteria are able to colonize the intestinal tract of chickens; they also are able to infect the oviducts, probably by invading the bloodstream of the chicken and traveling to the reproductive tract [162,163].

They are transmitted to the forming egg before the shell is deposited. The eggshells and the yolk can be contaminated with *Salmonella*; therefore, cleaning the eggshells is not effective in preventing transmission if the yolk is not cooked. Other common sources of infection are foods and utensils that become contaminated during the handling of uncooked chicken.

In contrast to *S. enteriditis,* typhi and paratyphi *Salmonella* colonize and infect only humans. These bacteria are transmitted by infected people (either acutely ill or asymptomatic chronic carriers), usually through contamination of

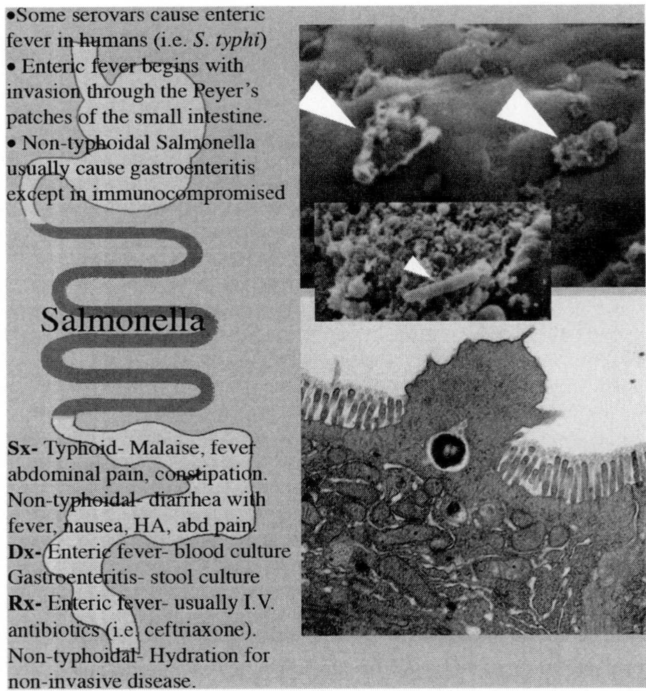

Fig. 4. Different *Salmonella* organisms cause invasive (enteric fever) and noninvasive (gastroenteritis) disease depending on host tropism and virulence factors. The invasive serovars enter the body through the small intestine at the Peyer's patches. Scanning electron micrograph (*top*) illustrates the uptake of *Salmonella* by specialized immune surveillance cells (M cells) located in the Peyer's patches of a mouse small intestine that was infected with *Salmonella* for 30 minutes. The large arrowheads show two M cells where *Salmonella* have adhered and caused rearrangements of the apical membrane. A second scanning electron micrograph (*middle*) is a close-up of an M cell with an adhered salmonella bacillus. Transmission electron micrograph (*bottom*) shows the entry of *Salmonella* into an M cell of the mouse Peyer's patch. Note the membrane projection of the M cell induced by invading *Salmonella*. Dx, diagnosis; HA, headache; Rx, treatment; Sx, symptoms. (*Scanning electron micrographs from* Jensen VB, Harty JT, Jones BD. Interactions of the invasive pathogens *Salmonella typhimurium, Listeria monocytogenes,* and *Shigella flexneri* with M cells and murine Peyer's patches. Infect Immun 1998;66:3758; with permission. Transmission electron micrograph courtesy of D. Monack.)

food or water with human feces. They are endemic in many countries and cause most serious disease in the young. Children younger than 1 year old and immunocompromised patients are susceptible to invasive complications. In the United States, invasive disease is fatal in 5% of patients [164].

The pathogenesis of enteric fever caused by typhi and paratyphi explains some of its clinical manifestations and results from direct invasion of lymphatics and the bloodstream to reach sterile organs. Many of the bacteria in an ingested inoculum perish in the stomach acid, and conditions that increase the stomach pH increase the numbers of infective bacteria able to reach the intestine. The relative hypochlorhydria and rapid gastric emptying of infants is thought to be a risk factor in developing disease [165,166]. When in the small intestine, *Salmonella,* similar to *Shigella,* have evolved a way to cross the epithelial barrier. They specifically invade mucosal cells overlying Peyer's patches termed M cells (Fig. 4) [167,168]. The function of M cells is to maintain immunologic surveillance by sampling the contents of the intestinal lumen. *Salmonella* in the intestinal lumen interact directly with M cells, inject bacterial proteins into them to induce their uptake, and cross the epithelial layer. When below the epithelium, the bacteria are ingested quickly by macrophages. From within the phagocytic vacuoles, the bacteria inject effector molecules into the cytoplasm, inducing macrophage cell death [169,170]. *Salmonella* are released and reingested by new macrophages recruited to the inflamed Peyer's patch. Infected macrophages transport viable *Salmonella* within the lymphatics and bloodstream to the mesenteric lymph nodes, liver, and spleen, where cycles of replication continue, resulting in the symptoms of enteric fever [170,171]. For most bacteria that cause bacteremia in humans, entering the bloodstream is a dead-end for the organisms because they either perish or kill their host without successful transmission. *Salmonella* take advantage of their ability to survive within sterile compartments of their hosts and somehow are able to exit into the lumen of the gut to become transmitted again to a new host.

Clinical manifestations and complications

Enteric fever

Asymptomatic infections are common, with 1% to 5% of the population in developing countries being carriers. In outbreaks with *S. typhi,* more than 50% of individuals infected may remain asymptomatic [172–174]. Enteric fever usually manifests with fever, malaise, headache, irritability, anorexia, mild joint pain, and abdominal pain. Constipation is more common than diarrhea. Blanching, erythematous, "rose" spots may appear in the second week of illness. Hepatomegaly and splenomegaly also are common, especially in infants. Life-threatening complications, such as intestinal perforation, osteomyelitis, pneumonia, meningitis, and pyelonephritis, may occur with typhoid fever. Infants and immunocompromised children are at highest risk of focal extraintestinal infections with *Salmonella,* particularly meningitis and osteomyelitis.

Gastroenteritis

Nontyphoidal *Salmonella* infections usually are self-limited and result in noninvasive gastroenteritis. Symptoms include fever, nausea, vomiting, headache, abdominal pain, and nonbloody or bloody diarrhea. Symptoms usually occur within 2 days of ingesting contaminated food or water. Diarrhea usually lasts for less than 1 week. Infants and children younger than 1 year old [175–178], immunocompromised patients [179], and patients with sickle cell anemia [180] also are at risk of bacteremia and invasive disease with nontyphoidal *Salmonella*.

Diagnosis and treatment

Diagnosis of enteric fever generally is made from blood culture, not stool studies. Enteric fever should be diagnosed promptly and treated with antibiotics according to the susceptibility of the bacterial isolate. Multidrug-resistant *S. typhi* is common in the developing world, but these strains are usually susceptible to ceftriaxone. In contrast, nontyphoidal *Salmonella* diarrhea in immunocompetent children beyond infancy does not benefit from antibiotic treatment, and antibiotics tend to prolong the carrier state [181,182].

Intestinal *Campylobacter*

Campylobacter are gram-negative, spiral-shaped bacilli with single polar flagella. Fourteen *Campylobacter* species are currently known, but *C. jejuni* and *C. coli* are the main human enteropathogens. Phylogenetically, *Campylobacter* are related closely to *Helicobacter* and are microaerophilic, fastidious in vitro, and adapted for life in the mucus layer near enterocytes.

Epidemiology and pathogenesis

Campylobacter are the most commonly isolated bacterial cause of gastroenteritis in developed countries. In contrast to *H. pylori,* which live exclusively in the human host, *Campylobacter* are commensals in the intestinal tracts of numerous birds and mammals, including chickens, domestic pets, pigs, and cattle. Despite being such a common cause of gastroenteritis in humans, campylobacteriosis is a zoonotic infection. *Campylobacter* have an optimal growth temperature of 42°C, which reflects their preferred host temperature in the gastrointestinal tract of birds, where they live without causing disease.

Transmission to humans occurs mostly through the consumption of contaminated food or water. Infection also can result from direct contact with farm animals or households pets [183]. Person-to-person transmission is uncommon. All natural sources of untreated water are contaminated with *Campylobacter* from animal feces. Campers and backpackers may be more likely to acquire *Campylobacter* than *Giardia* from natural water sources [184,185]. Unpasteurized milk has been the source of multiple outbreaks [186], but the most common source is chicken carcasses. *Campylobacter* can be cultured from 60% to 100% of chickens purchased in supermarkets [187–190]. In contrast to *Salmonella, Campylobacter* do not replicate substantially in food, especially at lower temperatures.

In developing countries, *Campylobacter*-related diarrhea tends to occur earlier in life; incidence drops as immunity is acquired [191]. Because travelers have poor immunity to foreign *Campylobacter* strains, *Campylobacter* infection is a common cause of traveler's diarrhea [192].

Campylobacter induce acute inflammatory enteritis with neutrophilic and monocytic infiltration of the mucosa in the colon and the small intestine. The pathogenesis of this inflammatory process is poorly understood because of a lack of animal models for the disease and difficulty in the genetic manipulation of *Campylobacter*. Currently, it is known that *Campylobacter* produce a toxin

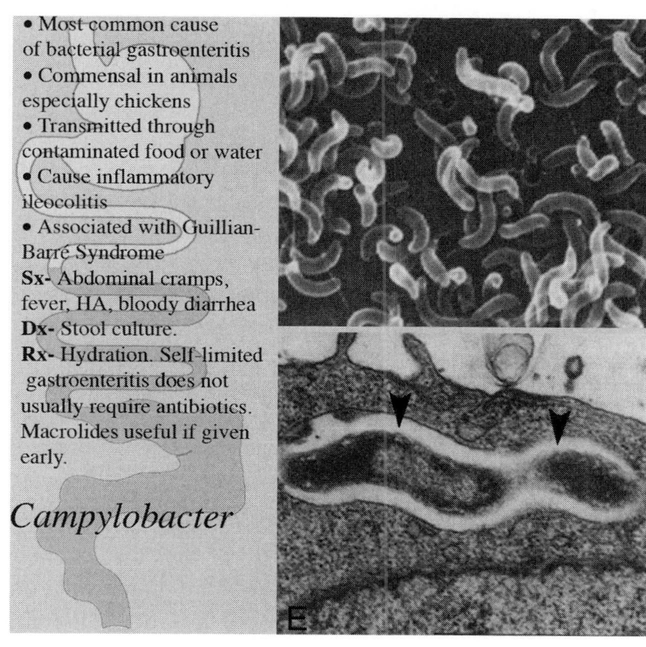

• Most common cause of bacterial gastroenteritis
• Commensal in animals especially chickens
• Transmitted through contaminated food or water
• Cause inflammatory ileocolitis
• Associated with Guillian-Barré Syndrome
Sx- Abdominal cramps, fever, HA, bloody diarrhea
Dx- Stool culture.
Rx- Hydration. Self-limited gastroenteritis does not usually require antibiotics. Macrolides useful if given early.
Campylobacter
E

Fig. 5. *Campylobacter* organisms live as commensals in the gastrointestinal tract of many animals, and cause inflammatory enteritis in children after ingestion of contaminated food or water. *Campylobacter* have a spiral shape seen on scanning electron micrograph (*top*) of an in vitro culture. They are able to invade and destroy epithelial cells in culture. Transmission electron micrograph (*bottom*) shows an example of *C. jejuni* inside a cultured epithelial cell. Arrowheads point to the intracellular bacterium within a vacuole (reproduced with permission from Fauchere et al, 1986 [60]) Dx, diagnosis; HA, headache; Rx, treatment; Sx, symptoms. (*Scanning electron micrograph from* Rollins DM, Colwell RR. Viable but nonculturable stage of *Campylobacter jejuni* and its role in survival in the natural aquatic environment. Appl Environ Microbiol 1986;52:531; with permission. *Transmission electron micrograph from* Fauchere JL, Rosenau A, Veron M, et al. Association with HeLa cells of *Campylobacter jejuni* and *Campylobacter coli* isolated from human feces. Infect Immun 1986;54:283; with permission.)

termed *cytolethal distending toxin,* which causes cells to enlarge and to stop dividing after cell cycle arrest [193]. The precise mechanism of action of this toxin and its contribution to gastroenteritis are not clear, however. In animal models, there is evidence that it has proinflammatory activity [194,195] and contributes to inflammatory diarrhea [196]. Mutant bacteria that lack the toxin are less invasive in immunocompromised mice [197]. *Campylobacter* also are able to invade intestinal epithelial cells in culture (Fig. 5) [198] and in animal models of infection [199]. This ability to breach and destroy cells in the colon is also a likely virulence factor involved in enterocolitis.

Clinical manifestations and complications

Campylobacter cause disease in all ages, with the peak incidence in children. An inoculum of 500 organisms may cause infection, and the incubation period ranges from 1 day to 1 week (mean 2.5 days) [200]. *Campylobacter* are sensitive to gastric acid, but when in the small intestine they are resistant to bile acids. Abdominal cramps and diarrhea are usually the first symptoms of infection, although about one third of patients report a flulike prodrome, with fever, headache, and myalgia [201,202]. In some people, abdominal pain is the only symptom, and diarrhea does not develop. Most people develop diarrhea, and blood in the stools is common, especially in children. The illness usually lasts 4 to 6 days with spontaneous resolution. Infants usually have milder disease, with less abdominal pain and fever, but they are more likely to have bloody stools. Although *Campylobacter* are a common cause of abortion in cattle, they rarely cause abortion in humans [203,204]. Occasionally, perinatal transmission occurs and may result in bacteremia and meningitis.

Campylobacter gastroenteritis also is associated with important late-onset sequelae, especially Guillain-Barré syndrome and postinfectious hypersensitivity syndromes, such as reactive arthritis, urticaria, and erythema nodosum. *Campylobacter* infection is the most commonly identified antecedent in Guillain-Barré syndrome and occurs in approximately 30 per 100,000 cases of campylobacter gastroenteritis [205]. The pathogenesis of Guillain-Barré syndrome is thought to be an autoimmune reaction to lipopolysaccharide antigens present in *Campylobacter* that mimic human gangliosides in peripheral nerve sheaths [206].

Diagnosis and treatment

Diagnosis of *Campylobacter* gastroenteritis is made from stool culture. Most episodes of gastroenteritis caused by *Campylobacter* usually are self-limited and should be treated with hydration. Antibiotic therapy generally is not necessary, although empirical antimicrobial treatment with ciprofloxacin is commonly used in adults. Because of the use of antibiotics in animal rearing, there is a rapidly increasing resistance to fluoroquinolones in *Campylobacter* strains, making ciprofloxacin empirical treatment of infectious enteritis less useful. Antibiotic therapy should be reserved for severe infection and for patients with HIV and other forms of immunosuppression. Macrolide antibiotics such as erythromycin and azithromycin are effective because they work against fluoroquinolone-resistant strains [207] and because these organisms are naturally resistant to cephalosporins, and clotrimazole.

Summary and clinical approach to a child with suspected bacterial infection of the gastrointestinal tract

In 1999, it was estimated that food-borne diseases cause approximately 76 million illnesses, 325,000 hospitalizations, and 5000 deaths yearly in the United States [208]. In the developing world, diarrhea is still a major killer of children younger than 5 years of age. Each year, 1.7 million deaths worldwide are due to infectious diarrhea. Ninety percent of these deaths are in children [209]. Hygienic practices in the developed world have reduced the prevalence of human-adapted pathogens, such as *H. pylori, Shigella,* and *Salmonella typhi*. Mass food production has introduced a tremendous amount of zoonotic infection in the developed world, however, caused by bacteria such as EHEC, *Salmonella enteriditis,* and *Campylobacter*.

Empirical management of childhood gastrointestinal tract infections should take into account the clinical presentation, travel and daycare history, immunologic status and age of host, and knowledge of the likely offending pathogens. Rehydration and electrolyte replacement is the most important aspect of treatment of most acute gastrointestinal illnesses. In addition, severely ill, immunocompromised, or very young children with suspected bacterial infections of the gastrointestinal tract should undergo further diagnostic workup and empirical therapy with antimicrobials.

The most common presentation of gastrointestinal infections is noninvasive, self-limited watery diarrhea that requires close attention to hydration and electrolyte management, but does not generally warrant antimicrobial therapy or further diagnosis. Either viral pathogens, such as rotavirus, or toxin-producing *E. coli* (ETEC) are usually responsible. At the cellular level, these syndromes show no destructive lesions of the mucosa or submucosa and have little accompanying inflammation. Antibiotics are not useful in viral infections and generally are not required for management of noninvasive bacterial infections except in the case of *Vibrio cholerae,* which causes massive watery diarrhea, and where antimicrobial therapy can reduce diarrheal output in half [210,211]. Other noninvasive bacterial infections may benefit from antimicrobials by reducing severity and duration of symptoms, such as in traveler's diarrhea caused by ETEC and chronic diarrhea caused by EPEC. Nevertheless, etiologic diagnosis is difficult to obtain for these infections, and empirical therapy with antimicrobials is not currently recommended.

Invasive bacterial illnesses of the gastrointestinal tract cause varying degrees of inflammation and gastrointestinal bleeding and can be recognized clinically or through stool examination. When invasive enteropathogens are suspected in a child who is likely to develop severe disease, stool cultures and blood cultures should be obtained so that an etiologic agent can be identified and appropriate antimicrobial therapy selected. Most laboratories routinely attempt to identify *Salmonella, Shigella,* and *Campylobacter* in stool samples. Some require special handling, such as *Yersinia,* which grows best at 25°C rather than at 37°C. Also, identification of the many different strains of pathogenic *E. coli* is not always available. Only EHEC (0157:H7) is routinely screened for because of its strong association with HUS.

Choosing outpatient empirical antimicrobial therapy for children with invasive bacterial gastroenteritis is not straightforward because many pathogenic strains have become resistant to first-line oral antibiotics used in pediatrics, such as amoxicillin and clotrimazole. Also, caution must be exercised when dealing with EHEC (0157:H7) because antibiotics may potentiate the release of toxin and, in some situations, increase the risk of HUS. It is generally more prudent to avoid empirical antibiotic therapy for mild cases of invasive gastroenteritis, obtain appropriate cultures, and perform follow-up before deciding on the treatment course.

For seriously ill patients in whom invasive disease with *Salmonella* (eg, enteric fever), *Shigella,* and *Yersinia* are suspected, empirical therapy with a third-generation cephalosporin (eg, ceftriaxone) would cover most isolates until identification and sensitivities are available. *Campylobacter* organisms are naturally resistant to cephalosporins, however.

Potentially invasive enteropathogens may cause only mild watery diarrhea, and these infections usually are missed on clinical grounds. These are usually self-limited illnesses, but in some cases, such as in early infancy, even mild enteric infections can lead to bacteremia (as with salmonellosis), and mild or even asymptomatic illness may lead to epidemic spread. Stool and blood cultures should be obtained in infants and young children with inflammatory diarrhea, when empirical antibiotic therapy is contemplated.

References

[1] Marshall BJ. The *Campylobacter pylori story*. Scand J Gastroenterol Suppl 1988;146:58–66.

[2] Drumm B, O'Brien A, Cutz E, et al. *Campylobacter pyloridis*-associated primary gastritis in children. Pediatrics 1987;80:192–5.

[3] Eastham EJ, Elliott TS, Berkeley D, et al. *Campylobacter pylori* infection in children. J Infect 1988;16:77–9.

[4] Imrie C, Rowland M, Bourke B, et al. Is *Helicobacter pylori* infection in childhood a risk factor for gastric cancer? Pediatrics 2001;107:373–80.

[5] Han SR, Zschausch HC, Meyer HG, et al. *Helicobacter pylori*: clonal population structure and restricted transmission within families revealed by molecular typing. J Clin Microbiol 2000; 38:515–24.

[6] Owen RJ, Xerry J. Tracing clonality of *Helicobacter pylori* infecting family members from analysis of DNA sequences of three housekeeping genes (ureI, atpA and ahpC), deduced amino acid sequences, and pathogenicity-associated markers (cagA and vacA). J Med Microbiol 2003;52:3646–51.

[7] Falush D, Wirth T, Linz B, et al. Traces of human migrations in *Helicobacter pylori* populations. Science 2003;299:1582–5.
[8] Deltenre M, de Koster E. How come I've got it? (A review of *Helicobacter pylori* transmission). Eur J Gastroenterol Hepatol 2000;12:479–82.
[9] Goodman KJ, Correa P. Transmission of *Helicobacter pylori* among siblings. Lancet 2000; 355:358–62.
[10] Miyaji H, Azuma T, Ito S, et al. *Helicobacter pylori* infection occurs via close contact with infected individuals in early childhood. J Gastroenterol Hepatol 2000;15:257–62.
[11] Malaty HM, El-Kasabany A, Graham DY, et al. Age at acquisition of *Helicobacter pylori* infection: a follow-up study from infancy to adulthood. Lancet 2002;359:931–5.
[12] Lindkvist P, Asrat D, Nilsson I, et al. Age at acquisition of *Helicobacter pylori* infection: comparison of a high and a low prevalence country. Scand J Infect Dis 1996;28:181–4.
[13] Kelly DJ. The physiology and metabolism of the human gastric pathogen *Helicobacter pylori*. Adv Microb Physiol 1998;40:3529–39.
[14] Merrell DS, Goodrich ML, Otto G, et al. pH-regulated gene expression of the gastric pathogen *Helicobacter pylori*. Infect Immun 2003;71:137–89.
[15] Foynes S, Dorrell N, Ward SJ, et al. *Helicobacter pylori* possesses two CheY response regulators and a histidine kinase sensor, CheA, which are essential for chemotaxis and colonization of the gastric mucosa. Infect Immun 2000;68:2016–23.
[16] Lee A. The microbiology and epidemiology of *Helicobacter pylori* infection. Scand J Gastroenterol Suppl 1994;201:2–6.
[17] Thomsen L, Tasman-Jones C, Morris A, et al. Ammonia produced by *Campylobacter pylori* neutralizes H+ moving through gastric mucus. Scand J Gastroenterol 1989;24:761–8.
[18] Eltumi M, Brueton MJ, Francis N. Diagnosis of *Helicobacter pylori* gastritis in children using the 13C urea breath test. J Clin Gastroenterol 1999;28:238–40.
[19] Kazi JL, Sinniah R, Zaman V, et al. Ultrastructural study of *Helicobacter pylori*-associated gastritis. J Pathol 1990;161:65–70.
[20] Wadstrom T, Hirmo S, Nilsson B. Biochemical aspects of *H. pylori* adhesion. J Physiol Pharmacol 1997;48:325–31.
[21] Backert S, Ziska E, Brinkmann V, et al. Translocation of the *Helicobacter pylori* CagA protein in gastric epithelial cells by a type IV secretion apparatus. Cell Microbiol 2000; 2:155–64.
[22] Odenbreit S, Puls J, Sedlmaier B, et al. Translocation of *Helicobacter pylori* CagA into gastric epithelial cells by type IV secretion. Science 2000;287:1497–500.
[23] Stein M, Rappuoli R, Covacci A. Tyrosine phosphorylation of the *Helicobacter pylori* CagA antigen after cag-driven host cell translocation. Proc Natl Acad Sci U S A 2000;97:1263–8.
[24] Censini S, Stein M, Covacci A. Cellular responses induced after contact with *Helicobacter pylori*. Curr Opin Microbiol 2001;4:41–6.
[25] Churin Y, Al-Ghoul L, Kepp O, et al. *Helicobacter pylori* CagA protein targets the c-Met receptor and enhances the motogenic response. J Cell Biol 2003;161:249–55.
[26] Higashi H, Tsutsumi R, Muto S, et al. SHP-2 tyrosine phosphatase as an intracellular target of *Helicobacter pylori* CagA protein. Science 2002;295:683–6.
[27] Stein M, Bagnoli F, Halenbeck R, et al. c-Src/Lyn kinases activate *Helicobacter pylori* CagA through tyrosine phosphorylation of the EPIYA motifs. Mol Microbiol 2002;43:971–80.
[28] Amieva MR, Vogelmann R, Covacci A, et al. Disruption of the epithelial apical-junctional complex by *Helicobacter pylori* CagA. Science 2003;300:1430–4.
[29] Camorlinga-Ponce M, Romo C, Gonzalez-Valencia G, et al. Topographical localisation of cagA positive and cagA negative *Helicobacter pylori* strains in the gastric mucosa:an in situ hybridisation study. J Clin Pathol 2004;57:822–8.
[30] Hazell SL, Lee A, Brady L, et al. *Campylobacter pyloridis* and gastritis: association with intercellular spaces and adaptation to an environment of mucus as important factors in colonization of the gastric epithelium. J Infect Dis 1986;153:658–63.
[31] Noach LA, Rolf TM, Tytgat GN. Electron microscopic study of association between *Helicobacter pylori* and gastric and duodenal mucosa. J Clin Pathol 1994;47:699–704.

[32] Terres AM, Pajares JM, Hopkins AM, et al. *Helicobacter pylori* disrupts epithelial barrier function in a process inhibited by protein kinase C activators. Infect Immun 1998;66:2943–50.
[33] van Amsterdam K, van der Ende A. Nutrients released by gastric epithelial cells enhance *Helicobacter pylori* growth. Helicobacter 2004;9:614–21.
[34] Yamashiro Y, Oguchi S, Otsuka Y, et al. *Helicobacter pylori* colonization in children with gastritis and peptic ulcer: II. ultrastructural change of the gastric mucosa. Acta Paediatr Jpn 1994;36:171–5.
[35] Amieva MR, Salama NR, Tompkins LS, et al. *Helicobacter pylori* enter and survive within multivesicular vacuoles of epithelial cells. Cell Microbiol 2002;4:677–90.
[36] Hulten K, Cars O, Hjelm E, et al. In-vitro activity of azithromycin in against intracellular *Helicobacter pylori*. J Antimicrob Chemother 1996;37:483–9.
[37] Ko GH, Kang SM, Kim YK, et al. Invasiveness of *Helicobacter pylori* into human gastric mucosa. Helicobacter 1999;4:77–81.
[38] Wyle FA, Tarnawski A, Schulman D, et al. Evidence for gastric mucosal cell invasion by *C. pylori*: an ultrastructural study. J Clin Gastroenterol 1990;12(Suppl 1):S92–8.
[39] de Bernard M, Cappon A, Del Giudice G, et al. The multiple cellular activities of the VacA cytotoxin of Helicobacter pylori. Int J Med Microbiol 2004;293:589–97.
[40] Nowak JA, Forouzandeh B. Estimates of *Helicobacter pylori* densities in the gastric mucus layer by PCR, histologic examination, and CLOtest. Am J Clin Pathol 1997;108:284–8.
[41] Ashorn M. What are the specific features of *Helicobacter pylori* gastritis in children? Ann Med 1995;27:617–20.
[42] Gormally SM, Prakash N, Durnin MT, et al. Association of symptoms with *Helicobacter pylori* infection in children. J Pediatr 1995;126:753–6.
[43] Kimia A, Zahavi I, Shapiro R, et al. The role of *Helicobacter pylori* and gastritis in children with recurrent abdominal pain. Isr Med Assoc J 2000;2:126–8.
[44] Kokkonen J, Haapalahti M, Tikkanen S, et al. Gastrointestinal complaints and diagnosis in children: a population-based study. Acta Paediatr 2004;93:880–6.
[45] Mittal SK, Mathew JL. *Helicobacter pylori* infection in children: a review. Trop Gastroenterol 2003;24:106–15.
[46] Prieto G, Polanco I, Larrauri J, et al. *Helicobacter pylori* infection in children: clinical, endoscopic, and histologic correlations. J Pediatr Gastroenterol Nutr 1992;14:420–5.
[47] Tolia V. *Helicobacter pylori* infection in pediatric patients. Curr Gastroenterol Rep 1999;1: 308–13.
[48] Kato S, Nishino Y, Ozawa K, et al. The prevalence of *Helicobacter pylori* in Japanese children with gastritis or peptic ulcer disease. J Gastroenterol 2004;39:734–8.
[49] Macarthur C, Saunders N, Feldman W. *Helicobacter pylori,* gastroduodenal disease, and recurrent abdominal pain in children. JAMA 1995;273:729–34.
[50] Ashorn M, Ruuska T, Karikoski R, et al. *Helicobacter pylori* gastritis in dyspeptic children: a long-term follow-up after treatment with colloidal bismuth subcitrate and tinidazole. Scand J Gastroenterol 1994;29:203–8.
[51] De Giacomo C, Valdambrini V, Lizzoli F, et al. A population-based survey on gastrointestinal tract symptoms and *Helicobacter pylori* infection in children and adolescents. Helicobacter 2002;7:356–63.
[52] Gunaid AA, Hassan NA, Murray-Lyon I. Prevalence and risk factors for *Helicobacter pylori* infection among Yemeni dyspeptic patients. Saudi Med J 2003;24:512–7.
[53] Hyams JS, Davis P, Sylvester FA, et al. Dyspepsia in children and adolescents: a prospective study. J Pediatr Gastroenterol Nutr 2000;30:413–8.
[54] Sherman PM, Macarthur C. Current controversies associated with *Helicobacter pylori* infection in the pediatric population. Front Biosci 2001;6:E187–92.
[55] Ando K, Shimamoto T, Tauchi T, et al. Can eradication therapy for *Helicobacter pylori* really improve the thrombocytopenia in idiopathic thrombocytopenic purpura? Our experience and a literature review. Int J Hematol 2003;77:239–44.
[56] Franchini M, Veneri D. *Helicobacter pylori* infection and immune thrombocytopenic purpura: an update. Helicobacter 2004;9:342–6.

[57] Huber MR, Kumar S, Tefferi A. Treatment advances in adult immune thrombocytopenic purpura. Ann Hematol 2003;82:723–37.
[58] Kurekci AE, Atay AA, Sarici SU, et al. Complete platelet recovery after treatment of *Helicobacter pylori* infection in a child with chronic immune thrombocytopenic purpura: a case report. Pediatr Hematol Oncol 2004;21:593–6.
[59] Michel M, Cooper N, Jean C, et al. Does *Helicobater pylori* initiate or perpetuate immune thrombocytopenic purpura? Blood 2004;103:890–6.
[60] Takahashi T, Yujiri T, Shinohara K, et al. Molecular mimicry by *Helicobacter pylori* CagA protein may be involved in the pathogenesis of *H. pylori*-associated chronic idiopathic thrombocytopenic purpura. Br J Haematol 2004;124:91–6.
[61] Ashorn M, Ruuska T, Makipernaa A. *Helicobacter pylori* and iron deficiency anaemia in children. Scand J Gastroenterol 2001;36:701–5.
[62] Takahashi T, Yujiri T, Tanizawa Y. *Helicobacter pylori* and chronic ITP: the discrepancy in the clinical responses to eradication therapy might be due to differences in the bacterial strains. Blood 2004;104:594.
[63] Barabino A, Dufour C, Marino CE, et al. Unexplained refractory iron-deficiency anemia associated with *Helicobacter pylori* gastric infection in children: further clinical evidence. J Pediatr Gastroenterol Nutr 1999;28:116–9.
[64] Choe YH, Kim SK, Hong YC. The relationship between *Helicobacter pylori* infection and iron deficiency: seroprevalence study in 937 pubescent children. Arch Dis Child 2003;88:178.
[65] Choi JW. Does *Helicobacter pylori* infection relate to iron deficiency anaemia in prepubescent children under 12 years of age? Acta Paediatr 2003;92:970–2.
[66] Seo JK, Ko JS, Choi KD. Serum ferritin and *Helicobacter pylori* infection in children: a sero-epidemiologic study in Korea. J Gastroenterol Hepatol 2002;17:754–7.
[67] Aggarwal A. Helicobacter pylori infection: a cause of growth delay in children. Indian Pediatr 1998;35:191–2.
[68] Bravo LE, Mera R, Reina JC, et al. Impact of *Helicobacter pylori* infection on growth of children: a prospective cohort study. J Pediatr Gastroenterol Nutr 2003;37:614–9.
[69] Ertem D, Pehlivanoglu E. *Helicobacter pylori* may influence height in children independent of socioeconomic factors. J Pediatr Gastroenterol Nutr 2002;35:232–3.
[70] Oderda G, Palli D, Saieva C, et al. Short stature and *Helicobacter pylori* infection in Italian children: prospective multicentre hospital based case-control study. The Italian Study Group on Short Stature and H pylori. BMJ 1998;317:514–5.
[71] Richter T, List S, Muller DM, et al. Five- to 7-year-old children with *Helicobacter pylori* infection are smaller than *Helicobacter*-negative children: a cross-sectional population-based study of 3,315 children. J Pediatr Gastroenterol Nutr 2001;33:472–5.
[72] Clemens J, Albert MJ, Rao M, et al. Impact of infection by *Helicobacter pylori* on the risk and severity of endemic cholera. J Infect Dis 1995;171:1653–6.
[73] Shmuely H, Samra Z, Ashkenazi S, et al. Association of *Helicobacter pylori* infection with *Shigella* gastroenteritis in young children. Am J Gastroenterol 2004;99:2041–5.
[74] Bhan MK, Bahl R, Sazawal S, et al. Association between *Helicobacter pylori* infection and increased risk of typhoid fever. J Infect Dis 2002;186:1857–60.
[75] Okuda M, Miyashiro E, Koike M, et al. Serodiagnosis of *Helicobacter pylori* infection is not accurate for children aged below 10. Pediatr Int 2002;44:387–90.
[76] Kato S, Ozawa K, Okuda M, et al. Accuracy of the stool antigen test for the diagnosis of childhood *Helicobacter pylori* infection: a multicenter Japanese study. Am J Gastroenterol 2003;98:296–300.
[77] Gold BD, Colletti RB, Abbott M, et al. *Helicobacter pylori* infection in children: recommendations for diagnosis and treatment. J Pediatr Gastroenterol Nutr 2000;31:490–7.
[78] Malfertheiner P, Megraud F, O'Morain C, et al. Current concepts in the management of *Helicobacter pylori* infection—the Maastricht 2–2000 Consensus Report. Aliment Pharmacol Ther 2002;16:167–80.
[79] Sherman P, Hassall E, Hunt RH, et al. Canadian Helicobacter Study Group Consensus

Conference on the approach to *Helicobacter pylori* infection in children and adolescents. Can J Gastroenterol 1999;13:553–9.

[80] Gottrand F, Kalach N, Spyckerelle C, et al. Omeprazole combined with amoxicillin and clarithromycin in the eradication of *Helicobacter pylori* in children with gastritis: a prospective randomized double-blind trial. J Pediatr 2001;139:664–8.

[81] Kato S, Konno M, Maisawa S, et al. Results of triple eradication therapy in Japanese children: a retrospective multicenter study. J Gastroenterol 2004;39:838–43.

[82] Rowland M, Kumar D, Daly L, et al. Low rates of *Helicobacter pylori* reinfection in children. Gastroenterology 1999;117:336–41.

[83] Wold AE, Caugant DA, Lidin-Janson G, et al. Resident colonic *Escherichia coli* strains frequently display uropathogenic characteristics. J Infect Dis 1992;165:46–52.

[84] Bonacorsi SP, Clermont O, Tinsley C, et al. Identification of regions of the *Escherichia coli* chromosome specific for neonatal meningitis-associated strains. Infect Immun 2000;68: 2096–101.

[85] Prasadarao NV, Wass CA, Kim KS. Identification and characterization of *S fimbria*-binding sialoglycoproteins on brain microvascular endothelial cells. Infect Immun 1997;65:2852–60.

[86] Kaper JB, Nataro JP, Mobley HL. Pathogenic *Escherichia coli*. Nat Rev Microbiol 2004;2: 123–40.

[87] Black RE, Merson MH, Huq I, et al. Incidence and severity of rotavirus and *Escherichia coli* diarrhoea in rural Bangladesh: implications for vaccine development. Lancet 1981;1:141–3.

[88] Todd EC. Epidemiology of foodborne diseases: a worldwide review. World Health Stat Q 1997; 50:30–50.

[89] Gaastra W, Svennerholm AM. Colonization factors of human enterotoxigenic *Escherichia coli* (ETEC). Trends Microbiol 1996;4:444–52.

[90] Nataro JP, Kaper JB. Diarrheagenic *Escherichia coli*. Clin Microbiol Rev 1998;11:142–201.

[91] Albano F, Brasitus T, Mann EA, et al. Colonocyte basolateral membranes contain *Escherichia coli* heat-stable enterotoxin receptors. Biochem Biophys Res Commun 2001;284:331–4.

[92] Vaandrager AB. Structure and function of the heat-stable enterotoxin receptor/guanylyl cyclase C. Mol Cell Biochem 2002;230:73–83.

[93] Thiagarajah JR, Verkman AS. CFTR pharmacology and its role in intestinal fluid secretion. Curr Opin Pharmacol 2003;3:594–9.

[94] Gabriel SE, Brigman KN, Koller BH, et al. Cystic fibrosis heterozygote resistance to cholera toxin in the cystic fibrosis mouse model. Science 1994;266:107–9.

[95] Fischer H, Machen TE, Widdicombe JH, et al. A novel extract SB-300 from the stem bark latex of Croton lechleri inhibits CFTR-mediated chloride secretion in human colonic epithelial cells. J Ethnopharmacol 2004;93:351–7.

[96] Ma T, Thiagarajah JR, Yang H, et al. Thiazolidinone CFTR inhibitor identified by high-throughput screening blocks cholera toxin-induced intestinal fluid secretion. J Clin Invest 2002;110:1651–8.

[97] Sonawane ND, Muanprasat C, Nagatani Jr R, et al. In vivo pharmacology and antidiarrheal efficacy of a thiazolidinone CFTR inhibitor in rodents. J Pharm Sci 2004;94:134–43.

[98] Thiagarajah JR, Broadbent T, Hsieh E, et al. Prevention of toxin-induced intestinal ion and fluid secretion by a small-molecule CFTR inhibitor. Gastroenterology 2004;126:511–9.

[99] Hill SM, Phillips AD, Walker-Smith JA. Enteropathogenic *Escherichia coli* and life threatening chronic diarrhoea. Gut 1991;32:154–8.

[100] Nougayrede JP, Fernandes PJ, Donnenberg MS. Adhesion of enteropathogenic *Escherichia coli* to host cells. Cell Microbiol 2003;5:359–72.

[101] DeVinney R, Gauthier A, Abe A, et al. Enteropathogenic *Escherichia coli*: a pathogen that inserts its own receptor into host cells. Cell Mol Life Sci 1999;55:961–76.

[102] Clarke SC, Haigh RD, Freestone PP, et al. Virulence of enteropathogenic *Escherichia coli,* a global pathogen. Clin Microbiol Rev 2003;16:365–78.

[103] Vallance BA, Finlay BB. Exploitation of host cells by enteropathogenic *Escherichia coli*. Proc Natl Acad Sci U S A 2000;97:8799–806.

[104] Dean P, Kenny B. Intestinal barrier dysfunction by enteropathogenic *Escherichia coli* is mediated by two effector molecules and a bacterial surface protein. Mol Microbiol 2004; 54:665–75.
[105] Bhan MK, Khoshoo V, Sommerfelt H, et al. Enteroaggregative *Escherichia coli* and *Salmonella* associated with nondysenteric persistent diarrhea. Pediatr Infect Dis J 1989; 8:499–502.
[106] Bhan MK, Raj P, Levine MM, et al. Enteroaggregative *Escherichia coli* associated with persistent diarrhea in a cohort of rural children in India. J Infect Dis 1989;159:1061–4.
[107] Knutton S, Shaw RK, Bhan MK, et al. Ability of enteroaggregative *Escherichia coli* strains to adhere in vitro to human intestinal mucosa. Infect Immun 1992;60:2083–91.
[108] Nishikawa Y, Zhou Z, Hase A, et al. Diarrheagenic *Escherichia coli* isolated from stools of sporadic cases of diarrheal illness in Osaka City, Japan between 1997 and 2000: prevalence of enteroaggregative E. coli heat-stable enterotoxin 1 gene-possessing E. coli. Jpn J Infect Dis 2002;55:183–90.
[109] Pabst WL, Altwegg M, Kind C, et al. Prevalence of enteroaggregative *Escherichia coli* among children with and without diarrhea in Switzerland. J Clin Microbiol 2003;41:2289–93.
[110] Sarantuya J, Nishi J, Wakimoto N, et al. Typical enteroaggregative *Escherichia coli* is the most prevalent pathotype among *E. coli* strains causing diarrhea in Mongolian children. J Clin Microbiol 2004;42:133–9.
[111] Canizalez-Roman A, Navarro-Garcia F. Fodrin CaM-binding domain cleavage by Pet from enteroaggregative *Escherichia coli* leads to actin cytoskeletal disruption. Mol Microbiol 2003; 48:947–58.
[112] Navarro-Garcia F, Canizalez-Roman A, Luna J, et al. Plasmid-encoded toxin of enteroaggregative *Escherichia coli* is internalized by epithelial cells. Infect Immun 2001;69:1053–60.
[113] Ostroff SM, Kobayashi JM, Lewis JH. Infections with *Escherichia coli* O157:H7 in Washington State: the first year of statewide disease surveillance. JAMA 1989;262:355–9.
[114] Garmendia J, Phillips AD, Carlier MF, et al. TccP is an enterohaemorrhagic *Escherichia coli* O157:H7 type III effector protein that couples Tir to the actin-cytoskeleton. Cell Microbiol 2004;6:1167–83.
[115] Friedrich AW, Bielaszewska M, Zhang WL, et al. *Escherichia coli* harboring Shiga toxin 2 gene variants: frequency and association with clinical symptoms. J Infect Dis 2002;185:74–84.
[116] Werber D, Fruth A, Buchholz U, et al. Strong association between shiga toxin-producing *Escherichia coli* O157 and virulence genes stx2 and eae as possible explanation for predominance of serogroup O157 in patients with haemolytic uraemic syndrome. Eur J Clin Microbiol Infect Dis 2003;22:726–30.
[117] Sandvig K. Shiga toxins. Toxicon 2001;39:1629–35.
[118] Waddell T, Head S, Petric M, et al. Globotriosyl ceramide is specifically recognized by the *Escherichia coli* verocytotoxin 2. Biochem Biophys Res Commun 1988;152:674–9.
[119] Heyderman RS, Soriani M, Hirst TR. Is immune cell activation the missing link in the pathogenesis of post-diarrhoeal HUS? Trends Microbiol 2001;9:262–6.
[120] Tesh VL, Ramegowda B, Samuel JE. Purified Shiga-like toxins induce expression of proinflammatory cytokines from murine peritoneal macrophages. Infect Immun 1994;62:5085–94.
[121] Thorpe CM, Smith WE, Hurley BP, et al. Shiga toxins induce, superinduce, and stabilize a variety of C–X-C chemokine mRNAs in intestinal epithelial cells, resulting in increased chemokine expression. Infect Immun 2001;69:6140–7.
[122] Stricklett PK, Hughes AK, Ergonul Z, et al. Molecular basis for up-regulation by inflammatory cytokines of Shiga toxin 1 cytotoxicity and globotriaosylceramide expression. J Infect Dis 2002;186:976–82.
[123] Fagundes-Neto U, Freymuller E, Gandolfi Schimitz L, et al. Nutritional impact and ultrastructural intestinal alterations in severe infections due to enteropathogenic *Escherichia coli* strains in infants. J Am Coll Nutr 1996;15:180–5.
[124] Fagundes-Neto U, Scaletsky IC. The gut at war: the consequences of enteropathogenic *Escherichia coli* infection as a factor of diarrhea and malnutrition. Sao Paulo Med J 2000;118:21–9.

[125] Zoja C, Morigi M, Remuzzi G. The role of the endothelium in hemolytic uremic syndrome. J Nephrol 2001;14(Suppl 4):S58–62.

[126] Tapper D, Tarr P, Avner E, et al. Lessons learned in the management of hemolytic uremic syndrome in children. J Pediatr Surg 1995;30:158–63.

[127] Yoshioka K, Yagi K, Moriguchi N. Clinical features and treatment of children with hemolytic uremic syndrome caused by enterohemorrhagic *Escherichia coli* O157:H7 infection: experience of an outbreak in Sakai City, 1996. Pediatr Int 1999;41:223–7.

[128] Begue RE, Mehta DI, Blecker U. *Escherichia coli* and the hemolytic-uremic syndrome. South Med J 1998;91:798–804.

[129] Dolezel Z, Kopecna L, Starha J, et al. Is it possible to influence the mortality in children with hemolytic uremic syndrome? Bratisl Lek Listy 2001;102:59–65.

[130] Senerwa D, Mutanda LN, Gathuma JM, et al. Antimicrobial resistance of enteropathogenic *Escherichia coli* strains from a nosocomial outbreak in Kenya. APMIS 1991;99:728–34.

[131] Thoren A. Antibiotic sensitivity of enteropathogenic *Escherichia coli* to mecillinam, trimethoprim-sulfamethoxazole and other antibiotics. Acta Pathol Microbiol Scand [B] 1980; 88:265–8.

[132] Welinder-Olsson C, Kjellin E, Badenfors M, et al. Improved microbiological techniques using the polymerase chain reaction and pulsed-field gel electrophoresis for diagnosis and follow-up of enterohaemorrhagic *Escherichia coli* infection. Eur J Clin Microbiol Infect Dis 2000;19:843–51.

[133] Thorpe CM. Shiga toxin-producing *Escherichia coli* infection. Clin Infect Dis 2004;38: 1298–303.

[134] Bell BP, Griffin PM, Lozano P, et al. Predictors of hemolytic uremic syndrome in children during a large outbreak of *Escherichia coli* O157:H7 infections. Pediatrics 1997;100:E12.

[135] Cimolai N, Basalyga S, Mah DG, et al. A continuing assessment of risk factors for the development of *Escherichia coli* O157:H7-associated hemolytic uremic syndrome. Clin Nephrol 1994;42:85–9.

[136] Proulx F, Turgeon JP, Delage G, et al. Randomized, controlled trial of antibiotic therapy for *Escherichia coli* O157:H7 enteritis. J Pediatr 1992;121:299–303.

[137] Ikeda K, Ida O, Kimoto K, et al. Effect of early fosfomycin treatment on prevention of hemolytic uremic syndrome accompanying *Escherichia coli* O157:H7 infection. Clin Nephrol 1999;52:357–62.

[138] Dundas S, Todd WT, Stewart AI, et al. The central Scotland *Escherichia coli* O157:H7 outbreak: risk factors for the hemolytic uremic syndrome and death among hospitalized patients. Clin Infect Dis 2001;33:923–31.

[139] Wong CS, Jelacic S, Habeeb RL, et al. The risk of the hemolytic-uremic syndrome after antibiotic treatment of *Escherichia coli* O157:H7 infections. N Engl J Med 2000;342:1930–6.

[140] Zhang X, McDaniel AD, Wolf LE, et al. Quinolone antibiotics induce Shiga toxin-encoding bacteriophages, toxin production, and death in mice. J Infect Dis 2000;181:664–70.

[141] Paton AW, Morona R, Paton JC. A new biological agent for treatment of Shiga toxigenic *Escherichia coli* infections and dysentery in humans. Nat Med 2000;6:265–70.

[142] Watanabe M, Matsuoka K, Kita E, et al. Oral therapeutic agents with highly clustered globotriose for treatment of Shiga toxigenic *Escherichia coli* infections. J Infect Dis 2004; 189:360–8.

[143] Trachtman H, Cnaan A, Christen E, et al. Effect of an oral Shiga toxin-binding agent on diarrhea-associated hemolytic uremic syndrome in children: a randomized controlled trial. JAMA 2003;290:1337–44.

[144] Tzipori S, Sheoran A, Akiyoshi D, et al. Antibody therapy in the management of shiga toxin-induced hemolytic uremic syndrome. Clin Microbiol Rev 2004;17:926–41.

[145] Levine OS, Levine MM. Houseflies (*Musca domestica*) as mechanical vectors of shigellosis. Rev Infect Dis 1991;13:688–96.

[146] Sansonetti PJ, Phalipon A. M cells as ports of entry for enteroinvasive pathogens: mechanisms of interaction, consequences for the disease process. Semin Immunol 1999;11:193–203.

[147] Tran Van Nhieu G, Bourdet-Sicard R, Dumenil G, et al. Bacterial signals and cell responses during *Shigella* entry into epithelial cells. Cell Microbiol 2000;2:187–93.
[148] High N, Mounier J, Prevost MC, et al. IpaB of *Shigella flexneri* causes entry into epithelial cells and escape from the phagocytic vacuole. EMBO J 1992;11:1991–9.
[149] Goldberg MB, Theriot JA. *Shigella flexneri* surface protein IcsA is sufficient to direct actin-based motility. Proc Natl Acad Sci U S A 1995;92:6572–6.
[150] Huskins WC, Griffiths JK, Faruque AS, et al. Shigellosis in neonates and young infants. J Pediatr 1994;125:14–22.
[151] Replogle ML, Fleming DW, Cieslak PR. Emergence of antimicrobial-resistant shigellosis in Oregon. Clin Infect Dis 2000;30:515–9.
[152] Ashkenazi S, Amir J, Waisman Y, et al. A randomized, double-blind study comparing cefixime and trimethoprim-sulfamethoxazole in the treatment of childhood shigellosis. J Pediatr 1993; 123:817–21.
[153] Eidlitz-Marcus T, Cohen YH, Nussinovitch M, et al. Comparative efficacy of two- and five-day courses of ceftriaxone for treatment of severe shigellosis in children. J Pediatr 1993;123:822–4.
[154] Basualdo W, Arbo A. Randomized comparison of azithromycin versus cefixime for treatment of shigellosis in children. Pediatr Infect Dis J 2003;22:374–7.
[155] Bhattacharya SK, Sur D. An evaluation of current shigellosis treatment. Expert Opin Pharmacother 2003;4:1315–20.
[156] Khan WA, Seas C, Dhar U, et al. Treatment of shigellosis: V. comparison of azithromycin and ciprofloxacin: a double-blind, randomized, controlled trial. Ann Intern Med 1997;126:697–703.
[157] Chan K, Baker S, Kim CC, et al. Genomic comparison of *Salmonella enterica* serovars and *Salmonella bongori* by use of an *S. enterica* serovar typhimurium DNA microarray. J Bacteriol 2003;185:553–63.
[158] Porwollik S, Boyd EF, Choy C, et al. Characterization of *Salmonella enterica* subspecies I genovars by use of microarrays. J Bacteriol 2004;186:5883–98.
[159] De Buck J, Van Immerseel F, Haesebrouck F, et al. Colonization of the chicken reproductive tract and egg contamination by *Salmonella*. J Appl Microbiol 2004;97:233–45.
[160] Davies R, Breslin M. Environmental contamination and detection of *Salmonella enterica* serovar enteritidis in laying flocks. Vet Rec 2001;149:699–704.
[161] Davies RH, Wray C. Mice as carriers of *Salmonella* enteritidis on persistently infected poultry units. Vet Rec 1995;137:337–41.
[162] Shivaprasad HL, Timoney JF, Morales S, et al. Pathogenesis of *Salmonella enteritidis* infection in laying chickens: I. studies on egg transmission, clinical signs, fecal shedding, and serologic responses. Avian Dis 1990;34:548–57.
[163] Timoney JF, Shivaprasad HL, Baker RC, et al. Egg transmission after infection of hens with *Salmonella* enteritidis phage type 4. Vet Rec 1989;125:600–1.
[164] Vugia DJ, Samuel M, Farley MM, et al. Invasive *Salmonella* infections in the United States, FoodNet, 1996–1999: incidence, serotype distribution, and outcome. Clin Infect Dis 2004; 38(Suppl 3):S149–56.
[165] Holt P. Severe salmonella infection in patients with reduced gastric acidity. Practitioner 1985; 229:1027–30.
[166] Khosla SN, Jain N, Khosla A. Gastric acid secretion in typhoid fever. Postgrad Med J 1993; 69:121–3.
[167] Neutra MR, Kraehenbuhl JP. The role of transepithelial transport by M cells in microbial invasion and host defense. J Cell Sci Suppl 1993;17:209–15.
[168] Penheiter KL, Mathur N, Giles D, et al. Non-invasive *Salmonella typhimurium* mutants are avirulent because of an inability to enter and destroy M cells of ileal Peyer's patches. Mol Microbiol 1997;24:697–709.
[169] Hueffer K, Galan JE. *Salmonella*-induced macrophage death: multiple mechanisms, different outcomes. Cell Microbiol 2004;6:1019–25.
[170] Monack DM, Bouley DM, Falkow S. *Salmonella typhimurium* persists within macrophages in the mesenteric lymph nodes of chronically infected Nramp1 + / + mice and can be reactivated by IFNgamma neutralization. J Exp Med 2004;199:231–41.

[171] Monack DM, Mueller A, Falkow S. Persistent bacterial infections: the interface of the pathogen and the host immune system. Nat Rev Microbiol 2004;2:747–65.

[172] Devi S, Murray CJ. *Salmonella* carriage rate amongst school children—a three year study. Southeast Asian J Trop Med Public Health 1991;22:357–61.

[173] Goh KT, Teo SH, Tay L, et al. Epidemiology and control of an outbreak of typhoid in a psychiatric institution. Epidemiol Infect 1992;108:221–9.

[174] Shinohara N, Tanaka H, Saito T, et al. Detection of carriers of typhoid bacilli by sewerage-tracing surveillance in Matsuyama City. Jpn J Med Sci Biol 1981;34:385–92.

[175] Lee SC, Yang PH, Shieh WB, et al. Bacteremia due to non-typhi *Salmonella*: analysis of 64 cases and review. Clin Infect Dis 1994;19:693–6.

[176] Lee WS, Puthucheary SD, Boey CC. Non-typhoid *Salmonella* gastroenteritis. J Paediatr Child Health 1998;34:387–90.

[177] Raucher HS, Eichenfield AH, Hodes HL. Treatment of *Salmonella* gastroenteritis in infants: the significance of bacteremia. Clin Pediatr (Phila) 1983;22:601–4.

[178] Torrey S, Fleisher G, Jaffe D. Incidence of *Salmonella* bacteremia in infants with *Salmonella* gastroenteritis. J Pediatr 1986;108:718–21.

[179] Lester A, Eriksen NH, Nielsen H, et al. Non-typhoid *Salmonella* bacteraemia in Greater Copenhagen 1984 to 1988. Eur J Clin Microbiol Infect Dis 1991;10:486–90.

[180] Onwubalili JK. Sickle cell disease and infection. J Infect 1983;7:2–20.

[181] Chiu CH, Lin TY, Ou JT. A clinical trial comparing oral azithromycin, cefixime and no antibiotics in the treatment of acute uncomplicated *Salmonella* enteritis in children. J Paediatr Child Health 1999;35:372–4.

[182] Sirinavin S, Garner P. Antibiotics for treating salmonella gut infections. Cochrane Database Syst Rev 2000;2:CD001167.

[183] Tenkate TD, Stafford RJ. Risk factors for *Campylobacter* infection in infants and young children: a matched case-control study. Epidemiol Infect 2001;127:399–404.

[184] Horman A, Rimhanen-Finne R, Maunula L, et al. *Campylobacter* spp., *Giardia* spp., *Cryptosporidium* spp., noroviruses, and indicator organisms in surface water in southwestern Finland, 2000–2001. Appl Environ Microbiol 2004;70:87–95.

[185] Taylor DN, McDermott KT, Little JR, et al. *Campylobacter* enteritis from untreated water in the Rocky Mountains. Ann Intern Med 1983;99:38–40.

[186] Centers for Disease Control and Prevention. Outbreak of *Campylobacter jejuni* infections associated with drinking unpasteurized milk procured through a cow-leasing program—Wisconsin, 2001. MMWR Morb Mortal Wkly Rep 2002;51:548–9.

[187] Denis M, Refregier-Petton J, Laisney MJ, et al. *Campylobacter* contamination in French chicken production from farm to consumers: use of a PCR assay for detection and identification of *Campylobacter jejuni* and *Camp. coli*. J Appl Microbiol 2001;91:255–67.

[188] Eyigor A, Dawson KA, Langlois BE, et al. Detection of cytolethal distending toxin activity and cdt genes in *Campylobacter* spp. isolated from chicken carcasses. Appl Environ Microbiol 1999;65:1501–5.

[189] Harrison WA, Griffith CJ, Tennant D, et al. Incidence of *Campylobacter* and *Salmonella* isolated from retail chicken and associated packaging in South Wales. Lett Appl Microbiol 2001;33:450–4.

[190] Zhao C, Ge B, De Villena J, et al. Prevalence of *Campylobacter* spp., *Escherichia coli*, and *Salmonella* serovars in retail chicken, turkey, pork, and beef from the Greater Washington, D.C., area. Appl Environ Microbiol 2001;67:5431–6.

[191] Taylor DN, Perlman DM, Echeverria PD, et al. *Campylobacter* immunity and quantitative excretion rates in Thai children. J Infect Dis 1993;168:754–8.

[192] Walz SE, Baqar S, Beecham HJ, et al. Pre-exposure anti-*Campylobacter jejuni* immunoglobulin A levels associated with reduced risk of *Campylobacter* diarrhea in adults traveling to Thailand. Am J Trop Med Hyg 2001;65:652–6.

[193] Whitehouse CA, Balbo PB, Pesci EC, et al. *Campylobacter jejuni* cytolethal distending toxin causes a G2-phase cell cycle block. Infect Immun 1998;66:1934–40.

[194] Fox JG, Rogers AB, Whary MT, et al. Gastroenteritis in NF-kappaB-deficient mice is produced with wild-type *Campylobacter jejuni* but not with *C. jejuni* lacking cytolethal distending toxin despite persistent colonization with both strains. Infect Immun 2004;72:1116–25.
[195] Hickey TE, McVeigh AL, Scott DA, et al. *Campylobacter jejuni* cytolethal distending toxin mediates release of interleukin-8 from intestinal epithelial cells. Infect Immun 2000;68:6535–41.
[196] Okuda J, Fukumoto M, Takeda Y, et al. Examination of diarrheagenicity of cytolethal distending toxin: suckling mouse response to the products of the cdtABC genes of *Shigella dysenteriae*. Infect Immun 1997;65:428–33.
[197] Purdy D, Buswell CM, Hodgson AE, et al. Characterisation of cytolethal distending toxin (CDT) mutants of *Campylobacter jejuni*. J Med Microbiol 2000;49:473–9.
[198] Everest PH, Goossens H, Butzler JP, et al. Differentiated Caco-2 cells as a model for enteric invasion by *Campylobacter jejuni* and *C. coli*. J Med Microbiol 1992;37:319–25.
[199] Russell RG, O'Donnoghue M, Blake Jr DC, et al. Early colonic damage and invasion of *Campylobacter jejuni* in experimentally challenged infant Macaca mulatta. J Infect Dis 1993; 168:210–5.
[200] Karmali MA, Fleming PC. *Campylobacter* enteritis. Can Med Assoc J 1979;120:1525–32.
[201] Blaser MJ, Berkowitz ID, LaForce FM, et al. *Campylobacter* enteritis: clinical and epidemiologic features. Ann Intern Med 1979;91:179–85.
[202] Drake AA, Gilchrist MJ, Washington 2nd JA, et al. Diarrhea due to *Campylobacter fetus* subspecies *jejuni*: a clinical review of 63 cases. Mayo Clin Proc 1981;56:414–23.
[203] Farrell DJ, Harris MT. A case of intrauterine fetal death associated with maternal *Campylobacter coli* bacteraemia. Aust N Z J Obstet Gynaecol 1992;32:172–4.
[204] Simor AE, Ferro S. *Campylobacter jejuni* infection occurring during pregnancy. Eur J Clin Microbiol Infect Dis 1990;9:142–4.
[205] McCarthy N, Giesecke J. Incidence of Guillain-Barre syndrome following infection with *Campylobacter jejuni*. Am J Epidemiol 2001;153:610–4.
[206] Sheikh KA, Ho TW, Nachamkin I, et al. Molecular mimicry in Guillain-Barre syndrome. Ann N Y Acad Sci 1998;845:307–21.
[207] Gomez-Garces JL, Cogollos R, Alos JL. Susceptibilities of fluoroquinolone-resistant strains of *Campylobacter jejuni* to 11 oral antimicrobial agents. Antimicrob Agents Chemother 1995; 39:542–4.
[208] Mead PS, Slutsker L, Dietz V, et al. Food-related illness and death in the United States. Emerg Infect Dis 1999;5:607–25.
[209] Ashbolt NJ. Microbial contamination of drinking water and disease outcomes in developing regions. Toxicology 2004;198:229–38.
[210] Khan WA, Begum M, Salam MA, et al. Comparative trial of five antimicrobial compounds in the treatment of cholera in adults. Trans R Soc Trop Med Hyg 1995;89:1722–7.
[211] Khan WA, Saha D, Rahman A, et al. Comparison of single-dose azithromycin and 12-dose, 3-day erythromycin for childhood cholera: a randomised, double-blind trial. Lancet 2002; 360:103–6.

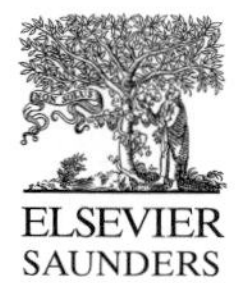

ELSEVIER
SAUNDERS

Pediatr Clin N Am 52 (2005) 779–794

PEDIATRIC CLINICS
OF NORTH AMERICA

Bone and Joint Infections in Children

Kathleen Gutierrez, MD

Department of Pediatrics, Division of Pediatric Infectious Disease, Stanford University School of Medicine, Stanford, CA 94305, USA

Bone and joint infections are a significant cause of morbidity in infants and young children. Although many principles regarding pathogenesis, diagnosis, and treatment of infection have remained constant over the years, other aspects of this important pediatric diagnosis are continuing to evolve. This article reviews current information regarding pathogenesis, epidemiology, and microbiology of pediatric bone and joint infections and the clinical presentation, diagnosis, and treatment of these infections.

Osteomyelitis

Osteomyelitis is inflammation of the bone caused by infection with bacterial or fungal organisms. Osteomyelitis often is categorized into three different types: (1) acute hematogenous osteomyelitis; (2) osteomyelitis secondary to contiguous spread of infection after trauma, puncture wounds, surgery, or joint replacement; and (3) osteomyelitis secondary to vascular insufficiency [1]. Acute hematogenous osteomyelitis is seen most often in children. Osteomyelitis caused by contiguous spread of infection is less common in children, and infection secondary to vascular insufficiency is rare in children.

Pathogenesis

Acute hematogenous osteomyelitis results from symptomatic or asymptomatic bacteremia. Because of its rich vascular supply, the metaphysis of the bone is most often involved. The infecting organism travels to metaphyseal capillary

E-mail address: mdkat@stanford.edu

doi:10.1016/j.pcl.2005.02.005 *pediatric.theclinics.com*

loops, where it replicates and causes local inflammation. As the bacteria replicate, they travel through vascular tunnels and adhere to cartilaginous matrix. *Staphylococcus aureus* is the most common cause of infection perhaps because of its capacity to express bacterial adhesions that promote attachment to extracellular bone matrix. This organism also is able to evade host defenses, attack host cells, and colonize bone persistently [1].

The bony metaphyses of children younger than 18 months are vascularized by the transphyseal vessels. Because these vessels enter the epiphysis and ultimately the joint space, young children are believed to have a higher risk of joint space infection complicating osteomyelitis. One clinical study found the incidence of adjacent joint involvement to be the same, however, in children older than 18 months compared with children younger than 18 months [2]. The authors speculated that some cases of joint involvement could be due to subperiosteal spread of infection into the joint space or that an adjacent site of osteomyelitis may predispose an adjacent joint to hematogenous seeding.

Animal models show that bone infection is more likely after bacteremic animals sustain trauma to the affected area. These animal models may explain why a history of trauma is elicited in approximately 30% children before onset of symptoms [3]. Contiguous osteomyelitis in children is seen in the setting of trauma; animal bites; puncture wounds; and direct extension of infection from an infected sinus, mastoid bone, or dental abscess.

Epidemiology

The exact incidence of childhood osteomyelitis in the United States is unknown. Other countries report a decrease in the diagnosis in recent years [4]. Approximately 50% of cases of osteomyelitis occur in the first 5 years of life. Boys are more likely than girls to be affected. The long bones of the lower extremities are most often involved, although any bone may be affected.

Microbiology

The type of infecting organism depends on the age of the child and underlying medical problem (Table 1). *S. aureus* is the most common cause of osteomyelitis in all age groups, accounting for 70% to 90% of infections. Infection caused by methicillin-resistant *S. aureus* (MRSA) is becoming an increasingly common problem. One group of investigators identified 59 patients with musculoskeletal infections caused by *S. aureus* over a 2-year period at their center. More than half of the patients described were infected with community-acquired MRSA (CA-MRSA) [5].

In addition to *S. aureus,* young infants may develop osteomyelitis caused by *Streptococcus agalactiae* or enteric gram-negative bacteria. Organisms other than *S. aureus* causing infection in older children include *Streptococcus pyogenes,*

Table 1
Usual infectious causes of pediatric osteomyelitis and pyogenic arthritis

Age	Organism
Infants 0–2 mo	*Staphylococcus aureus*
	Streptococcus agalactiae
	Gram-negative enteric bacteria
	Candida
≤5 y	*S. aureus*
	Streptococcus pyogenes
	Streptococcus pneumoniae
	Kingella kingae
	Haemophilus influenzae type b (if child not completely immunized with conjugate Hib vaccine)
>5 y	*S. aureus*
	S. pyogenes
Adolescent	*Neisseria gonorrhoeae*

Streptococcus pneumoniae, and *Kingella kingae* [6]. *S. pyogenes* causes approximately 10% of cases of acute hematogenous osteomyelitis with a peak incidence of disease in preschool-age and early school–age children [7]. Children with *S. pyogenes* osteomyelitis often have a recent history of varicella infection and present with higher fever and white blood cell (WBC) counts compared with children infected with *S. aureus*.

Children with osteomyelitis caused by *S. pneumoniae* are younger than children infected with *S. aureus* and *S. pyogenes*. They are more likely to have joint involvement [8]. The proportion of bone infections caused by *S. pneumoniae* is relatively small (approximately 1–4%); the impact of heptavalent pneumococcal conjugate vaccine on the incidence of osteomyelitis is limited.

K. kingae is reported as a pathogen with increasing frequency [9]. A cluster of bone and joint infections caused by *K. kingae* at a daycare center underscores the importance of this organism in children with musculoskeletal infections [10]. *K. kingae* is a fastidious gram-negative coccobacillary bacterium found in normal respiratory flora. Infection with this organism often is preceded by an upper respiratory tract infection or stomatitis; disrupted respiratory mucosa may facilitate invasion and hematogenous dissemination.

There has been a substantial decrease in musculoskeletal infections secondary to *Haemophilus influenzae* type b (Hib) as a result of an effective immunization program against this pathogen. Hib infection is rare in a completely immunized child, although other serotypes are reported to cause bone and joint infections.

Puncture wounds to the foot may result in osteomyelitis caused by mixed flora, including *Pseudomonas, S. aureus,* enteric gram-negative bacteria, and anaerobes. The source of bacteria is usually from moist colonized soles of tennis shoes. A series of cases describes osteomyelitis of the metatarsals occurring as a result of toothpick puncture injuries. The organisms isolated included skin and environmental organisms; others have reported infection with mouth organisms as a result of toothpick injuries [11].

Anaerobes are a rare cause of pyogenic osteomyelitis in healthy children. Predominant organisms are *Bacteroides, Fusobacterium, Clostridium,* and *Peptostreptococcus*. Anaerobic osteomyelitis can occur as the result of a bite, chronic sinusitis, mastoiditis, or dental infection.

Organisms causing bone infection in children with sickle cell disease include *Salmonella* and *S. aureus* and less commonly *Escherichia coli,* Hib, *Shigella,* and *S. pneumoniae*. Unusual causes of osteomyelitis include infection with *Mycobacterium, Bartonella, Coxiella burnetii,* or fungi (Table 2). The specific etiology of osteomyelitis is not determined in many cases; nonetheless, resolution after empirical therapy for *S. aureus* is usual [12].

Clinical manifestations

Most children with acute hematogenous osteomyelitis are symptomatic for less than 2 weeks. Symptoms include complaints of acute, persistent, and increasing pain over the affected bone. Osteomyelitis in an infant may present as irritability or reluctance to move the affected limb. Fever is usually present. Swelling or redness of the soft tissue over the affected bone may be seen. In one study, patients with culture-positive osteomyelitis were more likely than patients

Table 2
Other microbiologic causes of bone or joint infection in children

Risk Factors	Organism
Osteomyelitis	
Exposure to farm animals	*Coxiella burnetti*
Kitten exposure	*Bartonella*
Travel/contact	*Mycobacterium tuberculosis*
Sinusitis/mastoiditis/dental abscess	Anaerobes
Puncture wound foot	*Pseudomonas*, *Staphylococcus aureus*
Sickle cell disease	*Salmonella*, *S. aureus*
Travel or residence in endemic area ± immunosuppression	*Coccidioides immitis* *Blastomyces dermatitidis* *Histoplasma capsulatum* *Cryptococcus neoformans*
Chronic granulomatous disease	*Aspergillus*, *S. aureus*, *Serratia*
Arthritis	
Tick exposure in an endemic area	*Borrelia burgdorferi*
Travel/contact	*M. tuberculosis*
Rat exposure	*Streptobacillus moniliformis* *Spirillum minus*
Viral infection	Rubella, parvovirus B19, varicella zoster, hepatitis B
Travel or residence in an endemic area ± immunosuppression	*C. immitis* *B. dermatitidis* *H. capsulatum* *C. neoformans*
Newborn with intravascular line	*Candida*

with culture-negative osteomyelitis to have a history of antecedent trauma, changes in skin overlying the bone, associated cellulites, or high fever [12].

Pelvic osteomyelitis is reported in 1% to 11% of all cases of acute hematogenous osteomyelitis and typically affects older children [13]. Symptoms include hip, buttock, low back, or abdominal pain. Fever may be absent. Findings on physical examination include tenderness of the pelvic bones, pain with hip movement, decreased range of motion at the hip, and refusal or inability to bear weight. Any bone in the pelvis may be involved, but the ilium tends to be affected most often, presumably because of its rich blood supply. Symptoms and findings frequently are nonspecific and poorly localized and often are attributed to other diagnoses, such as pyogenic arthritis of the hip or appendicitis. Establishing the correct diagnosis often is delayed.

Osteomyelitis in a neonate is an uncommon but serious infection. It often results from hematogenous spread of microorganisms in patients with indwelling venous catheters. Presenting signs and symptoms include fever, irritability, refusal to move the affected limb, and redness and swelling over the affected area. Diagnosis may be delayed because of nonspecific signs of illness. Infection involving multiple bones and contiguous joints and soft tissue is common.

The differential diagnosis of bone pain in children includes trauma, malignancy, and bone infarction in patients with sickle cell disease. Differentiation between bone infection and infarction in a child with sickle cell anemia is difficult because in both cases the acute onset of fever and bone pain is common. In addition, a patient may have infarction that predisposes to infection.

Chronic recurrent multifocal osteomyelitis is a poorly understood inflammatory illness characterized by recurrent bone pain and fever. Girls are predominantly affected and have radiologic evidence of multiple, often symmetric bone lesions involving primarily the long bones and clavicles. Associated findings include psoriasis vulgaris and palmoplantar pustulosis.

Diagnosis

The diagnosis of osteomyelitis depends primarily on clinical findings and corroborative laboratory and radiographic results. The WBC count may be normal or increased. Erythrocyte sedimentation rate (ESR) is elevated in 80% to 90% of cases, and C-reactive protein (CRP) is elevated in 98% of cases. ESR generally peaks 3 to 5 days after admission, and CRP peaks within 48 hours of admission. CRP typically returns to normal 7 to 10 days after appropriate therapy. ESR may remain elevated for 3 or 4 weeks, even with appropriate therapy [14]. Patients who require surgical incision and drainage procedures may have prolonged time to normalization of ESR or CRP [15].

Every attempt should be made to establish a microbiologic diagnosis. A bacteriologic diagnosis can be made in 50% to 80% of cases if blood and bone cultures are obtained. In the case of culture-negative osteomyelitis that is not responding as expected to empirical therapy, a bone biopsy specimen should be obtained for histopathologic staining and for culture for bacteria, mycobacteria, and fungi. Inoculation of bone or abscess material directly into an aerobic blood culture bottle facilitates isolation of *K. kingae*. Cultures for *K. kingae* and other fastidious organisms may need to be incubated longer than usual laboratory protocol [6].

Plain films show soft tissue swelling in the first few days of illness. Periosteal and lytic changes in the bone generally are not seen until substantial bone destruction has occurred, usually 10 to 21 days after onset of symptoms. In some cases of proven bacterial osteomyelitis, bone changes are never seen on plain film, presumably because prompt diagnosis and treatment prevented extensive bone destruction.

The sensitivity of skeletal scintigraphy, using technetium-labeled methylene diphosphonate isotope, is 80% to 100%. Radionuclide bone scans usually are positive within 48 to 72 hours of onset of symptoms. In some cases of osteomyelitis, vascular supply to the bone is compromised, with decreased uptake of technetium to the affected area, resulting in a "cold scan." Some experts prefer bone scan as the initial study in the evaluation of suspected uncomplicated osteomyelitis of the long bones. It is less expensive than MR imaging, sedation of the child is generally not necessary, and it is particularly useful when multifocal osteomyelitis is suspected or the exact location of infection is not obvious on physical examination [16,17]. Radionuclide scans may be positive in other illnesses that result in increased osteoblastic activity, including malignancy, trauma, cellulitis, postsurgery, and arthritis.

MR imaging gives excellent resolution of bone and soft tissue. It is particularly useful for visualizing soft tissue abscess associated with osteomyelitis, bone marrow edema, and bone destruction. Contrast enhancement with gadolinium is used to look for areas of abscess formation [18]. If pelvic or vertebral body osteomyelitis is suspected, MR imaging is the imaging study of choice. MR imaging gives better spatial resolution than bone scan and is preferred if a surgical procedure to diagnose or drain an abscess is necessary. Limitations of MR imaging include the need for sedation in younger children, high cost, and inability to assess easily whether other bones are affected.

Differentiating bone infarction versus infection can be difficult in a child with sickle cell disease. In both situations, children present with fever and bone pain and have elevated inflammatory markers. Biopsy and culture of affected bone is often necessary to establish the diagnosis. Some authors have used the pattern of MR imaging contrast enhancement to distinguish acute medullary bone infarction from osteomyelitis [19].

Treatment

Successful treatment of osteomyelitis depends on the appropriate selection and administration of antibiotic therapy and surgical intervention as needed. Empirical selection of antibiotics depends on the age of the child and the clinical

Table 3
Empirical parenteral antibiotic therapy for pediatric bone and joint infections*

Infants 0–2 mo	Nafcillin* *plus* cefotaxime
Children ≤5 years†	Nafcillin* *plus* cefotaxime *or* ceftriaxone *or* Cefuroxime
Children >5 y	Nafcillin* *or* cefazolin*,‡

* If MRSA is a concern (if local rates of MRSA are >5–10%), use intravenous vancomycin or clindamycin as empirical therapy.

† Children who have been completely immunized against *Haemophilus influenzae* type b do not require antibiotic coverage for *H. influenzae* type b.

‡ Use ceftriaxone if *Neisseria gonorrhoeae* a consideration.

situation (Table 3). Infants 0 to 2 months old with osteomyelitis should be treated with antibiotics that have excellent coverage against *S. aureus, S. agalactaiae,* and enteric gram-negative bacteria.

Children 2 months to 5 years old should be treated empirically with antibiotics active against *S. aureus, S. pneumoniae, S. pyogenes, K. kingae,* and Hib (if not completely immunized with Hib vaccine). The American Academy of Pediatrics Committee on Infectious Diseases defines complete immunization for Hib as having had at least one dose of conjugate Hib vaccine at 15 months of age or older, two doses between 12 and 14 months of age, or a complete primary series when younger than 12 months with a booster dose at 12 months of age or older [20]. *K. kingae* generally is susceptible to most β-lactam antibiotics, including second-generation and third-generation cephalosporins. It often is resistant to clindamycin, and resistance to clotrimazole is reported [6].

When culture results are available, antibiotic therapy is modified depending on the organism and the susceptibility pattern. If no organism is isolated, but the patient is improving, initial empirical coverage is continued. If the patient is not improving, further diagnostic testing should be considered, including bone biopsy for histopathology and culture if not previously obtained or imaging studies to rule out areas of infection that may require surgical drainage or débridement.

Infection caused by MRSA is increasingly common in many communities. Many isolates of CA-MRSA are susceptible to clindamycin. Isolates of *S. aureus* that are erythromycin resistant and clindamycin susceptible should be evaluated for the presence of inducible macrolide-lincosamide-streptogramin B (MLS_B) resistance. This evaluation is done by means of a "D" test, performed by many hospital laboratories. Although some children treated with clindamycin for an infection with MRSA of the MLS_B phenotype clear their infection, it is recommended that in the setting of serious infection, clindamycin should not be used if this phenotype is identified [21].

Alternative drugs to consider for treatment of osteomyelitis caused by MRSA include intravenous vancomycin, trimethoprim-sulfamethoxasole, and linezolid. Bone and joint infections caused by MRSA should be managed in consultation with an expert in infectious disease. Empirical use of these antibiotics before organism identification and susceptibility testing depends on severity of illness and incidence of MRSA in the community.

In an open-label, noncomparative, nonrandomized, compassionate use study, linezolid was used to treat serious infections caused by resistant gram-positive bacteria. Microbiologic cure for the cases of osteomyelitis caused by MRSA was 72% [22]. Most patients in this study were adults. Side effects of linezolid include gastrointestinal symptoms and rash. Long-term use of linezolid has been associated with neutropenia, anemia, thrombocytopenia, and optic and peripheral neuropathies. Cases of lactic acidosis also have been reported with linezolid use. Linezolid was not effective in at least one animal study of experimental chronic *S. aureus* osteomyelitis [23].

The decision to change from parenteral to oral therapy depends on the availability of an appropriate oral antibiotic, the child's ability to take the medication by mouth, reliable caregivers, and the ability of the family to comply with frequent follow-up. Generally, oral therapy is begun when the child is afebrile, symptoms and signs of infection are resolving, and CRP is returning to normal. The availability of percutaneous central venous catheters has made home intravenous therapy of bone and joint infections an increasingly popular option. The prolonged presence of a central venous catheter increases the risk of infectious complications, including exit site infections and catheter-associated bacteremia [24]. Intravenous therapy should not be unduly prolonged after the child has shown significant improvement.

Sequential intravenous to oral therapy is proven to be effective and safe, provided that close follow-up of the patient is ensured. The dose of oral antibiotic is generally two to three times the usual dose for children if a β-lactam antibiotic, such as dicloxacillin or cephalexin, is used. The usual recommended oral doses of clindamycin, trimethoprim-sulfamethoxazole, fluoroquinolone antibiotics, and linezolid can be used because of the excellent bioavailability of these drugs (Table 4). Vancomycin always must be given intravenously.

Duration of therapy depends on extent of infection, clinical response, and presence of underlying risk factors. In general, 3 to 6 weeks of antibiotic therapy is given depending on the clinical response [14,25]. There is good evidence that treatment for less than 3 weeks results in an unacceptably high rate of relapse. Chronic infection is reported in 19% of children treated for less than 3 weeks compared with 2% in children treated longer than 3 weeks [26].

Table 4
Doses of oral antibiotics used for bone and joint infections

Antibiotic	Dose(mg/kg/d)	Interval
Cephalexin	100	q6–8h
Dicloxacillin	100	q6h
Clindamycin	30	q6–8h

Prognosis

Most children who receive appropriate therapy for osteomyelitis have no long-term sequelae. Recurrence of infection occurs in approximately 5% of cases. Risk factors for development of complications include delay in diagnosis, short duration of therapy, and young age at the time of initial illness. The reported incidence of sequelae in neonates with osteomyelitis ranges from 6% to 50%. Permanent abnormalities include disturbance in bone growth, limb-length discrepancies, arthritis, abnormal gait, and pathologic fractures.

There does not seem to be a significant difference in outcome for bone infections caused by MRSA compared with infections caused by methicillin-susceptible *S. aureus*. Children infected with MRSA tend to have longer duration of fever and prolonged hospitalization, however. Patients with complicated clinical courses, including patients with associated deep vein thrombosis, were found in one study more likely to be infected with MRSA with genes encoding for the Panton-Valentine leukocidin (PVL1) [5]. This strain of MRSA causes severe inflammatory lesions after intradermal injection in laboratory animals and has been associated with a poor prognosis in patients with pneumonia.

Chronic osteomyelitis develops in less than 5% of children after acute hematogeneous infection. It is observed more frequently after contiguous osteomyelitis. Bone necrosis occurs as a result of chronic inflammation and vascular compromise. Extensive fibrosis eventually results. Signs and symptoms of chronic osteomyelitis vary from chronic vague symptoms of swelling, pain, or intermittent drainage of the affected bone to acute exacerbations of fever, swelling, or redness over the bone. Effective management of chronic osteomyelitis usually requires surgical and medical management, with prolonged courses of antibiotics [27].

Pyogenic arthritis

Infection of the joint space in children usually is a complication of bacteremia. Viruses, fungal organisms, and *Mycobacterium tuberculosis* are uncommon causes of joint space infection (see Table 2). Children also may develop reactive arthritis as a consequence of bacterial infection elsewhere in the body.

Pathogenesis

Pyogenic arthritis usually occurs as a result of infection of the vascular synovium by means of hematogenous dissemination of bacteria. An acute inflammatory response follows, resulting in migration of polymorphonuclear WBCs, production of proteolytic enzymes, and cytokine secretion by chondrocytes. Degradation of articular cartilage begins 8 hours after onset of infection [28].

In children younger than 18 months of age, pyogenic arthritis can result from extension of a metaphyseal bone infection through transphyseal blood vessels.

The growth plate, the epiphysis, and eventually the joint space may be infected. Infection of the proximal femur and humerus often involves the hip and shoulder joints because the proximal metaphysis of each of these bones is intracapsular.

Epidemiology

Most cases of pyogenic arthritis occur in children 3 years old or younger. Cases are more frequent in boys. The joints of the lower extremities (hips, knees) are most often affected.

Microbiology

S. aureus is the most common cause of pyogenic arthritis in all age groups, and infection with CA-MRSA is becoming more common. Infants younger than 2 months of age also may have infection caused by *S. agalactiae, Neisseria gonorrhoeae,* and gram-negative enteric bacteria. Arthritis caused by *Candida* also is seen in the neonatal age group. *S. aureus, S. pyogenes, S. pneumoniae,* and *K. kingae* are predominant organisms in the 2-month to 5-year age range. Children older than 5 years are most likely to have arthritis caused by *S. aureus* and *S. pyogenes*. *N. gonorrhoeae* arthritis occurs in sexually active adolescents.

Before universal immunization of children with a conjugate Hib vaccine, Hib was a common cause of pyogenic arthritis in children younger than 5 years. Infection with Hib is now rare in immunized children. Arthritis caused by *K. kingae* has replaced Hib as the most common gram-negative arthritis in the child 2 months to 5 years old [6].

S. pneumoniae is reported to cause approximately 6% to 20% of all cases of pyogenic arthritis [29,30]. The impact of the recently licensed heptavalent pneumococcal vaccine on pneumococcal pyogenic arthritis is still being evaluated [31]. The vaccine confers immunity to the seven pneumococcal serotypes most frequently associated with invasive disease in children, but is not immunogenic against all serotypes. A surveillance study involving 157,471 children over a 3-year period after the vaccine was licensed revealed a significant decrease in the number of cases of invasive pneumococcal disease caused by serotypes in the vaccine or closely related to the serotypes in the vaccine [32]. There was no significant change in the incidence of disease caused by other serotypes. The types of invasive disease reported were primarily bacteremia and pneumonia. Because the incidence of pneumococcal arthritis after bacteremia is only about 0.6% [29], a significant decrease in the number of cases of pneumococcal bacteremia is likely to result in only a small reduction in cases of pyogenic arthritis.

Other causes of arthritis should be suspected on the basis of exposure history (see Table 2). *Borrelia burgdorferi* causes Lyme disease in endemic areas. Arthralgia is seen in early disseminated Lyme disease. Weeks to months after the initial infection, children may develop pauciarticular arthritis of the large joints, particularly the knees [33]. *N. gonorrhoeae* infection should be considered in a sexually active adolescent with joint infection. Hematogenous spread of the

Table 5
Infectious causes of reactive arthritis

Site of infection	Organism
Gastrointestinal tract	*Salmonella*
	Shigella
	Campylobacter
	Yersinia enterocolitica
Genitourinary tract	*Chlamydia trachomatis*
	*Neisseria gonorrhoeae**
Other	*Streptococcus pyogenes**
	*Neisseria meningiditis**

* These organisms also may infect the joint space directly.

organism can involve skin and joints (arthritis-dermatitis syndrome). The arthritis associated with *N. gonorrhoeae* also may be reactive in nature. Reactive arthritis is defined as inflammation of a joint after infection at some other site. Organisms that are associated with reactive arthritis are listed in Table 5.

Clinical manifestations

Trauma or upper respiratory tract infection often precedes joint symptoms. Symptoms of pyogenic arthritis include acute onset of joint pain, fever, irritability, and limp. Pain associated with pyogenic arthritis of the hip may be referred to the groin, thigh, or knee. Findings on physical examination include redness, swelling, and warmth over the affected joint. The child complains of pain with movement of the joint and restricted range of motion. Patients should be evaluated for signs of pharyngitis, rash, heart murmur, hepatosplenomegaly, and evidence of other joint or bone involvement.

Differential diagnosis

The most common cause of hip pain in childhood is transient synovitis. Transient synovitis predominates in children 5 to 10 years old. The child generally has low-grade fever or is afebrile. Pain is usually unilateral, but may be bilateral in some cases. Pain ranges from mild to severe enough to wake the child up at night. Physical examination generally reveals a non–ill-appearing child with decreased range of motion of the hip joint.

Other causes of joint pain and swelling include reactive arthritis, juvenile rheumatoid arthritis, trauma, and malignancy. Legg-Calvé-Perthes disease is an idiopathic avascular necrosis of the capital femoral epiphysis and may cause mild pain and limp in boys (mean age 7 years). Slipped capital femoral epiphysis is the most common hip disorder of adolescents; symptoms may include abnormal gait, pain, and abnormal range of motion of the hip joint.

Diagnosis

Diagnosis of pyogenic arthritis must be made promptly to prevent damage to the articular cartilage. Every attempt should be made to establish a microbiologic diagnosis. Blood and joint fluid should be obtained for aerobic and anaerobic cultures. Joint fluid should be inoculated directly into blood culture bottles to enhance identification of fastidious organisms such as *K. kingae*. Gram stain and cell count also should be performed on joint fluid. A WBC count of 50,000/mm^3 or greater with a predominance of polymorphonuclear cells is consistent with bacterial infection, but also is seen sometimes with rheumatologic disease. The peripheral WBC count, ESR, and CRP are generally elevated, although occasionally CRP is normal, especially with infection caused by *K. kingae*. If *N. gonorrhoeae* is suspected, cultures of joint fluid, blood, pharynx, skin lesion, cervix, urethra, vagina, and rectum should be obtained and inoculated onto special media. *N. gonorrhoeae* also can be detected by nucleic acid amplification techniques using urine, urethral, cervical, or vaginal specimens. A throat culture for *S. pyogenes* should be sent if the patient has signs or symptoms of pharyngitis. Antibody titers to antistreptolysin O and anti-DNase B also may be useful to diagnose infection with *S. pyogenes*. Lyme disease serology (including Western blot) is used to diagnose Lyme arthritis in a patient with the appropriate exposure history. Plain radiographs of adjacent bone are useful in evaluating for other causes of joint pain and swelling, including trauma, malignancy, and osteomyelitis.

The prompt diagnosis of pyogenic arthritis of the hip is important to prevent serious permanent long-term sequelae. Untreated infection of the hip can result in vascular compromise and ischemic necrosis of the femoral head. Differentiation between pyogenic arthritis and transient synovitis of the hip is challenging. Several studies have shown that a combination of clinical and laboratory features can assist in differentiating these diagnoses (Table 6). Kocher et al [34] found that

Table 6
Differentiation of pyogenic arthritis from transient synovitis of the hip

Study	Predictors analyzed	No. predictors present (+):Predictive probability of pyogenic arthritis (%)*
Kocher et al [34]	History of fever	4 +: 99.8%
	Non–weight bearing	3 +: 93–95.2%
	ESR ≥40 mm/h	2 +: 33.8–62.2%
	WBC >12,000/mm^3	1 +: 2.1–5.3%
		0 +: 0.1%
Jung et al [36]	Body temperature >37°C	5 +: 99.1%
	ESR >20 mm/h	4 +: 84.8–97.3%
	CRP >1 mg/dL	3 +: 24.3–77.2%
	WBC >11,000/mm^3	2 +: 4.3–22.7%
	Increased hip joint space >2 mm	1 +: 0.3–9.9%
		0 +: 0.1%

* Exact predictive probability depends on which multivariate predictor was positive.

if a child with hip pain had all four diagnostic variables of fever, refusal to walk, elevated ESR ($\geq$40 mm/h) and elevated WBC count (>12,000/mm^3), the probability of pyogenic arthritis was greater than 99%.

Kocher's criteria have been applied restrospectively to patients with a known diagnosis of pyogenic arthritis. In one study, the predictive probability of presence of fever, refusal to walk, and elevated ESR and WBC count was found to be considerably less reliable (60%) in predicting pyogenic arthritis [35]. Of patients within the group defined as having proven or presumed septic arthritis who had positive cultures, however, 35% were diagnosed with infection with coagulase-negative staphylococci. This organism is not a usual cause of pediatric pyogenic arthritis and is more often considered a contaminant. This study underscores, however, the fact that the validity of clinical prediction algorithms may vary among studies.

Other investigators have used similar methods in an attempt to differentiate pyogenic arthritis and transient synovitis. Jung et al [36] evaluated children with hip pain using fever (>37°C), ESR (>20 mm/h), CRP (>1 mg/dL), WBC count (>11,000/mm^3), and plain radiographs to determine if there was widening of the joint space (>2 mm) to predict the presence of pyogenic arthritis. If four or five of these criteria were present, the child had a high likelihood (predictive probability >99.1%) of septic arthritis and was a candidate for joint aspiration.

Although most clinicians use fever and elevated inflammatory markers to guide their management of children with hip pain, there is considerable overlap in the clinical and laboratory findings in children with pyogenic arthritis and transient synovitis [37]. Close follow-up of patients in whom the diagnosis is unclear is crucial. Plain radiographs are obtained to rule out fracture, malignancy, or osteomyelitis as the cause of pain. Ultrasound is useful in determining whether fluid is present in the hip joint and is used to guide joint aspiration. Ultrasound cannot differentiate infected from noninfected fluid.

Management

The successful management of pyogenic arthritis depends on timely decompression of the joint space and institution of appropriate antibiotic therapy. Children with pyogenic arthritis should be managed in collaboration with an orthopedic surgeon experienced in the treatment of pediatric bone and joint infections. Aspiration of the affected joint usually is performed for diagnostic and therapeutic purposes. In the case of hip and shoulder joint infections, prompt surgical drainage of infected joint fluid usually is required. The initial choice of empirical antibiotic therapy (see Table 3) depends on the age of the child, clinical presentation, and local patterns of antibiotic resistance. In general, infants younger than 2 months old are treated with nafcillin and a third-generation cephalosporin to cover *S. aureus* and enteric gram-negative bacteria. Older children should receive antibiotic therapy active against *S. aureus, S. pyogenes,* and *K. kingae*. If *N. gonorrhoeae* is suspected, ceftriaxone should be used. Clindamycin is an appropriate antibiotic for most gram-positive bacteria, including some strains of CA-MRSA. It is not active, however, against *K. kingae*. If MRSA is suspected, vancomycin should be used empirically until culture and susceptibility results are available. If cultures are positive for MRSA, clindamycin is an appropriate drug if the isolate is susceptible, and there is no evidence of the MLS_B phenotype (see the section on osteomyelitis). Intra-articular injection of antibiotics is not appropriate. Most antibiotics achieve high synovial fluid concentrations, and the antibiotic may cause a chemical synovitis when directly injected into the joint. As with osteomyelitis, a child should be treated with intravenous antibiotics until there is significant clinical improvement, inflammatory markers are returning to normal, and the child's oral intake is normal. The doses of oral antibiotics used are the same as doses used to treat osteomyelitis (Table 4).

Some centers have found the use of guidelines helpful in standardizing care of uncomplicated cases of pyogenic arthritis. Use of short courses of intravenous therapy (3–4 days) followed by the appropriate oral antibiotic decreased the duration of hospitalization at one center [38]. Compared with patients who were treated before implementation of guidelines, there was no increase in the risk of adverse outcomes in patients followed a minimum of 1 year. Although clinical guidelines may be useful as a framework for evaluation and treatment of pyogenic arthritis, strict guidelines are not appropriate for children with underlying risk factors for severe disease or for children not responding to initial therapy.

The duration of therapy for uncomplicated pyogenic arthritis depends on the response to therapy and the suspected organism [39]. Generally, infections with *S. pneumoniae, K. kingae,* Hib, and *N. gonorrhoeae* are treated for 2 to 3 weeks. Infections caused by *S. aureus* or gram-negative enteric bacteria are treated 3 to 4 weeks.

Prognosis

Complications of pyogenic arthritis include abnormal bone growth, limp, unstable articulation of the affected joint, and decreased range of motion. Complications are reported in approximately 10% to 25% of all cases. Risk factors for sequelae include delay in time to diagnosis of more than 4 or 5 days, onset of disease in infancy, infection with *S. aureus* or gram-negative bacteria, and infection of adjacent bone. In one study from Costa Rica, a 4-day course of dexamethasone given with appropriate antimicrobial and surgical therapy decreased the duration of symptoms and long-term joint dysfunction. [40]. Further studies are needed to confirm the benefits and risks of this treatment approach.

Summary

The numbers of bone and joint infections resulting from vaccine-preventable infections, such as Hib and *S. pneumoniae,* have decreased in recent years. *S. aureus* remains an important cause of pyogenic arthritis and osteomyelitis, and the prevalence of CA-MRSA is increasing. Transition from intravenous to oral antibiotic therapy remains the treatment of choice for uncomplicated pediatric bone and joint infections if the family is reliable and close follow-up can be ensured.

References

[1] Lew DP, Waldvogel FA. Osteomyelitis. Lancet 2004;364:369–79.

[2] Perlman MH, Patzakis MJ, Kumar PJ, Holtom P. The incidence of joint involvement with adjacent osteomyelitis in pediatric patients. J Pediatr Orthop 2000;20:40–3.

[3] Morrissy RT, Haynes DW. Acute hematogenous osteomyelitis: a model with trauma as an etiology. J Pediatr Orthop 1989;9:447–56.

[4] Blyth MJ, Kincaid R, Craigen MA, Bennet GC. The changing epidemiology of acute and subacute haematogenous osteomyelitis in children. J Bone Joint Surg Br 2001;83:99–102.

[5] Martinez-Aguilar G, Avalos-Mishaan A, Hulten K, et al. Community-acquired, methicillin-resistant and methicillin-susceptible *Staphylococcus aureus* musculoskeletal infections in children. Pediatr Infect Dis J 2004;23:701–6.

[6] Yagupsky P. *Kingella kingae*: from medical rarity to an emerging paediatric pathogen. Lancet Infect Dis 2004;4:358–67.

[7] Ibia EO, Imoisili M, Pikis A. Group A beta-hemolytic streptococcal osteomyelitis in children. Pediatrics 2003;112(1 Pt 1):e22–6.

[8] Tan TQ, Mason Jr EO, Barson WJ, et al. Clinical characteristics and outcome of children with pneumonia attributable to penicillin-susceptible and penicillin-nonsusceptible *Streptococcus pneumoniae*. Pediatrics 1998;102:1369–75.

[9] Centers for Disease Control and Prevention. *Kingella kingae* infections in children—United States, June 2001–November 2002. MMWR Morb Mortal Wkly Rep 2004;53:244.

[10] Centers for Disease Control and Prevention. Osteomyelitis/septic arthritis caused by *Kingella kingae* among day care attendees—Minnesota, 2003. MMWR Morb Mortal Wkly Rep 2004;53: 241–3.

[11] Imoisili MA, Bonwit AM, Bulas DI. Toothpick puncture injuries of the foot in children. Pediatr Infect Dis J 2004;23:80–2.

[12] Floyed RL, Steele RW. Culture-negative osteomyelitis. Pediatr Infect Dis J 2003;22:731–6.

[13] Davidson D, Letts M, Khoshhal K. Pelvic osteomyelitis in children: a comparison of decades from 1980–1989 with 1990–2001. J Pediatr Orthop 2003;23:514–21.

[14] Peltola H, Unkila-Kallio L, Kallio MJ. Simplified treatment of acute staphylococcal osteomyelitis of childhood. The Finnish Study Group. Pediatrics 1997;99:846–50.

[15] Khachatourians AG, Patzakis MJ, Roidis N, Holtom PD. Laboratory monitoring in pediatric acute osteomyelitis and septic arthritis. Clin Orthop 2003;409:186–94.

[16] Connolly LP, Connolly SA. Skeletal scintigraphy in the multimodality assessment of young children with acute skeletal symptoms. Clin Nucl Med 2003;28:746–54.

[17] Connolly LP, Connolly SA, Drubach LA, Jaramillo D, Treves ST. Acute hematogenous osteomyelitis of children: assessment of skeletal scintigraphy-based diagnosis in the era of MRI. J Nucl Med 2002;43:1310–6.

[18] Chung T. Magnetic resonance imaging in acute osteomyelitis in children. Pediatr Infect Dis J 2002;21:869–70.

[19] Umans H, Haramati N, Flusser G. The diagnostic role of gadolinium enhanced MRI in distinguishing between acute medullary bone infarct and osteomyelitis. Magn Reson Imaging 2000;18:255–62.

[20] American Academy of Pediatrics. Haemophilus influenzae infection. In: Pickering LK, editor. Red Book: 2003 report of the Committee on Infectious Diseases. 26th edition. Elk Grove Village (IL): American Academy of Pediatrics; 2003. p. 293–301.

[21] Martinez-Aguilar G, Hammerman WA, Mason Jr EO, Kaplan SL. Clindamycin treatment of invasive infections caused by community-acquired, methicillin-resistant and methicillin-susceptible *Staphylococcus aureus* in children. Pediatr Infect Dis J 2003;22:593–8.
[22] Birmingham MC, Rayner CR, Meagher AK, Flavin SM, Batts DH, Schentag JJ. Linezolid for the treatment of multidrug-resistant, gram-positive infections: experience from a compassionate-use program. Clin Infect Dis 2003;36:159–68.
[23] Patel R, Piper KE, Rouse MS, Steckelberg JM. Linezolid therapy of *Staphylococcus aureus* experimental osteomyelitis. Antimicrob Agents Chemother 2000;44:3438–40.
[24] Maraqa NF, Gomez MM, Rathore MH. Outpatient parenteral antimicrobial therapy in osteoarticular infections in children. J Pediatr Orthop 2002;22:506–10.
[25] Nelson JD. Toward simple but safe management of osteomyelitis. Pediatrics 1997;99:883–4.
[26] Dich VQ, Nelson JD, Haltalin KC. Osteomyelitis in infants and children: a review of 163 cases. Am J Dis Child 1975;129:1273–8.
[27] Ramos OM. Chronic osteomyelitis in children. Pediatr Infect Dis J 2002;21:431–2.
[28] Shaw BA, Kasser JR. Acute septic arthritis in infancy and childhood. Clin Orthop 1990;257: 212–25.
[29] Ross JJ, Saltzman CL, Carling P, Shapiro DS. Pneumococcal septic arthritis: review of 190 cases. Clin Infect Dis 2003;36:319–27.
[30] Bradley JS, Kaplan SL, Tan TQ, et al. Pediatric pneumococcal bone and joint infections. The Pediatric Multicenter Pneumococcal Surveillance Study Group (PMPSSG). Pediatrics 1998; 102:1376–82.
[31] Schutze GE, Tucker NC, Mason Jr EO. Impact of the conjugate pneumococcal vaccine in Arkansas. Pediatr Infect Dis J 2004;23:1125–9.
[32] Black S, Shinefield H, Baxter R, et al. Postlicensure surveillance for pneumococcal invasive disease after use of heptavalent pneumococcal conjugate vaccine in Northern California Kaiser Permanente. Pediatr Infect Dis J 2004;23:485–9.
[33] Shapiro ED, Gerber MA. Lyme disease. Clin Infect Dis 2000;31:533–42.
[34] Kocher MS, Zurakowski D, Kasser JR. Differentiating between septic arthritis and transient synovitis of the hip in children: an evidence-based clinical prediction algorithm. J Bone Joint Surg Am 1999;81:1662–70.
[35] Luhmann SJ, Jones A, Schootman M, Gordon JE, Schoenecker PL, Luhmann JD. Differentiation between septic arthritis and transient synovitis of the hip in children with clinical prediction algorithms. J Bone Joint Surg Am 2004;86:956–62.
[36] Jung ST, Rowe SM, Moon ES, Song EK, Yoon TR, Seo HY. Significance of laboratory and radiologic findings for differentiating between septic arthritis and transient synovitis of the hip. J Pediatr Orthop 2003;23:368–72.
[37] Del Beccaro MA, Champoux AN, Bockers T, Mendelman PM. Septic arthritis versus transient synovitis of the hip: the value of screening laboratory tests. Ann Emerg Med 1992;21:1418–22.
[38] Kocher MS, Mandiga R, Murphy JM, et al. A clinical practice guideline for treatment of septic arthritis in children: efficacy in improving process of care and effect on outcome of septic arthritis of the hip. J Bone Joint Surg Am 2003;85:994–9.
[39] Syrogiannopoulos GA, Nelson JD. Duration of antimicrobial therapy for acute suppurative osteoarticular infections. Lancet 1988;1:37–40.
[40] Odio CM, Ramirez T, Arias G, et al. Double blind, randomized, placebo-controlled study of dexamethasone therapy for hematogenous septic arthritis in children. Pediatr Infect Dis J 2003; 22:883–8.

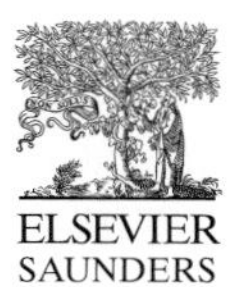
ELSEVIER
SAUNDERS

PEDIATRIC CLINICS
OF NORTH AMERICA

Pediatr Clin N Am 52 (2005) 795–810

Bacterial Meningitis in Children

Susana Chávez-Bueno, MD*, George H. McCracken, Jr, MD

Department of Pediatrics, Division of Pediatric Infectious Diseases, University of Texas Southwestern Medical Center of Dallas, 5323 Harry Hines Boulevard, Dallas, TX 75390-9063, USA

Meningitis is defined as inflammation of the membranes that surround the brain and spinal cord. Microbiologic causes include bacteria, viruses, fungi, and parasites. Before routine use of pneumococcal conjugate vaccine, bacterial meningitis affected almost 6000 people every year in the United States; about half of all cases occurred in children 18 years old or younger [1]. Approximately 10% of patients with bacterial meningitis die [2], and 40% have sequelae including hearing impairment and other neurologic sequelae [3].

Epidemiology

The etiology of bacterial meningitis is affected most by the age of the patient. In neonates, the most common etiologic agents are group B streptococci (GBS) and gram-negative enteric bacilli. Although the incidence of early-onset neonatal GBS disease decreased by two thirds after implementation of the Centers for Disease Control and Prevention revised guidelines for intrapartum antibiotic prophylaxis in 2002 [4,5], GBS remains an important cause of late-onset disease, typically manifest as meningitis. *Escherichia coli* and other gram-negative enteric bacilli, including *Klebsiella, Enterobacter,* and *Salmonella,* cause sporadic disease except in nosocomial outbreaks and in developing countries [6–8]. Other pathogens that occasionally cause meningitis in neonates, especially during outbreaks, include *Listeria monocytogenes, Enterobacter sakazakii* [9,10], and *Citrobacter koseri* (formerly *Citrobacter diversus*). A unique feature of neonatal

* Corresponding author.
E-mail address: Susana.Chavez-Bueno@UTSouthwestern.edu (S. Chávez-Bueno).

doi:10.1016/j.pcl.2005.02.011 **pediatric.theclinics.com**

meningitis caused by *C. koseri* is a high association with the development of brain abscesses [11]. Other rare causes of meningitis in neonates include staphylococci, enterococci, and viridans streptococci.

In infants and young children worldwide, S*treptococcus pneumoniae, Neisseria meningitides,* and *Haemophilus influenzae* type b (Hib) are the most common causes of bacterial meningitis. Among children older than 5 years of age and adolescents, *S. pneumoniae* and *N. meningitidis* are the predominant causes of bacterial meningitis [1,12]. Most of the bacteria responsible for invasive disease, including meningitis, in children have a polysaccharide capsule [13,14].

The incidence of meningitis caused by Hib has decreased markedly in areas of the world where Hib conjugate vaccines are routinely used [15]. Replacement with the other capsular types (*H. influenzae* types a and c to f) has not occurred after the widespread use of Hib vaccines [16]. The incidence of meningitis caused by *S. pneumoniae* and *N. meningitidis* (serotype C) also have been reduced in areas where conjugated vaccines against these pathogens have been introduced.

The highest risk of bacterial meningitis caused by *S. pneumoniae* is in children younger than 2 years old. In 1995, before universal immunization against this pathogen, the estimated incidence of pneumococcal meningitis was more than 20 cases per 100,000 US population in this age group [1]. The seven most common serotypes that cause invasive disease in the United States are 4, 6B, 9V, 14, 19, 18C, and 23 [17]. These serotypes are included in the heptavalent pneumococcal conjugate vaccine, PCV7, which is licensed in the United States. The incidence of invasive disease, including bacterial meningitis, caused by *S. pneumoniae* has been reduced by greater than 90% after the implementation of universal use of this vaccine [18], beginning in infancy.

Most cases of invasive meningococcal disease in the United States are caused by serogroups B, C, Y, and W-135 [19]. Serogroup A strains account for most epidemics, especially in sub-Saharan Africa [20]. Serogroup C predominates in England. The incidence of meningococcal meningitis is greatest in infants younger than 1 year old; a second peak incidence is observed at age 15 to 17 years [21,22]. A conjugate vaccine against menigococcal serogroup C was introduced into the routine immunization schedule in 1999 in England. The use of this vaccine was associated with an overall 81% reduction of serogroup C disease within 2 years of implementation [23]. Continued surveillance has raised concerns about long-term effectiveness in infants vaccinated before 6 months of age [24].

Factors that increase the risk for bacterial meningitis include immunosuppresive states, such as HIV infection, asplenia [25], terminal complement deficiencies, and immunoglobulin deficiencies. Penetrating head injuries, neurosurgical procedures, or the presence of cerebrospinal fluid (CSF) leaks are other risk factors for meningitis. Patients with ventriculoperitoneal shunts are at risk of meningitis caused by staphylococci (especially coagulase-negative strains) and gram-negative organisms, including *Pseudomonas* [26]. Patients with cochlear implants have more than a 30-fold increased incidence of pneumococcal meningitis [27].

Pathogenesis

Bacteria reach the CNS either by hematogenous spread or by direct extension from a contiguous site. In neonates, pathogens are acquired from nonsterile maternal genital secretions. In infants and children, many of the organisms that cause meningitis colonize the upper respiratory tract. Direct inoculation of bacteria into the CNS can result from trauma, skull defects with CSF leaks, congenital dura defects such as a dermal sinuses or meningomyelocele, or extension from a suppurative parameningeal focus.

After bacteremia, pathogens penetrate the blood-brain barrier to enter the subarachnoid space. Surface bacterial proteins known to facilitate invasion of the blood-brain barrier include *E coli* proteins IbeA, IbeB, and ompA; *S. pneumoniae* protein CbpA; and *N. meningitidis* proteins Opc, Opa, and PilC, a pili protein [28]. Transcellular penetration has been shown for *S. pneumoniae*, GBS, *L. monocytogenes,* and *E coli*.

The intense inflammation elicited by bacterial products, such as gram-negative lipopolysaccharide or gram-positive peptidoglycan, persists after bacteria are destroyed by the host responses and antibiotic therapy [29]. These substances induce production of different inflammatory mediators by CNS astrocytes and ependymal, glial, and endothelial cells. The inflammatory mediators include tumor necrosis factor-α; interleukin (IL)-1, IL-6, IL-8, and IL-10; macrophage induced proteins 1 and 2; and other mediators including nitric oxide, matrix metalloproteinase-2, and prostaglandins [30–32]. The ensuing granulocyte influx and altered blood-brain barrier permeability result in the release of proteolytic products and toxic oxygen radicals. Accompanying cerebral edema and increased intracranial pressure contribute to neuronal damage and death. Neuronal death is believed to be caused by apoptosis through caspase-dependent and independent pathways [33,34].

Clinical features

Manifestations of bacterial meningitis depend on the age of the patient. Fever, neck stiffness, and mental status changes are present in less than 50% [35], and Kernig and Brudzinski signs are present in only about 5% of adults with bacterial meningitis [36]. These manifestations are observed even less frequently in children with bacterial meningitis. Signs of meningeal irritation, such as neck stiffness, Brudzinski and Kernig signs, or the tripod phenomenon, in children also are not specific for bacterial meningitis. In one study, bacterial meningitis was present in only about one third of children with signs of meningeal irritation [37]. Seizures occur as the presenting symptom in one third of cases of bacterial meningitis in children. Seizures are more common in children with meningitis caused by *S. pneumoniae* and Hib compared with children with meningococcal meningitis [38]. Petechiae and purpura may accompany meningitis caused by any bacteria, but they are more common in patients with meningococcal meningitis than patients with meningitis caused by *S. pneumoniae* or *H. influenzae*. Symptoms may be subtle in infants and include fever only, irritability, lethargy, and difficulty feeding. Signs include fever, apnea, seizures, a bulging fontanel, and a rash.

Diagnosis

A lumbar puncture is necessary for the definitive diagnosis of bacterial meningitis. Analysis of CSF should include Gram stain and cultures, white blood cell (WBC) count and differential, and glucose and protein concentrations. Cytocentrifugation of the CSF enhances the ability to detect bacteria and perform a more accurate determination of the WBC differential.

Typical findings in the CSF in bacterial meningitis include pleocytosis, usually with a WBC count greater than 1000 cells/mm^3 and predominance of polymorphonuclear leukocytes. In some cases, especially when performed early in the disease, the WBC count can be normal [39], and there may be a lymphocyte predominance. It is common for the polymorphonuclear leukocyte count to increase after 48 hours of diagnosis and then to decrease thereafter [40]. Glucose concentration usually is decreased with a CSF-to-serum glucose ratio of 0.6 or less in neonates and 0.4 or less in children older than 2 months of age, whereas protein concentration usually is elevated [41]. A reduced absolute CSF concentration of glucose is as sensitive as the CSF-to-serum glucose ratio in the diagnosis of bacterial meningitis.

A traumatic lumbar puncture, which introduces blood into the spinal fluid during the procedure, makes interpretation of the CSF cell count difficult. Several methods have been used to distinguish peripheral blood WBCs from true CSF leukocytosis, but none have proved accurate. Caution is recommended when interpreting traumatic lumbar punctures [42,43].

The Gram-stained smear of CSF has a lower limit of detection of about 10^5 colony-forming units/mL. Of patients with untreated bacterial meningitis, 80% to 90% have a positive CSF Gram stain. Unless unusual pathogens, such as anaerobes, are suspected, agar plate cultures of CSF are preferred to liquid media. Routine inoculation of CSF into broth culture is not recommended because isolates recovered by this technique are frequently contaminants [44,45].

With the exception of meningitis caused by gram-negative enteric bacilli, the yield of bacterial CSF cultures decreases soon after antibiotic therapy has been started [46]. The CSF WBC count and glucose and protein concentrations generally remain abnormal for several days, however, after initiating appropriate antibiotic therapy. Some authors recommend using latex agglutination tests to detect bacterial capsular antigens in patients with suspected bacterial meningitis who have been receiving antibiotics at the time the lumbar puncture is performed. These tests are not specific, however, and they identify very few cases of bacterial meningitis not already detected by CSF culture [47]. In the future, more sensitive techniques, such as amplification of the 16S rRNA gene by polymerase chain reaction, may help to diagnose cases of bacterial meningitis in patients pretreated with antibiotics. Broad-range polymerase chain reaction has shown a sensitivity of 86% and specificity of 97% in detecting multiple organisms simultaneously compared with culture [48]. Real-time polymerase chain reaction techniques are even more sensitive in the clinical setting [49].

The presence of focal neurologic signs, cardiovascular instability, or papilledema in a patient with suspected bacterial meningitis raises the suspicion of increased intracranial pressure. In such cases, neuroimaging should be done before performing a lumbar puncture to avoid possible herniation [50,51]. Blood cultures and antibiotic administration should be done while awaiting results of neuroimaging studies to avoid substantial delays in the initiation of treatment.

Management

Antibiotic selection

Factors to consider when selecting the appropriate antibiotic for treating bacterial meningitis include its activity against the causative pathogen and its ability to penetrate and attain effective bactericidal concentrations in the CSF. The integrity of the blood-brain barrier is compromised during meningitis, resulting in increased permeability to most antibiotics. β-Lactam antibiotics achieve concentrations of 5% to 20% of concomitant serum values. Even in the absence of substantial inflammation, penetration of highly lipid-soluble antibiotics, such as rifampin, chloramphenicol, and quinolones, is 30% to 50% of serum concentrations. In contrast, the concentration of vancomycin is less than 5% of the serum concentrations. Experimental models of bacterial meningitis suggest that prompt bacteriologic cure is predictable if antibiotic concentrations that are 10-fold to 30-fold greater than the minimal bactericidal concentration (MBC) for a specific microorganism are attained in CSF.

The pharmacodynamic properties of different antibiotics affect their bacteriologic efficacy. Aminoglycosides and fluoroquinolones exhibit concentration-dependent activity. Their effectiveness is determined by the ratio between the peak concentration or area under the concentration curve of the antibiotic and the MBC of the pathogen [52]. In contrast, the β-lactam antibiotics and vancomycin show concentration-independent activity. The time over the MBC during which the drug concentration exceeds the minimum inhibitory concentration (MIC) seems to determine drug effectiveness. These drugs need to be administered at frequent dosing intervals [53].

Empirical therapy

Empirical regimens are selected to cover the most likely etiologic agents. Therapy should be modified when the offending organism and its antimicrobial susceptibilities are known. In neonates, during the first 2 to 3 weeks of life, ampicillin with either an aminoglycoside or cefotaxime is commonly used as initial empirical therapy. For neonates with late-onset meningitis, a regimen containing an antistaphylococcal antibiotic, such as nafcillin or vancomycin, *plus* cefotaxime *or* ceftazidime with or without an aminoglycoside is recommended [54].

Recommendations for empirical therapy of bacterial meningitis have been published as a practice guideline by the Infectious Disease Society of America [55]. For children older than 1 month of age, vancomycin plus a third-generation cephalosporin (ceftriaxone or cefotaxime) are recommended for initial therapy. In patients with predisposing factors, such as penetrating trauma, postneurosurgery, or CSF shunt, empirical therapy should include vancomycin *plus* cefepime *or* ceftazidime *or* meropenem. In cases of basilar skull fracture, a regimen containing vancomycin *plus* ceftriaxone *or* cefotaxime usually provides adequate empirical therapy.

Pathogen-specific antimicrobial therapy

Penicillin G or ampicillin remains the standard therapy for susceptible (MIC $\leq$0.06 μg/mL) strains of *S. pneumoniae* or *N. meningitidis*; a third-generation cephalosporin is a reasonable alternative. A third-generation cephalosporin (ceftriaxone or cefotaxime) is indicated to treat either of these organisms if they are not susceptible to penicillin (MIC $\geq$0.1 μg/mL), but are susceptible to the cephalosporin (MIC $\leq$0.5 μg/mL). Isolates that are not susceptible to penicillin and have a MIC to the third-generation cephalosporin that is 1 μg/mL or

Table 1
Recommended antimicrobial therapy for selected pathogens in children with bacterial meningitis

Bacteria	Antimicrobial of choice	Alternative therapy
Haemophilus influenzae		
β-lactamase negative	Ampicillin	Ceftriaxone, cefotaxime, cefepime, chloramphenicol*, fluoroquinolone
β-lactamase positive	Ceftriaxone or cefotaxime	Cefepime, chloramphenicol*, fluoroquinolone
Streptococcus agalactiae	Penicillin G ± gentamicin or ampicillin ± gentamicin	Ceftriaxone or cefotaxime
Listeria monocytogenes	Ampicillin ± gentamicin	Trimethoprim-sulfamethoxazole
Escherichia coli and other Enterobacteriaceae	Ceftriaxone or cefotaxime ± aminoglycoside	Cefepime or meropenem
Pseudomonas aeruginosa	Ceftazidime + aminoglycoside or cefepime + aminoglycoside	Meropenem ± aminoglycoside
Staphylococcus aureus		
Methicillin susceptible	Nafcillin or oxacillin	Vancomycin
Methicillin resistant	Vancomycin ± rifampin	—
Enterococcus		
Ampicillin susceptible	Ampicillin + gentamicin	—
Ampicillin resistant	Vancomycin + gentamicin	—

* 50% of *H. influenzae* isolates are resistant in certain areas of the world.

greater should be treated with vancomycin *plus* a third-generation cephalosporin (ceftriaxone or cefotaxime); and the addition of rifampin should be considered. Cefepime and meropenem are alternative therapies for *S. pneumoniae* with intermediate resistance to penicillin (MIC 0.1–1 μg/mL); a fluoroquinolone, either gatifloxacin or moxifloxacin, is an effective alternative for penicillin-resistant or cephalosporin-resistant isolates.

Vancomycin and rifampin are usually active against cefotaxime-resistant or ceftriaxone-resistant *S. pneumoniae,* although vancomycin-tolerant strains have been described. Vancomycin tolerance is thought to arise from a defect in the bacterium's endogenous cell death pathway that results in defective autolysis. In one study, these isolates represented almost 4% of *S. pneumoniae* nasopharyngeal isolates from children and 10% of meningitis isolates from adults and children. These isolates were associated with increased mortality in the infected children [56].

Antibiotics recommended for other pathogens causing bacterial meningitis in children are summarized in Table 1. Dosages of the most commonly used intravenous antibiotics for therapy of bacterial meningitis in children are presented in Table 2.

Table 2
Dosages of antibiotics administered intravenously for pediatric patients with bacterial meningitis

	Total daily dose (dosing interval in hours)		
	Neonates, age in days*		
Antibiotic	0–7	8–28	Infants and children
Amikacin**	15–20 mg/kg (12)	30 mg/kg (8)	20–30 mg/kg (8)
Ampicillin	150 mg/kg (8)	200 mg/kg (6–8)	200–300 mg/kg (6)
Cefepime	—	—	150 mg/kg (8)
Cefotaxime	100–150 mg/kg (8–12)	150–200 mg/kg (6–8)	200–300 mg/kg (6–8)
Ceftazidime	100–150 mg/kg (8–12)	150 mg/kg (8)	150 mg/kg (8)
Ceftriaxone	—	—	80–100 mg/kg (12–24)
Chloramphenicol	25 mg/kg (24)	50 mg/kg (12–24)	75–100 mg/kg (6)
Gentamicin**	5 mg/kg (12)	7.5 mg/kg (8)	7.5 mg/kg (8)
Meropenem	—	—	120 mg/kg (8)
Nafcillin	75 mg/kg (8–12)	100–150 mg/kg (6–8)	200 mg/kg (6)
Oxacillin	75 mg/kg (8–12)	150–200 mg/kg (6–8)	200 mg/kg (6)
Penicillin G	0.15 mU/kg (8–12)	0.2 mU/kg (6–8)	0.3 mU/kg (4–6)
Rifampin	—	10–20 mg/kg (12)	10–20 mg/kg (12–24)
Tobramycin**	5 mg/kg (12)	7.5 mg/kg (8)	7.5 mg/kg (8)
Trimethoprim-sulfamethoxazole	—	—	10–20 mg/kg (6–12)
Vancomycin***	20–30 mg/kg (8–12)	30–45 mg/kg (6–8)	60 mg/kg (6)

* For neonates weighing <2000 g, refer to Bradley JS, Pocket book of pediatric antimicrobial therapy. 15th edition; ** Need to monitor peak and trough serum concentrations; *** Maintain serum trough concentrations of 15–20 μg/mL.

Adapted from Tunkel AR, Hartman BJ, Kaplan SL, et al. Practice guidelines for the management of bacterial meningitis. Clin Infect Dis 2004;39:1267–84.

With the use of antibiotics to which the organism exhibits in vitro susceptibility, CSF cultures become sterile in most cases within 24 to 36 hours after initiating therapy [57]. In some cases, a repeat lumbar puncture is indicated 24 to 48 hours after start of therapy because of lack of clinical improvement or when meningitis is caused by resistant *S. pneumoniae* strains or by gram-negative enteric bacilli. The authors also recommend a second lumbar puncture in all neonates because the clinical findings are not helpful in judging success of therapy in this age group, and delayed sterilization of CSF is common.

Duration of therapy depends on the age of the patient, the causative pathogen, and the clinical course. The duration of antibiotic treatment is individualized, and longer regimens than the ones suggested herein might be required for complicated cases. For neonates with GBS meningitis, 14 to 21 days is recommended; for *L. monocytogenes* meningitis, 10 to 14 days is usually satisfactory; and for gram-negative enteric meningitis, a minimum of 3 weeks of therapy usually is provided. Meningococcal meningitis usually is treated for 4 to 7 days; *H. influenzae,* for 7 to 10 days; and *S. pneumoniae,* for 10 to 14 days. Neuroimaging (head CT or MR imaging) is recommended in neonates to determine whether intracranial complications require prolonged therapy or whether surgical intervention is required.

Adjunctive and supportive therapy

Dexamethasone

Animal models of bacterial meningitis have shown beneficial effects of dexamethasone administration, including decreasing inflammation, reducing cerebral edema and increased intracranial pressure, and lessening brain damage [53]. In adults with bacterial meningitis, a recently published prospective, randomized, placebo-controlled, double-blind multicenter trial showed that dexamethasone recipients had a lower percentage of unfavorable outcomes, including death, compared with subjects who received placebo. Benefits were evident in the subgroup with pneumococcal meningitis, but not in others [58]. In pediatric patients, several double-blind, placebo-controlled studies to evaluate the use of adjunctive dexamethasone in bacterial meningitis have been conducted. These studies showed a reduction of indices of meningeal inflammatory and decreased audiologic and neurologic sequelae in patients who received dexamethasone compared with patients who received placebo. These beneficial effects were greatest in cases of *H. influenzae* meningitis, especially in regards to hearing outcomes. Clinical benefit was less evident in cases of pneumococcal meningitis; dexamethasone was most beneficial when given with or shortly before the first dose of parenteral antibiotic therapy [59].

Because dexamethasone can decrease antibiotic penetration into the CNS, concerns have been raised that the use of steroids may impede the eradication of highly resistant pneumococcal strains from the CSF [38,60,61]. Clinical data do not support this hypothesis, however, when the combination of vancomycin and a third-generation cephalosporin is used as initial empirical therapy.

Current recommendations support the use of dexamethasone in infants and children with Hib meningitis [55]. For infants and children 6 weeks old and older with pneumococcal meningitis, adjunctive therapy with dexamethasone should be considered after weighing the potential benefits and possible risks. Data are insufficient to recommend dexamethasone therapy in neonates with bacterial meningitis [55].

Recommended dexamethasone dosing regimens range from 0.6 to 0.8 mg/kg daily in two or three divided doses for 2 days to 1 mg/kg in four divided doses for 2 to 4 days [41,55]. For optimal results, the first dose of dexamethasone should be administered before or concomitant with the first parenteral antibiotic dose.

Other adjunctive therapies, such as different anti-inflammatory drugs and compounds including lipopolysaccharide-neutralizing proteins, anticytokine antibodies [62], and anticytotoxic agents [63], have been tested in animal models of bacterial meningitis with varied success [32]. None of these compounds has been evaluated in patients with bacterial meningitis.

Supportive therapy

Maintenance of adequate cerebral perfusion and management of increased intracranial pressure are crucial to the prevention of potential life-threatening complications of bacterial meningitis. Maintaining normal blood pressure may require infusion of a vasoactive agent, such as dopamine or dobutamine. Fluid restriction is advised only in patients who are not dehydrated and have evidence of inappropriate antidiuretic hormone secretion (hyponatremia). There is no evidence that fluid restriction reduces cerebral edema in children with bacterial meningitis. Fluid restriction in the presence of hypovolemia could result in decreased systemic blood pressure that could compromise cerebral perfusion [64].

Strategies used to reduce increased intracranial pressure include antipyretic agents, avoiding frequent and vigorous procedures such as intubation and tracheal suction, 30° bed head elevation, short-term hyperventilation, mannitol administration, and high-dose barbiturate therapy. Control and prevention of seizures can be attained with anticonvulsant medications; benzodiazepines, phenytoin, and phenobarbital are commonly used for this purpose.

Complications

The mortality rate for bacterial meningitis in children ranges from 4% to 10% in more recent studies. Case-fatality rate and incidence of neurologic sequelae are greatest in pneumococcal meningitis. Approximately 15% of children with pneumococcal meningitis present in shock [65]. Shock also is a common presentation in cases of meningococcal meningitis, and it can be associated with disseminated intravascular coagulation.

Seizures are a common complication of bacterial meningitis, affecting one third of patients. Seizures that persist for longer than 4 days after diagnosis or arise for the first time late in the course of the disease are more likely to be associated with neurologic sequelae. Focal seizures have a worse prognosis.

Subdural effusions are present in one third of patients with bacterial meningitis and are associated more commonly with *H. influenzae* and *S. pneumoniae* than with meningococcal meningitis. They are asymptomatic and resolve spontaneously without permanent neurologic sequelae in most cases [66]. Subdural empyema should be suspected when prolonged fever and irritability with or without CSF leukocytosis are present. This is an uncommon complication of bacterial meningitis in infants, occurring in less than 2% of cases. Management consists of surgical drainage and appropriate antibiotic therapy [67].

Brain abscesses are an uncommon complication of bacterial meningitis; they are more likely to occur in newborns infected with *C. koseri* or *Proteus* species. Hydrocephalus, hemorrhage, and infarctions resulting from thromboses are other potential complications of bacterial meningitis in children.

Persistent fevers often are related to nosocomially acquired infection, including infections caused by viruses or infected intravenous catheters. Drug fever, which is commonly associated with β-lactam antibiotics and anticonvulsant therapy, should be suspected when other causes of persistent fever have been excluded. Cranial imaging with CT or MR imaging with gadolinium should be performed in cases of prolonged obtundation, seizures persisting for more than 72 hours after the start of treatment, continued excessive irritability, persistently abnormal CSF indices, and focal neurologic findings and in newborn infants.

Prognosis

Factors that can affect outcome from bacterial meningitis are age; etiology; CSF findings at the time of diagnosis, including concentration of bacteria or bacterial products, WBC count, and glucose concentration; and the time to sterilization of CSF after start of therapy. Decreased level of consciousness and seizures occurring during hospitalization have been associated with increased mortality and neurologic sequelae in several studies [2,65]. Seizures that are focal or are difficult to control imply an underlying vascular disturbance, such as venous thrombosis or infarction, and are associated with epilepsy and other neurologic sequelae [68].

The most common neurologic sequela of bacterial meningitis is hearing impairment. Some degree of hearing loss occurs in about 25% to 35% of patients with meningitis caused by *S. pneumoniae* and in 5% to 10% of patients with *H. influenzae* and *N. meningitidis* infection. Low glucose concentration in CSF has been shown to correlate with the development hearing impairment in several studies [2,61,69]. Approximately 10% of children develop neuromotor and learning disabilities and speech and behavioral problems as a consequence of bacterial meningitis [70,71].

Prevention

Vaccines

Antibodies directed against the bacterial capsular components of *H. influenzae, N. meningitides,* and *S. pneumoniae* play a major role in development of immunity against these organisms. Immunization with the *Haemophilus,* pneumococcal, and meningococcal conjugate vaccines has had a significant impact on the incidence of invasive diseases in children caused by these organisms.

The routine use of conjugated Hib vaccines in children has been associated with a reduction of more than 99% of invasive disease, including meningitis, in developed countries. Rates of Hib disease have been affected modestly in other areas of the world where the vaccine is not routinely available [14,72].

The heptavalent conjugate pneumococcal vaccine, PCV7, was approved for routine use in infants in 2000. Initial clinical trials showed a reduction of more than 90% in invasive pneumococcal infections in children [73]. Subsequent clinical studies have confirmed the efficacy of conjugated pneumococcal vaccine in children and a concomitant reduction in the incidence of invasive pneumococcal disease in adults, attributed to reduced circulation of the bacteria [18,29, 74,75]. Children older than 2 years of age who are at risk of developing invasive pneumococcal disease, such as children with sickle hemoglobinopathy, should receive the conjugate vaccine followed by the 23-valent polysaccharide vaccine. This includes patients with cochlear implants [75].

A quadrivalent meningococcal polysaccharide vaccine against serogroups A, C, Y, and W-135 strains is recommended in the United States for high-risk children older than 2 years, such as children with asplenia or terminal complement deficiencies. In 2000, the Advisory Committee on Immunization Practices recommended that health care providers inform all college students about the risks of meningococcal disease in this population and to make this vaccine available to individuals who want to reduce their risk for meningococcal disease, which is highest in freshmen living in dormitories [76]. Immunogenicity of the vaccines developed against serogroup B meningococci is poor. A major problem of vaccine development for this serogroup is the homology of this bacterium's capsular polysaccharide with components of human neural tissue. Current research is ongoing to improve the immune response to vaccines designed against this serogroup, which is endemic in North America and Europe [77]. A meningococcal serogroup C conjugate vaccine is routinely being administered in the United Kingdom and Canada. The Vaccines and Related Biological Products Advisory Committee of the US Food and Drug Administration voted to recommend licensure of a quadrivalent conjugate meningococcal vaccine (groups A, C, Y, and W-135) for protection against invasive meningococcal disease in adolescents and adults age 11 to 55 years. Clinical trials with this vaccine showed modest immunogenicity in infants [78].

Maternal immunization with GBS (*Streptococcus agalactiae*) conjugate vaccine may represent a future strategy to reduce neonatal GBS streptococcal disease. Maternal administration of prophylactic antibiotics has an impact on preventing only early-onset GBS disease [79].

Chemoprophylaxis

Administration of prophylactic antibiotics to asymptomatic contacts of meningitis index cases is indicated to decrease carriage and prevent spread of the disease. Recommendations for chemoprophylaxis in cases of *H. influenzae* and *N. menigitidis* meningitis are provided in Table 3 [80].

Table 3
Chemoprophylaxis of *Haemophilus influenzae* type b and meningococcal meningitis (*Neisseria meningitidis*)

	H. influenzae	*N. meningitidis*
Individuals for whom chemoprophylaxis is recommended	All members of the household* with: ≥1 contact <4 years old incompletely immunized, including infants < 12 months old without the primary series Immunocompromosed child in household, even if >4 years old and fully immunized All susceptible nursery/childcare center contacts when ≥2 cases of Hib invasive disease have occurred within 60 d Index case treated with ampicillin or chloramphenicol if <2 years of age or with a susceptible household contact	All household contacts Childcare/nursery school contacts during 7 d before onset of illness Direct exposure to index case's secretions—kissing, sharing of eating utensils, toothbrushes, close social contact—during 7 d before onset of illness Health care workers who performed unprotected mouth-to-mouth resuscitation, intubation, suction Frequently slept or ate in same dwelling as index case during 7 d before onset of illness
Recommended agents/dosage	Rifampin 20 mg/kg orally once daily × 4 d. Decrease dose to 10 mg/kg/d for infants <1 month old[†]	Rifampin 10 mg/kg orally once daily × 2 d. Decrease dose to 5 mg/kg/d for infants ≤1 month old[†] *or* Ceftriaxone 125 mg for ≤15 years olds or 250 mg for >15 years olds intramuscularly, single dose *or* Ciprofloxacin 500 mg orally in ≥18 years old, singe dose

* Includes people residing with the index case or nonresidents who spent ≥4 hours with the index case for at least 5 of the 7 days preceeding the hospital admission day of the index case.

[†] Maximum daily dose of 600 mg. Not recommended in pregnant women.

Summary

Prompt and accurate diagnosis and adequate treatment of bacterial meningitis in children remains a major challenge, as reflected by the continued high morbidity and case-fatality rates of the disease worldwide. Appropriate use of antibiotics, along with adjunctive therapies, such dexamethasone, has proved helpful in the prevention of neurologic sequelae in children with bacterial meningitis. Better understanding of pathophysiologic mechanisms likely would result in more effective therapies in the future. Use of conjugate vaccines against the most common pathogens has been crucial in preventing bacterial meningitis in children.

References

[1] Schuchat A, Robinson K, Wenger JD, et al. Bacterial meningitis in the United States in 1995. Active Surveillance Team. N Engl J Med 1997;337:970–6.

[2] Arditi M, Mason Jr EO, Bradley JS, et al. Three-year multicenter surveillance of pneumococcal meningitis in children: clinical characteristics, and outcome related to penicillin susceptibility and dexamethasone use. Pediatrics 1998;102:1087–97.

[3] Grimwood K, Anderson VA, Bond L, et al. Adverse outcomes of bacterial meningitis in school-age survivors. Pediatrics 1995;95:646–56.

[4] Schrag S, Gorwitz R, Fultz-Butts K, Schuchat A. Prevention of perinatal group B streptococcal disease: revised guidelines from CDC. MMWR Morb Mortal Wkly Rep 2002;51:1–22.

[5] Centers for Disease Control and Prevention. Diminishing racial disparities in early-onset neonatal group B streptococcal disease—United States, 2000–2003. MMWR Morb Mortal Wkly Rep 2004;53:502–5.

[6] Moreno MT, Vargas S, Poveda R, Saez-Llorens X. Neonatal sepsis and meningitis in a developing Latin American country. Pediatr Infect Dis J 1994;13:516–20.

[7] Laving AM, Musoke RN, Wasunna AO, Revathi G. Neonatal bacterial meningitis at the newborn unit of Kenyatta National Hospital. East Afr Med J 2003;80:456–62.

[8] Osrin D, Vergnano S, Costello A. Serious bacterial infections in newborn infants in developing countries. Curr Opin Infect Dis 2004;17:217–24.

[9] Centers for Disease Control and Prevention. *Enterobacter sakazakii* infections associated with the use of powdered infant formula—Tennessee, 2001. JAMA 2002;287:2204–5.

[10] Stoll BJ, Hansen N, Fanaroff AA, Lemons JA. *Enterobacter sakazakii* is a rare cause of neonatal septicemia or meningitis in VLBW infants. J Pediatr 2004;144:821–3.

[11] Doran TI. The role of *Citrobacter* in clinical disease of children: review. Clin Infect Dis 1999; 28:384–94.

[12] Dawson KG, Emerson JC, Burns JL. Fifteen years of experience with bacterial meningitis. Pediatr Infect Dis J 1999;18:816–22.

[13] Schoendorf KC, Adams WG, Kiely JL, Wenger JD. National trends in *Haemophilus influenzae* meningitis mortality and hospitalization among children, 1980 through 1991. Pediatrics 1994;93: 663–8.

[14] Centers for Disease Control and Prevention. Progress toward eliminating *Haemophilus influenzae* type b disease among infants and children—United States, 1998–2000. MMWR Morb Mortal Wkly Rep 2002;51:234–7.

[15] Martin M, Casellas JM, Madhi SA, et al. Impact of *Haemophilus influenzae* type b conjugate vaccine in South Africa and Argentina. Pediatr Infect Dis J 2004;23:842–7.

[16] Kelly DF, Moxon ER, Pollard AJ. *Haemophilus influenzae* type b conjugate vaccines. Immunology 2004;113:163–74.

[17] Feikin DR, Klugman KP. Historical changes in pneumococcal serogroup distribution: implications for the era of pneumococcal conjugate vaccines. Clin Infect Dis 2002;35:547–55.
[18] Black S, Shinefield H, Baxter R, et al. Postlicensure surveillance for pneumococcal invasive disease after use of heptavalent pneumococcal conjugate vaccine in Northern California Kaiser Permanente. Pediatr Infect Dis J 2004;23:485–9.
[19] Rosenstein NE, Perkins BA, Stephens DS, Popovic T, Hughes JM. Meningococcal disease. N Engl J Med 2001;344:1378–88.
[20] Robbins JB, Schneerson R, Gotschlich EC, et al. Meningococcal meningitis in sub-Saharan Africa: the case for mass and routine vaccination with available polysaccharide vaccines. Bull World Health Organ 2003;81:745–55.
[21] Neuman HB, Wald ER. Bacterial meningitis in childhood at the Children's Hospital of Pittsburgh: 1988–1998. Clin Pediatr (Phila) 2001;40:595–600.
[22] Pollard AJ. Global epidemiology of meningococcal disease and vaccine efficacy. Pediatr Infect Dis J 2004;23:S274–9.
[23] Miller E, Salisbury D, Ramsay M. Planning, registration, and implementation of an immunisation campaign against meningococcal serogroup C disease in the UK: a success story. Vaccine 2001;20(Suppl 1):S58–67.
[24] Trotter CL, Andrews NJ, Kaczmarski EB, Miller E, Ramsay ME. Effectiveness of meningococcal serogroup C conjugate vaccine 4 years after introduction. Lancet 2004;364:365–7.
[25] Schutze GE, Mason Jr EO, Barson WJ, et al. Invasive pneumococcal infections in children with asplenia. Pediatr Infect Dis J 2002;21:278–82.
[26] Odio C, McCracken Jr GH, Nelson JD. CSF shunt infections in pediatrics: a seven-year experience. Am J Dis Child 1984;138:1103–8.
[27] Reefhuis J, Honein MA, Whitney CG, et al. Risk of bacterial meningitis in children with cochlear implants. N Engl J Med 2003;349:435–45.
[28] Huang SH, Jong AY. Cellular mechanisms of microbial proteins contributing to invasion of the blood-brain barrier. Cell Microbiol 2001;3:277–87.
[29] Kaplan SL, Mason Jr EO, Wald ER, et al. Decrease of invasive pneumococcal infections in children among 8 children's hospitals in the United States after the introduction of the 7-valent pneumococcal conjugate vaccine. Pediatrics 2004;113:443–9.
[30] Ramilo O, Saez-Llorens X, Mertsola J, et al. Tumor necrosis factor alpha/cachectin and interleukin 1 beta initiate meningeal inflammation. J Exp Med 1990;172:497–507.
[31] Leib SL, Tauber MG. Pathogenesis of bacterial meningitis. Infect Dis Clin North Am 1999;13: 527–48.
[32] van der Flier M, Geelen SP, Kimpen JL, Hoepelman IM, Tuomanen EI. Reprogramming the host response in bacterial meningitis: how best to improve outcome? Clin Microbiol Rev 2003;16: 415–29.
[33] Meli DN, Christen S, Leib SL, Tauber MG. Current concepts in the pathogenesis of meningitis caused by *Streptococcus pneumoniae*. Curr Opin Infect Dis 2002;15:253–7.
[34] Mitchell L, Smith SH, Braun JS, Herzog KH, Weber JR, Tuomanen EI. Dual phases of apoptosis in pneumococcal meningitis. J Infect Dis 2004;190:2039–46.
[35] van de Beek D, de Gans J, Spanjaard L, Weisfelt M, Reitsma JB, Vermeulen M. Clinical features and prognostic factors in adults with bacterial meningitis. N Engl J Med 2004;351:1849–59.
[36] El Bashir H, Laundy M, Booy R. Diagnosis and treatment of bacterial meningitis. Arch Dis Child 2003;88:615–20.
[37] Oostenbrink R, Moons KG, Theunissen CC, Derksen-Lubsen G, Grobbee DE, Moll HA. Signs of meningeal irritation at the emergency department: how often bacterial meningitis? Pediatr Emerg Care 2001;17:161–4.
[38] Kaplan SL. Clinical presentations, diagnosis, and prognostic factors of bacterial meningitis. Infect Dis Clin North Am 1999;13:579–94.
[39] Freedman SB, Marrocco A, Pirie J, Dick PT. Predictors of bacterial meningitis in the era after *Haemophilus influenzae*. Arch Pediatr Adolesc Med 2001;155:1301–6.
[40] Straussberg R, Harel L, Nussinovitch M, Amir J. Absolute neutrophil count in aseptic and bacterial meningitis related to time of lumbar puncture. Pediatr Neurol 2003;28:365–9.

[41] Saez-Llorens XM. Acute bacterial meningitis beyond the neonatal period. In: Long SS, editor. Principles and practice of pediatric infectious diseases. 2nd ed. Philadelphia: Churchill Livingstone; 2003. p. 264–71.
[42] Bonadio WA, Smith DS, Goddard S, Burroughs J, Khaja G. Distinguishing cerebrospinal fluid abnormalities in children with bacterial meningitis and traumatic lumbar puncture. J Infect Dis 1990;162:251–4.
[43] Mazor SS, McNulty JE, Roosevelt GE. Interpretation of traumatic lumbar punctures: who can go home? Pediatrics 2003;111:525–8.
[44] Meredith FT, Phillips HK, Reller LB. Clinical utility of broth cultures of cerebrospinal fluid from patients at risk for shunt infections. J Clin Microbiol 1997;35:3109–11.
[45] Sturgis CD, Peterson LR, Warren JR. Cerebrospinal fluid broth culture isolates: their significance for antibiotic treatment. Am J Clin Pathol 1997;108:217–21.
[46] Kanegaye JT, Soliemanzadeh P, Bradley JS. Lumbar puncture in pediatric bacterial meningitis: defining the time interval for recovery of cerebrospinal fluid pathogens after parenteral antibiotic pretreatment. Pediatrics 2001;108:1169–74.
[47] Nigrovic LE, Kuppermann N, McAdam AJ, Malley R. Cerebrospinal latex agglutination fails to contribute to the microbiologic diagnosis of pretreated children with meningitis. Pediatr Infect Dis J 2004;23:786–8.
[48] Schuurman T, de Boer RF, Kooistra-Smid AM, van Zwet AA. Prospective study of use of PCR amplification and sequencing of 16S ribosomal DNA from cerebrospinal fluid for diagnosis of bacterial meningitis in a clinical setting. J Clin Microbiol 2004;42:734–40.
[49] Bryant PA, Li HY, Zaia A, et al. Prospective study of a real-time PCR that is highly sensitive, specific, and clinically useful for diagnosis of meningococcal disease in children. J Clin Microbiol 2004;42:2919–25.
[50] Rennick G, Shann F, de Campo J. Cerebral herniation during bacterial meningitis in children. BMJ 1993;306:953–5.
[51] Shetty AK, Desselle BC, Craver RD, Steele RW. Fatal cerebral herniation after lumbar puncture in a patient with a normal computed tomography scan. Pediatrics 1999;103:1284–7.
[52] Craig WA. Pharmacokinetic/pharmacodynamic parameters: rationale for antibacterial dosing of mice and men. Clin Infect Dis 1998;26:1–12.
[53] Saez-Llorens X, McCracken Jr GH. Antimicrobial and anti-inflammatory treatment of bacterial meningitis. Infect Dis Clin North Am 1999;13:619–36.
[54] Saez-Llorens X, McCracken Jr GH. Bacterial meningitis in children. Lancet 2003;361:2139–48.
[55] Tunkel AR, Hartman BJ, Kaplan SL, et al. Practice guidelines for the management of bacterial meningitis. Clin Infect Dis 2004;39:1267–84.
[56] Rodriguez CA, Atkinson R, Bitar W, et al. Tolerance to vancomycin in pneumococci: detection with a molecular marker and assessment of clinical impact. J Infect Dis 2004;190:1481–7.
[57] Bonadio WA. The cerebrospinal fluid: physiologic aspects and alterations associated with bacterial meningitis. Pediatr Infect Dis J 1992;11:423–31.
[58] de Gans J, van de Beek D. Dexamethasone in adults with bacterial meningitis. N Engl J Med 2002;347:1549–56.
[59] McIntyre PB, Berkey CS, King SM, et al. Dexamethasone as adjunctive therapy in bacterial meningitis: a meta-analysis of randomized clinical trials since 1988. JAMA 1997;278:925–31.
[60] Martinez-Lacasa J, Cabellos C, Martos A, et al. Experimental study of the efficacy of vancomycin, rifampicin and dexamethasone in the therapy of pneumococcal meningitis. J Antimicrob Chemother 2002;49:507–13.
[61] Wald ER, Kaplan SL, Mason Jr EO, et al. Dexamethasone therapy for children with bacterial meningitis. Meningitis Study Group. Pediatrics 1995;95:21–8.
[62] Paris MM, Friedland IR, Ehrett S, et al. Effect of interleukin-1 receptor antagonist and soluble tumor necrosis factor receptor in animal models of infection. J Infect Dis 1995;171:161–9.
[63] Bifrare YD, Kummer J, Joss P, Tauber MG, Leib SL. Brain-derived neurotrophic factor protects against multiple forms of brain injury in bacterial meningitis. J Infect Dis 2005;191:40–5.
[64] Moller K, Larsen FS, Bie P, Skinhoj P. The syndrome of inappropriate secretion of antidiuretic

hormone and fluid restriction in meningitis—how strong is the evidence? Scand J Infect Dis 2001;33:13–26.

[65] Kornelisse RF, Westerbeek CM, Spoor AB, et al. Pneumococcal meningitis in children: prognostic indicators and outcome. Clin Infect Dis 1995;21:1390–7.

[66] Snedeker JD, Kaplan SL, Dodge PR, Holmes SJ, Feigin RD. Subdural effusion and its relationship with neurologic sequelae of bacterial meningitis in infancy: a prospective study. Pediatrics 1990;86:163–70.

[67] Jacobson PL, Farmer TW. Subdural empyema complicating meningitis in infants: improved prognosis. Neurology 1981;31:190–3.

[68] Pomeroy SL, Holmes SJ, Dodge PR, Feigin RD. Seizures and other neurologic sequelae of bacterial meningitis in children. N Engl J Med 1990;323:1651–7.

[69] Fortnum HM. Hearing impairment after bacterial meningitis: a review. Arch Dis Child 1992; 67:1128–33.

[70] Bedford H, de Louvois J, Halket S, Peckham C, Hurley R, Harvey D. Meningitis in infancy in England and Wales: follow up at age 5 years. BMJ 2001;323:533–6.

[71] Koomen I, Grobbee DE, Roord JJ, Donders R, Jennekens-Schinkel A, van Furth AM. Hearing loss at school age in survivors of bacterial meningitis: assessment, incidence, and prediction. Pediatrics 2003;112:1049–53.

[72] Peltola H. Worldwide *Haemophilus influenzae* type b disease at the beginning of the 21st century: global analysis of the disease burden 25 years after the use of the polysaccharide vaccine and a decade after the advent of conjugates. Clin Microbiol Rev 2000;13:302–17.

[73] Black S, Shinefield H, Fireman B, et al. Efficacy, safety and immunogenicity of heptavalent pneumococcal conjugate vaccine in children. Northern California Kaiser Permanente Vaccine Study Center Group. Pediatr Infect Dis J 2000;19:187–95.

[74] Whitney CG, Farley MM, Hadler J, et al. Decline in invasive pneumococcal disease after the introduction of protein-polysaccharide conjugate vaccine. N Engl J Med 2003;348:1737–46.

[75] Pneumococcal Vaccination for Cochlear Implant Candidates and Recipients. Updated recommendations of the Advisory Committee on Immunization Practices. MMWR Morb Mortal Wkly Rep 2003;52:1–2.

[76] Meningococcal Disease and College Students. Recommendations of the Advisory Committee on Immunization Practices (ACIP). MMWR Morb Mortal Wkly Rep 2000;49:11–20.

[77] Danzig L. Meningococcal vaccines. Pediatr Infect Dis J 2004;23:S285–92.

[78] Rennels M, King Jr J, Ryall R, Papa T, Froeschle J. Dosage escalation, safety and immunogenicity study of four dosages of a tetravalent meninogococcal polysaccharide diphtheria toxoid conjugate vaccine in infants. Pediatr Infect Dis J 2004;23:429–35.

[79] Paoletti LC, Madoff LC. Vaccines to prevent neonatal GBS infection. Semin Neonatol 2002; 7:315–23.

[80] American Academy of Pediatrics. Committee on Infectious Diseases. Red book. Elk Grove Village (IL): American Academy of Pediatrics; 2003.

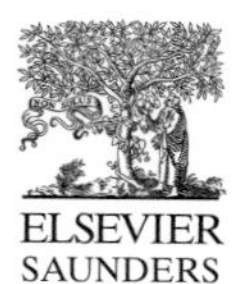

PEDIATRIC CLINICS
OF NORTH AMERICA

Pediatr Clin N Am 52 (2005) 811–835

Distinguishing Among Prolonged, Recurrent, and Periodic Fever Syndromes: Approach of a Pediatric Infectious Diseases Subspecialist

Sarah S. Long, MD[a,b,*]

[a]*Department of Pediatrics, Drexel University College of Medicine, Philadelphia, PA 19134, USA*
[b]*Section of Infectious Diseases, St. Christopher's Hospital for Children, Erie Avenue at Front Street, Suite 1112, Philadelphia, PA 19134, USA*

Approaching the differential diagnosis of a child with a prolonged, recurrent, or periodic fever requires an extensive interview with disciplined dissection of the history. Diagnoses are considered and supported or excluded. Review of systems is used to understand the totality of the condition and to seek certain occurrences specific to diagnoses considered. A careful and complete physical examination is systems based, beginning with growth and ending with a thorough neurologic examination. Laboratory tests rarely establish an unexpected diagnosis. They are used to support or confirm a diagnosis, or to establish "wellness" of major organ systems as predicted by history and physical examination. This article discusses three objectives for the clinician: (1) to categorize patterns of fever illnesses and prioritize differential diagnoses; (2) to diagnose and manage the most frequently encountered prolonged fever syndrome, deconditioning; and (3) to expand knowledge and approach to diagnosing periodic fever syndromes. The approach described in this article represents the honed, 30-year experience of a pediatric infectious diseases subspecialist. Definitions of fever syndromes are shown in Box 1. Figs. 1 and 2 are algorithms to help the pediatrician manage confidently

* Section of Infectious Diseases, St. Christopher's Hospital for Children, Erie Avenue at Front Street, Suite 1112, Philadelphia, PA 19134.

E-mail address: sarah.long@drexelmed.edu

doi:10.1016/j.pcl.2005.02.007

pediatric.theclinics.com

Box 1. Defining fever patterns*

Prolonged fever: A single illness in which duration of fever exceeds that expected for the clinical diagnosis (eg, > 10 days for viral upper respiratory tract infections; >3 weeks for mononucleosis)

or

A single illness in which fever was an initial major symptom and subsequently is low grade or only a perceived problem

Fever of unknown origin: A single illness of at least 3 weeks' duration in which fever >38.3°C is present on most days, and diagnosis is uncertain after 1 week of intense evaluation

Recurrent fever: A single illness in which fever and other signs and symptoms wane and wax (sometimes in relationship to discontinuation of antimicrobial therapy)

or

Repeated unrelated febrile infections of the same organ system (eg, sinopulmonary, urinary tract)

or

Multiple illnesses occurring at irregular intervals, involving different organ systems in which fever is one, variable component.

Periodic fever: Recurring episodes of illness for which fever is the cardinal feature, and other associated symptoms are similar and predictable, and duration is days to weeks, with intervening intervals of weeks to months of complete well-being. Episodes can have either ''clockwork'' or irregular periodicity.

* Categories are not diagnoses. Definitions are useful only as they help weight a differential diagnosis (see Figs. 1 and 2) and prioritize investigation and referral.

most patients with prolonged or recurrent fever and recognize patients who require subspecialty consultation.

History

The most frequent outpatient consultation performed by this subspecialist is to evaluate children with the predominant complaint of fever or of a prolonged illness that includes fever. The first step is to categorize the illness according to the pattern and duration of the elevated temperature. The accompanying features

Fig. 1. Primary practitioner's decision tree for a child or adolescent with prolonged fever. GI, gastrointestinal; Hem/Onc, hematology/oncology; ID, infectious disease; PE, physical examination; Rheum, rheumatology.

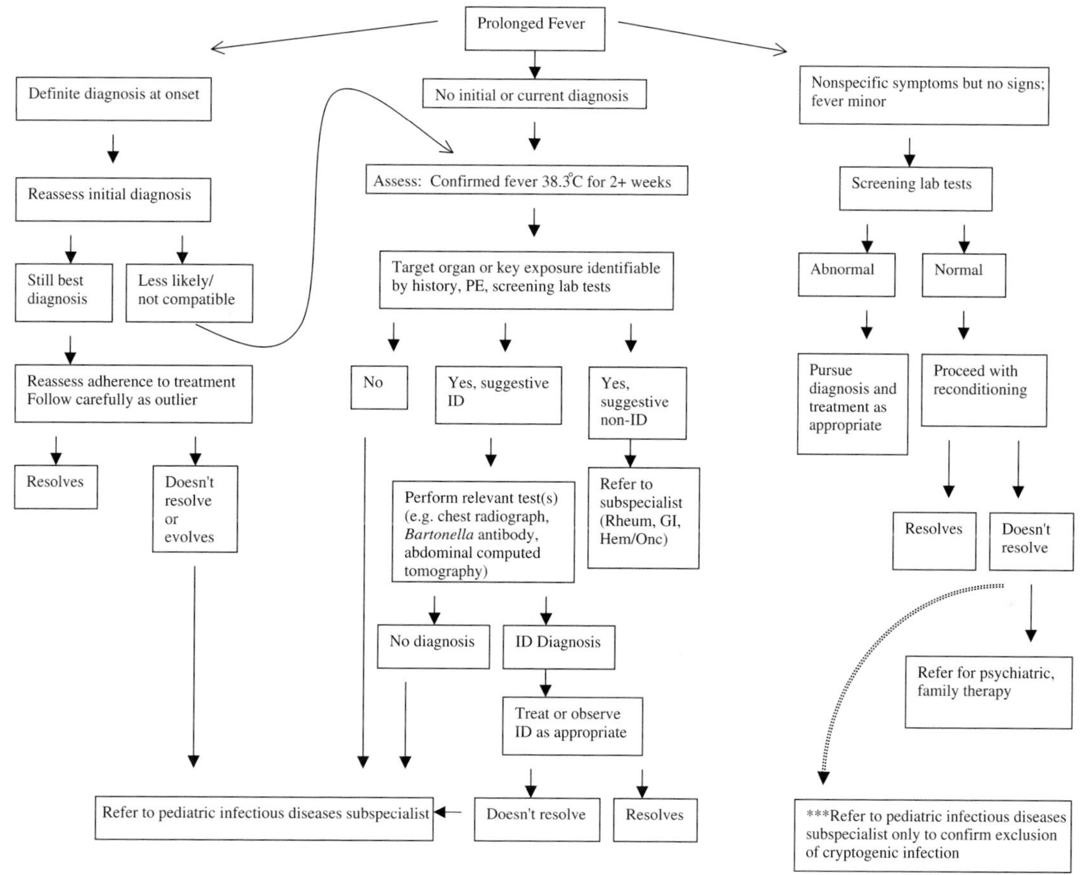
Prolonged Fever
Definite diagnosis at onset
No initial or current diagnosis
Nonspecific symptoms but no signs; fever minor
Reassess initial diagnosis
Assess: Confirmed fever 38.3°C for 2+ weeks
Screening lab tests
Still best diagnosis
Less likely/ not compatible
Target organ or key exposure identifiable by history, PE, screening lab tests
Abnormal
Normal
Reassess adherence to treatment Follow carefully as outlier
No
Yes, suggestive ID
Yes, suggestive non-ID
Pursue diagnosis and treatment as appropriate
Proceed with reconditioning
Resolves
Doesn't resolve or evolves
Perform relevant test(s) (e.g. chest radiograph, *Bartonella* antibody, abdominal computed tomography)
Refer to subspecialist (Rheum, GI, Hem/Onc)
Resolves
Doesn't resolve
No diagnosis
ID Diagnosis
Refer for psychiatric, family therapy
Treat or observe ID as appropriate
Refer to pediatric infectious diseases subspecialist
Doesn't resolve
Resolves
***Refer to pediatric infectious diseases subspecialist only to confirm exclusion of cryptogenic infection

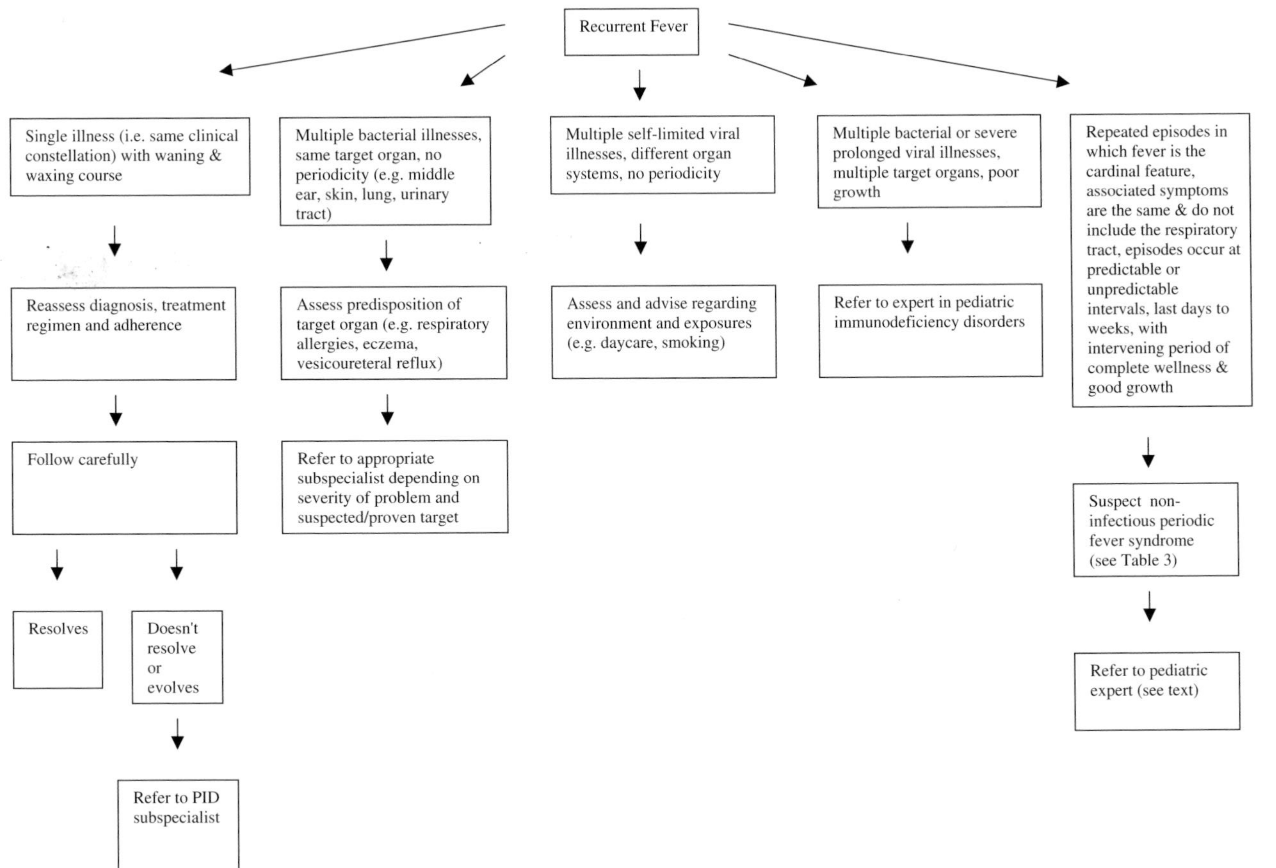

Recurrent Fever
Single illness (i.e. same clinical constellation) with waning & waxing course
Reassess diagnosis, treatment regimen and adherence
Follow carefully
Resolves
Doesn't resolve or evolves
Refer to PID subspecialist
Multiple bacterial illnesses, same target organ, no periodicity (e.g. middle ear, skin, lung, urinary tract)
Assess predisposition of target organ (e.g. respiratory allergies, eczema, vesicoureteral reflux)
Refer to appropriate subspecialist depending on severity of problem and suspected/proven target
Multiple self-limited viral illnesses, different organ systems, no periodicity
Assess and advise regarding environment and exposures (e.g. daycare, smoking)
Multiple bacterial or severe prolonged viral illnesses, multiple target organs, poor growth
Refer to expert in pediatric immunodeficiency disorders
Repeated episodes in which fever is the cardinal feature, associated symptoms are the same & do not include the respiratory tract, episodes occur at predictable or unpredictable intervals, last days to weeks, with intervening period of complete wellness & good growth
Suspect non-infectious periodic fever syndrome (see Table 3)
Refer to pediatric expert (see text)

of the illness, environmental exposures, and genetic background often are important clues to the diagnosis.

Fever of unknown origin

By convention, fever of unknown origin (FUO) is defined as a single illness that has lasted for 3 or more weeks, with temperature greater than 38.3°C on most days and with uncertain diagnosis after 1 week of intense evaluation (formerly to include hospitalization; now to include CT of the abdomen). Attention to uncovering exposures, symptoms, signs, or laboratory findings that target an organ or multiple organs is the most fruitful approach to making the correct diagnosis. Excellent reviews of FUO are published [1–3]. A thoughtful differential diagnosis and performance of the crucial laboratory test is a more successful approach than is "running a list." General principles of diagnosis of infectious diseases pertain to FUO—that is, the patient is more likely to have an uncommon presentation (ie, prolonged fever) of a common disease than an uncommon disease [4]. The frequent diagnosis of visceral cat-scratch disease as a cause of FUO is an example, and a history of exposure to kittens is the clue [3,5]. Table 1 provides examples in which the obvious findings of conditions may be absent, but subtle findings can lead to a simple test to confirm the diagnosis, the best working diagnosis, or the site for biopsy.

There are a few infectious diseases for which fever and nonspecific symptoms and signs may be the only findings, such as endocarditis, tuberculosis, and chronic meningococcemia. Blood cultures for routine bacteriology and isolation of mycobacteria should be performed in patients with FUO. There are numerous cases of FUO that are not infectious diseases. Inflammatory diseases and neoplasms are prominent among the noninfectious etiologies. Follow-up for development of specific organ or laboratory abnormalities may be the only way to diagnose some malignancies. Removing exposures to "medicinal" products can be diagnostic and therapeutic.

Prolonged illness with fever

One of the most frequent referrals to pediatric infectious disease subspecialists for "prolonged fever" is an adolescent with low-grade or falsely perceived fever who generally feels unwell and is unable to attend school and social activities – the adolescent has the so called "dwindles". Such patients require the same disciplined performance of history and examination as those with true FUO. Referral to a pelvic inflammatory disease subspecialist frequently is one of many. For the subspecialist to offer a definitive opinion, the family must perceive that a thorough and thoughtful consultation has occurred. All laboratory test results, actual imaging studies, and biopsy slides should be reviewed. The

Fig. 2. Primary practitioner's decision tree for a child or adolescent with recurrent fever. PID, pediatric infectious diseases.

Table 1
Clues to diagnosis in enigmatic cases of fever of unknown origin*

Disorder	History	Examination	Abnormal screening laboratory test
Inflammatory bowel disease	Vague intermittent abdominal discomfort or loose stools	Mild abdominal tenderness or guarding; perianal skin tag; erythema nodosum; decreased velocity of growth	Hypochromic, microcytic anemia; elevated ESR or CRP; occult blood test on stool; pANCA test
Bacterial endocarditis	Fatigue	Cardiac murmur, splenomegaly, splinter hemorrhages	Anemia, thrombocytopenia; urinalysis with RBCs; elevated ESR; decreased complement
Visceral cat-scratch disease	Kitten exposure	Papular skin lesion; abdominal tenderness; hepatomegaly, splenomegaly	Elevated ESR
EBV infection	Fatigue, periorbital edema	Splenomegaly	Reactive lymphocytes; elevated serum hepatic enzymes; elevated direct bilirubin
HIV infection	Mononucleosis-like (rash, sore throat, myalgia, arthralgia), night sweats	Lymphadenopathy, pharyngitis	Reactive lymphocytes, leukopenia, thrombocytopenia

Salmonella, *Yersinia* infection	Exposure; no appetite → rapid weight loss	Mild lower or right upper quadrant abdominal tenderness or guarding	Left shift neutrophils; mildly elevated serum hepatic enzymes; ESR >60 mm/h
sJIA	Fatigue; broad daily fever swings	Truncal rash during fever	ESR >60 mm/h, frequently ≥ 100 mm/h
Malignancy	Fatigue, excessive weight loss unrelated to appetite	Unusual node enlargement (eg, supraclavicular, post-cervical, asymmetric tonsillar enlargement)	Neutropenia or all blood cell lines decreased; elevated serum uric acid
Nephrogenic diabetes insipidus	Morning fever; "excess" fluid intake	Normal	Normal CBC and ESR; hypernatremia, elevated BUN
Drug hypersensitivity	History of use of nonprescription, prescription or alternative medicine product	Normal	Mild eosinophilia
Chronic inflammatory pseudotumor	Mild, persistent abdominal discomfort; poor appetite	Mild abdominal tenderness or guarding	Anemia of chronic inflammation; elevated ESR (<60 mm/h)

Abbreviations: CRP, C-reactive protein; EBV, Epstein-Barr virus; ESR, estimated sedimentation rate; pANCA, perinuclear antineutrophil cytoplasmic antibody; RBCs, red blood cells; sJIA, systemic-onset juvenile idiopathic arthritis.

* Clues on history, examination, or a laboratory test result that frequently are subtle or have been overlooked. Usually present singly; notation can lead to a narrow differential diagnosis or focused confirmatory test.

findings listed in Box 2 taken together suggest that no cryptogenic infection or serious medical condition is present. Deconditioning (ie, diminution of physical strength, stamina, and vitality), loss of self-esteem, fear of failure to perform at previous expectation, and secondary gain all may play into the clinical state of affairs.

Before the illness, the patient usually was a super-energetic athlete or super-achieving student. Self and family expectations are high. Self-esteem or place in the family rests on achievement. An acute illness occurred, with clear date of onset and objective findings—frequently fever, headache, congestion, muscle aches, poor appetite, and excessive sleeping—which precluded usual activities and which attracted concern of parents, extended family, schoolmates, coaches, or teachers. The acute illness is self-limited, but the adolescent does not feel "100%" well and does not return to school or activities. All interested parties become more concerned. The primary practitioner recommends rest.

A family *modus operandi* ensues that centers around the patient despite lack of objective abnormalities. Over the next 4 to 6 weeks, the patient becomes increasingly sedentary. Temperature infrequently exceeds 38°C after the first week. Review of systems usually elicits multiple subjective positive responses. Weight that was lost in the first 2 weeks has been regained; sometimes there is excessive weight gain. Prodded recitation of a typical 24-hour period of activity reveals late morning awakening, snacking, lounging, hours of television and computer activity, performance of home-delivered or e-mail-delivered schoolwork, and no or little daytime sleep despite constant feeling of tiredness. Evening activity is talking with family or friends (by telephone or computer) and early retirement to room but difficulty (and often late) falling asleep, which is then uninterrupted. There is no physical exertion or exercise. Forays into social events or school frequently are avoided or aborted for fear of or for feeling of tiredness

Box 2. Typical findings in patients with deconditioning

- Age >12 years
- Preillness achievement high
- Family expectations high
- Acute febrile illness with onset easily dated
- Family and outside attention high
- Lengthy list, but vague complaints
- Odd complaints (eg, "shooting" pains; 30-second "blindness"; stereotypic sporadic, brief unilateral tremors, jerks, or "paralysis")
- No daytime sleep
- Preserved weight
- Extreme cooperation with examination
- Normal physical and neurologic examination
- Normal results of screening laboratory tests (see text and Box 4)

or faintness. When the adolescent is asked what physical problem precluded attending school the day before, there is no concrete answer. There may be a family model of chronic illness, mental illness, or recent loss of a person important to the patient. The patient is dispassionate at least or is highly animated while enumerating symptoms and expresses hopes and plans for the future when queried. (If this is not the observed affect, depression is a possible diagnosis.) The patient and parent should be interviewed alone to inquire about disruptive family events or possible abuse.

Physical and neurologic examinations and growth are normal. Laxity of joints has been a finding in some patients with prolonged fatigue [6]. Screening laboratory tests (complete blood count; serum chemistry tests of electrolytes, blood urea nitrogen and creatinine, hepatic enzymes, uric acid, calcium and glucose; erythrocyte sedimentation rate and C-reactive protein; urinalysis) are normal; when extensive laboratory testing has been performed, an unimportant finding out of the normal range may be present. Sometimes Epstein-Barr virus, cytomegalovirus, or Lyme serologic testing has been interpreted incorrectly.

It is a disservice to diagnose "chronic fatigue syndrome" in such a patient or to infer a need for or to refer to another subspecialist for targeted symptoms when they are minor, such as congestion or headache. Two precise conclusions of the consultation should be addressed with the parents and patient: what the diagnosis is not and what it is. After oral summation of the history, it is concluded that maintenance of weight, abnormal pattern but not excessive sleeping, normal physical examination (naming the organ systems evaluated), and normal screening laboratory tests (naming the organ systems evaluated) so many weeks after onset of illness virtually exclude cryptogenic infection and serious medical conditions. Pointing out the discordance of the lengthy list of symptoms versus the normal matching physical and test findings of critical organ function helps segue to the assessment of the problem as deconditioning rather than ongoing disease. Treatment includes forced, incremental return to school and other activities (with any day's decision to stay home requiring examination by the pediatrician) and promises from family members to levy no expectation of productivity and to focus on health rather than illness. Finally, the thoughtful physician needs to validate that the patient truly feels ill and will have to work through increased feeling of fatigue during the reconditioning process. The pediatrician needs to assume the leadership role in setting the pace of activity and determining the need for professional family therapy or psychiatric care.

Recurrent fever

Children normally have 10 or fewer self-limited viral illnesses per year for the first 2 to 3 years of life. Children attending daycare have more. Many of these illnesses are associated with fever, especially when complicated by otitis media (or especially in the "otitis-prone child"). A child with multiple, self-limited illnesses, no serious or unusual infections, and good growth and development should not be pursued for a defect in host immune response or cryptogenic

Table 2
Differentiating features in the history that help to categorize the problem in children with recurrent fever

	Self-limited infections in healthy child	Compromised host*	Child with a periodic fever syndrome
Periodicity of episodes	Irregular	Relapse/recurrence of bacterial infection quickly after discontinuation of antibiotics	Clockwork periodicity or irregularly frequent or occasional
Characteristics of episodes	Waning and waxing course of a single illness (eg, EBV); multiple simple illnesses (ie, different symptoms, exanthems, diagnoses)	Slow response to treatment of bacterial infections (eg, sinopulmonary); some episodes require hospitalization/parenteral antibiotic therapy	Abrupt onset and cessation; fever dominant; no respiratory tract symptoms
Clustering of episodes	Concurrent illness in contacts (home, daycare, school); few-to-no episodes in summer	Ill during all seasons, when others are and are not	Episodes during all seasons; contacts are not ill before or after
Course of episodes	Each as expected for infectious agent	Even simple infections (eg, AOM, skin and soft tissue infections) are protracted; skin infections heal with scarring	Identical, symptoms predictable course
History of identifiable childhood illnesses	Expected course (eg, chickenpox, HSV stomatitis, gastroenteritis)	Severe and protracted course; hospitalization	Expected course (often notably less ill, less frequently than peers)
Interval between episodes	Completely well (or frequently atopic symptoms)	Never well generally; lingering specific symptoms	Completely well
Catch-up growth and energy	Excellent	Poor	Excellent

Abbreviations: AOM, acute otitis media; EBV, Epstein-Barr virus; HSV, herpes simplex virus.

* Conditions such as acquired (HIV-associated) or congenital immunodeficiency, cystic fibrosis, or ciliary dyskinesia.

Box 3. Targeted questions in history of episodes for children with suspected periodic fever syndrome

- Prodrome and first symptoms of episode
- Cadence of appearance of other symptoms
- Peak of fever
- Duration of fever
- Associated symptoms and signs (eg, exanthem; mouth ulcers; pain in abdomen, chest, or joints; mood change)
- Duration of associated symptoms and signs
- Similarity of symptoms and course for each episode

infection. Although most children with recurrent fevers have had a series of self-limited infections, other infectious disease considerations include recurrent urinary tract infection, sinopulmonary infection, and occult dental infection. With history of certain exposures, brucellosis, borreliosis, and malaria are considered. Autoimmune diseases (eg, systemic lupus erythematosus) and especially autoinflammatory diseases (eg, inflammatory bowel disease and systemic-onset juvenile idiopathic arthritis) also can manifest as recurrent fever [7,8]. Additional targeted questions help to sort through common recurring, self-limited viral illnesses in healthy children to uncover the unusual child with a periodic fever syndrome or the rare child with a congenital or acquired defect in immune function (Table 2). Most importantly, the exact features of the episodes, the rapidity of return to health at the conclusion of episodes, time interval between episodes, and family history should be determined. Key elements of periodic fever syndromes are that fever is the cardinal feature of the illness, episodes recur after symptom-free intervals, and episodes have a predictable course (ie, the same constellation of symptoms) and lack respiratory tract symptoms. Specific features of episodes are identified (Box 3). Family history includes genetic background and history in family members or siblings of similar problems, autoimmune or autoinflammatory illness, or amyloidosis. It is important to query whether immunizations elicit a highly febrile response or trigger a typical episode.

Physical examination

The physical examination and laboratory evaluation are important components of the evaluation of children with prolonged, recurrent, or periodic fever (Box 4). A great deal of reassurance can be obtained if evaluation of the growth chart reveals recovery of weight between episodes of fever and steady velocity of height and weight increments over time. Inflammatory bowel disease can present with recurring fevers (that typically are "low grade" and of variable periodicity). Examination is aimed at excluding abnormalities in target organs that might be affected if infection is the cause of prolonged fever and to ascertain the presence

Box 4. Physical examination and laboratory testing in children with prolonged, recurrent, or periodic fever

Physical examination

- Growth chart
- Thorough general examination
- Careful organ-specific examination
- Notation of mouth ulcers, exanthem, joint abnormalities, lymph nodes

Tests

- Simple (during episode and interval, if periodic fever)
- Complete blood count with manual differential count of white blood cells
- Erythrocyte sedimentation rate and C-reactive protein
- Screening serum chemistry tests (and uric acid level if prolonged fever)
- Serum quantitative immunoglobulin levels
- Urinalysis
- Urine culture
- Chest plain radiograph (if prolonged or recurrent fever)
- Other imaging only as directed by examination
- Blood culture (if prolonged fever)

of signs consistent with noninfectious diseases, such as malignancies and autoimmune, endocrine, and metabolic disorders. Special attention should be given to the presence of mouth ulcers, gingivitis, or rashes; abnormalities of joints or lymph nodes; or findings on abdominal examination in patients being assessed for a periodic fever syndrome.

Laboratory evaluations and imaging studies

Laboratory testing for patients with prolonged or recurrent fever are simple and should be targeted to specific organs (see Box 4) [1,2,4]. The main goal of performing laboratory tests in children with periodic fever is to lead the clinician toward a specific disorder (eg, recurrent urinary tract infection) or to support the diagnosis of a noninfectious periodic fever syndrome. Simple tests rarely *confirm* a specific noninfectious periodic fever syndrome. Tests for unusual infectious causes of recurrent fever rarely are diagnostic in the absence of a specific exposure history.

The initial tests to consider in the workup of patients with prolonged or recurrent fever include complete blood count with manual examination of white blood cells; erythrocyte sedimentation rate and C-reactive protein; screening serum chemistry tests, including hepatic enzymes and albumin; quantitative immunoglobulins, including IgA, IgD, and IgE. Bacterial cultures of blood and urine should be performed during at least two febrile episodes, and culture of a throat specimen for *Streptococcus pyogenes* should be obtained if pharyngitis symptoms or signs have been present.

Differential diagnosis of periodic fever

Periodic fever is defined as recurrent episodes of illness in which fever is the cardinal feature and is associated with a predictable and similar set of symptoms that last days to weeks. Each episode is separated by symptom-free intervals ranging from weeks to months. In some instances, the episodes have *consistent, clockwork periodicity,* whereas in others, they do not. Patients with autoinflammatory disorders in which recurrent urticaria, arthritis, and multiorgan dysfunction are the prominent feature of the febrile episodes are not likely to be referred to infectious diseases consultants [9,10]. These disorders include Muckle-Wells syndrome, familial cold autoinflammatory syndrome, neonatal-onset multisystem disease, and chronic infantile neurologic cutaneous and articular syndrome. These disorders are not discussed further. Disorders that are discussed all have the cardinal feature of periodic fever; they are considered in order of their frequency (Table 3).

Periodic fever, aphthous stomatitis, pharyngitis, and cervical adenopathy (PFAPA) is the most common disorder with periodic fever, it has no defined etiology, and no confirmatory laboratory tests are available. Other syndromes are uncommon, and each syndrome is associated with a specific genetic mutation that can be diagnosed. Only cyclic neutropenia has a simple confirming laboratory test finding (neutropenia) and confirming genetic mutation. Several excellent reviews of the hereditary periodic fever syndromes are published [11–14]. With genetic testing becoming available (http://www.genedx.com), disorders previ-

Table 3
Periodic fever syndromes*

Syndrome	Cause
PFAPA syndrome	Unknown
Cyclic neutropenia	Enzyme defect
Familial Mediterranean fever	Protein defect
HIDS	Enzyme defect
TRAPS	Protein defect

Abbreviations: HIDS, hyperImmunoglobulinemia D; TRAPS, tumor necrosis factor receptor–associated syndrome.

* Conditions for which the patient is likely to be referred to an infectious diseases subspecialist.

Table 4
Differentiating features of periodic fever syndromes

	PFAPA	Cyclic neutropenia	Familial Mediterranean fever	HIDS	TRAPS
Onset <5 y	Expected	Usual; often <1 year old	Common; peak onset middle of first decade	Expected; often <1 year old	Variable
Length fever episode	4 d	5–7 d	2 d	4 d	Weeks; sometimes days
Periodicity of episodes	q3–6 wk (28 d)	q21 d in >90%	Irregular intervals: weekly, q3–4 mo or less often	q4–8 wk or irregular	Irregular intervals; varies weeks to years
Associated symptoms/signs	Pharyngitis 65–70%; aphthous stomatitis 65–70%; cervical adenopathy 75–85%	Ulcers, gingivitis, periodontitis; otitis media and sinusitis; rare peritonitis; rare gram-negative bacillary or clostridial septicemia	Polyserositis; erysipelas-like rash; scrotal pain and swelling	Abdominal pain, diarrhea in young; arthralgia; rashes; splenomegaly; mood swings; immunizations trigger	Migratory myalgia; pseudocellulitis; conjunctivitis, periorbital edema; other
Ethnic/geographic	None; rare in siblings	No ethnic	Jewish, Armenian, Arab, Turkish	Dutch, French, others	Irish and Scottish but variable including Mediterranean descent

Inheritance	None; parent may have history of excessive high fevers as child	Autosomal dominant	Autosomal recessive	Autosomal recessive	Autosomal dominant
Laboratory findings	Mild neutrophila; ESR elevated <60 mm/h during episode only	Absolute neutrophil count <200 cells/mm^3 for 3–5 d	Elevated acute-phase reactants	Elevated acute-phase reactants; variable ↓ serum cholesterol; variable ↑ IgA and IgD	Elevated acute-phase reactants
Etiology/diagnosis	Unknown; clinical diagnosis	Chromosome 19; *ELA2* mutations leading to mutant neutrophil elastase; apoptosis marrow myeloid cells	Chromosome 16; *MEFV* missense mutations leading to ↓ pyrin	Chromosome 12; *MVK* mutations leading to ↓ mevalonate kinase and isoprenoids	Chromosome 12; *TNFRSF1A* mutations leading to ↓ soluble TNF receptor superfamily type 1A
Treatment	None established (see text)	Recombinant G-CSF; aggressive periodontal care; aggressive treatment suspected septicemia	Colchicine	Simvastatin (preliminary) Etanercept (preliminary)	Corticosteroid Etanercept (preliminary)

Abbreviations: ESR, erythrocyte sedimentation rate; G-CSF, granulocyte colony stimulating factor.

Modified from Long S. Periodic fever. In: Pollard AJ, Finn A, editors. Hot topics in infection and immunity in children. New York: Kluver Academic/Plenum Publishers; 2005. p. 101–15.

ously believed to be rare are being diagnosed increasingly, and spectra of clinical findings are being broadened. Differentiating features of periodic fever syndromes are shown in Table 4 [15].

Periodic fever, aphthous stomatitis, pharyngitis, and cervical adenopathy

PFAPA is a nonhereditary, autoinflammatory disorder first described in 12 children from Tennessee and Alabama in 1987 [16]. Now more than 200 cases have been described or anecdotally reported representing all racial backgrounds and continents except South America and Africa. Europe, and the Middle East account for most cases outside the United States. No case definition or diagnostic test has been universally agreed on. Population-based incidence figures do not exist. There may be underrepresentation in the United States of African American and Hispanic children; referral bias cannot be excluded as a reason. In the United States, the diagnosis of PFAPA is much more common than the diagnoses of cyclic neutropenia and other genetically determined periodic fever syndromes. In 1992, Feder [17] reported a beneficial effect of cimetidine on the manifestations of individual episodes and frequency of recurrent disease. In 1989, Abramson et al [18] reported unexpected resolution of PFAPA after tonsillectomy in three cases. Except for two anecdotal cases, in which Epstein-Barr virus infection with aberrant antibody response was reported [19] and disseminated *Mycobacterium chelonae* infection was proved in a normal child [20], no infectious or autoimmune cause of this disorder has been established. Marshall et al [16] noted dramatic resolution of individual episodes of illness after a single-dose corticosteroid; subsequent reports supported this observation [21–23].

Clinical features

Based on numerous case series, a constellation of signs and symptoms has emerged that distinguish PFAPA as a syndrome, separate from others (see Table 4). Slight male predominance and onset before 3 years old (almost always before 5 years old) are typical. The child has a brief prodrome of clinginess and "glassy eyes," then suddenly temperature increases to 39°C to 40.5°C followed by poor appetite, low energy, and chills but no rigors. Fever typically is poorly responsive to acetaminophen or ibuprofen and lasts 3 to 4 days. During the episode, a few shallow, mildly painful ulcers may appear in the mouth. All symptoms and signs cease after 4 to 5 days. Episodes occur at intervals of 21 to 36 days (typically 28 days). The only laboratory abnormalities are mildly elevated white blood cells during episodes (typically approximately 13,000/mm^3) with neutrophilia and sometimes a modest left shift. Platelets are normal or modestly elevated (<400,000/mm^3); erythrocyte sedimentation rate is elevated (usually <60 mm/h). Hemoglobin characteristically is unaffected; urinalysis is normal; serum hepatic enzymes, albumin, and immunoglobulins are normal.

Between episodes, children have no lingering symptoms, seem uncommonly energetic, and have good appetite. They do not have recurrent, unusual, or severe infections. Parents report fewer "regular colds" than siblings or peers. Any laboratory abnormality reverts to normal between episodes.

In most cases, the syndrome is typical, and the working diagnosis is made with confidence. PFAPA should not be the working diagnosis if age of onset is older than 5 years, the child is not completely healthy outside of episodes, "extra symptoms" exist (eg, repeated or severe gastrointestinal or neurobehavioral symptoms) during episodes, or when a sibling also has a periodic fever syndrome.

PFAPA is considered to be an autoinflammatory syndrome. It has no known cause, and there is no confirming diagnostic test. Sometimes a single dose of prednisone at the onset of an episode may be useful as a "test." Although rapid resolution is expected in PFAPA, the specificity of this response is unknown.

Treatment and outcome

In 1999, Thomas et al [21] reported a follow-up study of 94 children cared for in Tennessee and Connecticut over a 10-year period. Mean age at follow-up was 8.9 years. Mean duration of PFAPA was 4.5 years; only 41% of children had resolution over the mean follow-up of 3.3 years, and episodes retained characteristics as on diagnosis. Cimetidine, which was used in less than one third of the children for either treatment or prophylaxis, was judged to be "somewhat-to-very effective" in 43%. Prednisone (most often given as one or two doses of 1–2 mg/kg/d) was judged to be somewhat-to-very effective in 90%. Inexplicably, but consistent with the experience of most experts, prednisone often was associated with more frequent episodes of illness. Tonsillectomy and adenoidectomy was performed in 47 of the 94 children and was judged to be somewhat-to-very effective in 86%. Characteristics of febrile episodes do not change in PFAPA, although wellness interval may lengthen as a harbinger of resolution. The working diagnosis should be revisited over time because other periodic fever syndromes evolve over years, and sometimes initial features could mimic PFAPA.

Cyclic neutropenia

Cyclic neutropenia is a rare hematologic disorder characterized by regular cycling of the peripheral neutrophil count (to nadir of <200 cells/mm^3), and a symptom complex manifesting during the neutropenic nadirs. Because blood monocytes, reticulocytes, platelets, and lymphocytes can have similar periodic oscillations as neutrophils, the disorder sometimes is called *cyclic hematopoiesis*.

Cyclic neutropenia was first recognized almost a century ago. The autosomal dominant pattern of inheritance, natural history, and clinical associations of mucosal ulcerations and skin infections were described half a century ago. In 1989, Hammond et al [24] reported the favorable response to granulocyte colony-stimulating factor, and 10 years later mutations of the gene for neutrophil elastase (*ELA2*) were identified [25]. All cases of cyclic neutropenia and most cases of severe congenital neutropenia are due to mutations of *ELA2*. In 2001, Aprikyan et al [26] hypothesized that accelerated cellular apoptosis was the cause for cyclic neutropenia.

Clinical features

Diagnosis of cyclic neutropenia usually is established early in childhood. Cardinal features include recurrent fever with clockwork periodicity, pharyngitis, mouth ulcers, and lymphadenopathy. Some cases are diagnosed because of recurrent cellulitis or furunculosis. Compared with the mild oral manifestations of PFAPA syndrome, children with cyclic neutropenia complain of deep and painful mouth ulcers that often last more than 1 week. In contrast to PFAPA, gingivitis and periodontitis are common in patients with cyclic neutropenia. Recurrent bacterial otitis media, sinusitis, and pharyngitis are frequent. Recurrent cellulitis and furunculosis after insect bites, minor cuts, or abrasions distinguish cyclic neutropenia from other periodic fever syndromes. Some patients have few and relatively minor associated bacterial infections, but acute bacterial peritonitis and septic shock and overwhelming gram-negative bacillary or clostridial septicemia resulting from colonic ulcers during the period of neutropenia have been described. Bacterial complications occur only during the periods of neutropenia. Although ulcers, gingivitis, and periodontal disease linger, the child usually is well before the onset of the next episode.

Etiology and diagnostic tests

During the neutropenic period, peripheral neutrophils are reduced to less than 200 cells/mm^3 for 3 to 5 days. The count then usually increases to about 2000 cells/mm^3, where it remains until the next neutropenic period. If bone marrow is examined at the onset of neutropenia, early myeloid precursors are present, but postmitotic neutrophils are absent. Recovery is rapid, with cells from promyelocytic to band neutrophilic forms. Because neutropenia appearing in the peripheral blood may be resolving by the time the clinical features of fever, stomatitis, and tender lymphadenopathy appear, children with a history compatible with cyclic neutropenia should have twice-weekly complete blood counts performed beginning during the interval of wellness and continuing through the next febrile episode.

Cyclic neutropenia is inherited as an autosomal dominant disorder with full penetrance but varying severity of clinical manifestations. Commonly an affected parent of a child with cyclic neutropenia has not been recognized because of milder clinical and laboratory manifestations. The genetic abnormality is localized to chromosome 19p13.3, resulting in mutation of *ELA2* and its neutrophil elastase protein product. Diagnosis is confirmed by genetic testing.

Treatment and outcome

Adverse effects of cyclic neutropenia include pain and discomfort, periodontal disease frequently resulting in decidual tooth extractions in childhood, recurrent common bacterial infections, and serious or life-threatening bacterial infections. Increased rates of spontaneous abortion in women with cyclic neutropenia have been reported. No tendency toward malignancy has been noted in children with cyclic neutropenia.

Most children with cyclic neutropenia should be treated with recombinant granulocyte colony-stimulating factor daily or on alternate days ($\leq$5 μg/kg/d) [27]. More than 90% of children respond to this therapy with a reduced frequency of episodes of neutropenia and associated complications.

Familial Mediterranean fever

Familial Mediterranean fever (FMF) is an inherited autoinflammatory syndrome in which seemingly unprovoked or minor stress or trauma causes fever and inflammatory serositis/synovitis without autoantibodies or autoreactive T lymphocytes. FMF is an autosomal recessive disease and the most prevalent inherited periodic fever syndrome, affecting more than 10,000 individuals worldwide. FMF is almost completely restricted to non-Ashkenazi Jews, Armenians, Arabs, and Turks [28]. More than 90% of Jewish FMF patients are of Sephardic or Middle Eastern origin. The high heterozygous carrier frequency (>1 in 10 North African Jews and Armenians) is speculated to have conferred survival advantage, probably against an infectious pathogen [29]. In 1997, the International Familial Mediterranean Fever Consortium and the French Familial Mediterranean Fever Consortium independently cloned the mutant *MEFV* gene, the former group naming the protein product *pyrin* (indicating relationship to fever) and the latter group calling it *marenostrin* (meaning "our sea," indicating relationship to the Mediterranean Sea). Pyrin protein is a member of the death-domain-fold superfamily, which provides critical biochemical pathways of apoptosis and innate immunity [30,31].

MEFV mutations are more varied and complex than originally described. Single genotype-phenotype correlations are not solid, and multiple genotypes exist. Description of manifestations as if FMF were a single disease are valuable only as generalities.

Clinical features

Symptoms of FMF begin before age 2 years in 20% of patients; two thirds of affected individuals have manifestations before 10 years of age. Less than 10% have onset after age 30. Episodes do not have predictable periodicity. A typical attack is heralded by abdominal pain, then an increase in temperature to 40°C followed by chills. Fever lasts 12 hours to 3 days and is rarely the only manifestation. Abdominal pain, which is sometimes accompanied by diarrhea, is present in greater than 90% of patients, begins suddenly a few hours before fever, and persists 1 to 2 days after defervescence. This presentation can simulate other causes of "acute abdomen," and attacks can follow surgical trauma to the peritoneal serosa. Pleuritic chest pain occurs in 25% to 80% of patients; it is the presenting manifestation in less than 10% of patients. Pericarditis is less common (<1% of cases). Small fluid collections can be detected by various imaging techniques when serosal involvement occurs. Arthritis is common and varies in nature by ethnic origin. Acute pain and effusion in the wrists, ankles, or knees, occurring asymmetrically and resolving completely over days, is typical. An erysipelas-like exanthem reported in 7% to 40% of patients almost invariably affects the extensor surface of the lower leg and dorsum of the foot. It usually is unilateral and fades spontaneously within 2 to 3 days. Splenomegaly occurs in 30% to 50% of patients.

Etiology and diagnostic tests

There is no specific laboratory marker for FMF. During febrile attacks, nonspecific elevations in inflammatory mediators, fibrinogen, C-reactive protein, neutrophils, and erythrocyte sedimentation rate occur. If sampled, serosal or synovial fluid shows neutrophilic pleocytosis. Proteinuria (> 0.5 g protein/24 h) in patients with FMF suggests amyloidosis. At least 28 mutations in the *MEFV,* most clustered in one exon, have been described on the short arm of chromosome 16. Genetic testing is the confirmatory test for FMF, with some limitations. Genetics laboratories usually screen for the five most frequent mutations (accounting for 85% of FMF). Also, single mutant-allele disease and double mutant-allele nondisease are described.

Treatment and outcome

Colchicine is the treatment of choice. The drug is concentrated in neutrophils, where it acts on microtubules, possibly by up-regulating *MEFV* gene expression. Colchicine prevents attacks in 60% of individuals with FMF and significantly reduces the number of attacks in an additional 20% to 30%. Adherence to therapy is important because attacks can follow within days of discontinuance. Regardless of efficacy in prevention of attacks, colchicine therapy arrests or prevents amyloidosis, the life-threatening complication of FMF.

Hyperimmunoglobulinemia D and periodic fever syndrome

Hyperimmunoglobulinemia D and periodic fever syndrome (HIDS) was first described in several Dutch patients by van der Meer et al in 1984 [32]. Most patients with HIDS are white and from western European countries; 60% are Dutch or French. The HIDS registry in the Netherlands currently has data on more than 200 patients worldwide. In 1999, the defect in HIDS patients was mapped to mutations in the *MVK* gene on the long arm of chromosome 12 that encodes mevalonate kinase [33,34]. HIDS is inherited as an autosomal recessive trait; most affected patients are compound heterozygotes for missense mutations in the *MVK* gene. In most patients with HIDS, the activity of mevalonate kinase is 5% to 15% of normal. Less than 1% of patients have complete deficiency of the enzyme, which is associated with mevalonic aciduria. Mevalonic aciduria is characterized by dysmorphic features, failure to thrive, mental retardation, ataxia, recurrent fever attacks, and death in early childhood. Five adults with neurologic signs and symptoms and mevalonate kinase deficiency have been described, suggesting that there may be overlap syndromes and a continuum of disease [35].

Clinical features

Recurrent attacks of fever usually begin in the first year of life [36]. Periodicity can vary, but recurrence every 4 to 6 weeks is typical. Characteristically, some attacks are triggered by immunization, injury, or stress and heralded by chills followed by a rapid increase of temperature to 39°C or greater. Fever usually lasts 4 to 6 days. Headache, abdominal pain, vomiting, and diarrhea may accompany attacks. Some children with HIDS display irritable or aggressive behavior during febrile attacks.

Prominent cervical lymphadenopathy is common. Arthralgias or arthritis of medium joints (knees, ankles, wrists) and an erythematous macular, popular, or petechial rash predominantly on extremities are less common. Painful aphthous ulcers in the mouth or vagina occur in some patients. Orchitis has been described. Patients are well between attacks, and growth is unimpaired. With increasing age, frequency and severity of febrile episodes tend to decrease.

Etiology and diagnostic tests

HIDS should be suspected when periodic fever begins in infancy. Elevated serum levels of IgD (>100 IU/dL) and IgA (> 5 times upper limit of normal) are characteristic but not universally present, especially in children younger than 3 years old [36,37]. Screening for *MVK* mutations is confirmatory. More than 20 mutations have been identified, but one mutation, *V377I,* is present in more than 80% of patients. Screening for this mutation is an important first step. If the mutation is not found, and suspicion remains high, sequencing of the gene to detect other mutations is indicated. Measurement of mevalonate kinase activity in leukocytes or urine has intrinsic limitations and is not recommended as a diagnostic test.

Treatment and outcome

There is no established treatment for HIDS. Beneficial effect of simvastatin, which acts by inhibiting hydroxymethylglutaryl-coA reductase in the isoprenoid pathway, has been reported [38]. Although abnormalities of tumor necrosis factor (TNF)-α are not the primary cause of HIDS, plasma TNF-α levels are elevated in HIDS patients during attacks. Treatment with etanercept has been reported [39]. Although HIDS previously was not thought to be associated with increased mortality or amyloidosis, the first case of amyloidosis in a patient with HIDS was reported in 2004 [40].

Tumor necrosis factor receptor–associated periodic syndrome

The TNF receptor–associated periodic syndrome (TRAPS) was first described in 1982 in a large Irish family. It was called familial Hibernian fever [41]. Although most of the reported families with TRAPS are of Irish and Scottish descent, a wide range of ethnic origins have been reported [42]. Although inheritance is autosomal dominant, there is variable penetrance, and sporadic cases appear occasionally. The susceptibility gene for this familial periodic fever syndrome had been mapped to the short arm of chromosome 12. It results from a missense mutation in the *TNFRSF1A* gene, from which the name *TRAPS* arises [43,44]. The hypothesized pathogenesis of TRAPS is that missense mutations lead to structural abnormalities that cause failure of shedding of TNF-α receptor from its intracellular site to the extracellular circulation, where binding to TNF-α would prevent ongoing induction of inflammation.

Clinical features

The prototypic clinical syndrome described in familial Hibernian fever is only one manifestation of the ever-growing group of genotypes and phenotypes of TRAPS. Some cases are FMF-like, some are HIDS-like, and kindreds have been described with combined defects. Age of onset varies from a few weeks to older than 40 years. Siblings may be affected. Most often, symptoms first occur in school-age children. Attacks of fever are heralded by severe localized pain and tightness of one muscle group, which is migratory, in most patients. Skin rashes—tender, raised erythematous plaques simulating cellulitis—occur most frequently on the extremities and migrate distally. Painful conjunctivitis and periorbital edema also distinguish TRAPS from the other periodic fever syndromes. Less specific but frequent symptoms include abdominal pain, arthralgia, testicular pain, and pleuritic chest pain. Duration of fever and other symptoms usually is greater than 1 week, but shorter and milder, nonspecific symptoms or fever alone are described.

The case report of genetic diagnosis of TRAPS in a man who had been diagnosed with PFAPA (with atypical features) at age 8 years highlights situations in which gene analysis would be invaluable [45,46]. MR imaging has suggested involvement of subcutaneous tissue, fascia, and muscles; biopsy specimens have shown mononuclear cell infiltration of fascia without myositis in one [47] and panniculitis with small vessel vasculitis in another [48]. Attacks occur at irregular intervals weeks to years apart and can be triggered by minor infections, physical stress, or emotional stress. Neutrophilia and elevated C-reactive protein and erythrocyte sedimentation rate are typical findings during attacks. Elevated serum immunoglobulins, including IgA and IgD, can be present.

Etiology and diagnostic tests

In patients with symptoms suggesting TRAPS, identification of mutations in the *TNFRSF1A* gene is the definitive diagnostic test. More than 28 described mutations lead to qualitative or quantitative abnormalities in TNF receptor-family type 1A proteins. Most are in exons 2 to 4 in the extracellular domains. In 2003, Aganna et al [49] showed heterogeneous gene defects in patients with familial TRAPS-like syndromes, but found that *TNFRSF1A* mutations were not commonly associated with sporadic (nonfamilial) TRAPS-like cases. In "classic" TRAPS, soluble *TNFSFR1A* is low (<1 mg/mL). During attacks, serum levels may increase to within normal limits. If gene analysis is not available, measurement of serum soluble *TNFSFR1A* level between attacks can be used as a screening test.

Treatment and outcome

Attacks of TRAPS respond dramatically to high-dose oral prednisone (>20 mg in adults), but response wanes over time. Colchicine has no effect. Etanercept is highly effective; it was reported to result in long-term remissions in some patients after a single course [50]. Prognosis is related mainly to presence or absence of amyloidosis, which is reported to occur in 10% to 25% of affected families. Certain mutations in *TNFRSF1A* and other modifier genes may influence occurrence of amyloidosis.

Summary

Most children with the perceived problem of prolonged, recurrent, or periodic fever are healthy and have self-limited, common illnesses. With careful delineation of specific features of the illness, confirmation of maintenance of growth and sense of well-being, and reassurance of normal findings on physical examination, the primary care practitioner usually can reassure families and continue to reassess the patient as circumstances dictate. For a child with true fever of unknown origin, a pediatric infectious diseases subspecialist should be consulted. For the unusual child with a course compatible with a noninfectious periodic fever syndrome, referral to a subspecialist is important because condition-specific diagnostic tests and interventions are available or are under study, genetic counseling may be important, and follow-up for evolution of disease or sequelae is crucial. The consultant might be a pediatric immunologist, rheumatologist, infectious diseases consultant, or hematologist depending on findings and expertise of available consultants. For the rare child with a suspected immunologic defect, referral to an immunologist (or infectious diseases subspecialist in some geographic areas) is necessary to begin complex evaluations, which often lead to lifesaving therapies.

References

[1] deKleijn EM, Vandenbroucke JP, van der Meer JW. Fever of unknown origin (FUO): I. a prospective multicenter study of 167 patients with FUO, using fixed epidemiologic entry criteria. The Netherlands FUO Study Group. Medicine 1997;76:392–400.

[2] deKleijn EM, van Lier HJ, van der Meer JW. Fever of unknown origin (FUO): II. diagnostic procedures in a prospective multicenter study of 167 patients. The Netherlands FUO Study Group. Medicine 1997;76:401–14.

[3] Jacobs RF, Schutze GE. *Bartonella henselae* as a cause of prolonged fever and fever of unknown origin in children. Clin Infect Dis 1998;26:80–4.

[4] Long SS, Edwards KM. Fever of unknown origin and periodic fever syndromes. In: Long SS, Pickering LK, Prober CG, editors. Principles and practice of pediatric infectious diseases. 2nd edition. New York: Churchill Livingstone; 2003. p. 114–22.
[5] Arisoy ES, Correa AG, Wagner ML, Kaplan SL. Hepatosplenic cat-scratch disease in children: selected clinical features and treatment. Clin Infect Dis 1999;28:778–84.
[6] Barron DF, Cohen BA, Geraghty MT, Violand R, Rowe PC. Joint hypermobility is more common in children with chronic fatigue syndrome than in healthy controls. J Pediatr 2002;141:421–5.
[7] John CC, Gilsdorf JR. Recurrent fever in children. Pediatr Infect Dis J 2002;21:1071–80.
[8] Knockaert DC, Vanneste LJ, Bobbaers HJ. Recurrent or episodic fever of unknown origin. Medicine 1993;72:184–95.
[9] Frenkel J. Overt and occult rheumatic diseases: the child with chronic fever. Best Pract Res Clin Rheum 2002;16:443–69.
[10] Hoffman HM, Rosengren S, Boyle DL, et al. Prevention of cold-associated acute inflammation in familial cold autoinflammatory syndrome by interleuken-1 receptor antagonist. Lancet 2004;364:1779–85.
[11] Grateau G. Clinical and genetic aspects of the hereditary periodic fever syndromes. Rheumatology 2004;43:410–5.
[12] Centola M, Aksentijevich I, Kastner DL. The hereditary periodic fever syndromes: molecular analysis of a new family of inflammatory diseases. Hum Mol Genet 1998;7:1581–8.
[13] McDermott MF. Genetic clues to understanding periodic fevers, and possible therapies. Trends Mol Med 2002;8:550–4.
[14] Drenth JPH, van der Meer JWM. Hereditary periodic fever. N Engl J Med 2001;345:1748–58.
[15] Long S. Periodic fever. In: Pollard AJ, Finn A, editors. Hot topics in infection and immunity in children. New York: Kluver Academic/Plenum Publishers; 2005. p. 101–15.
[16] Marshall GS, Edwards KM, Butler J, Lawton AR. Syndrome of periodic fever, pharyngitis, and aphthous stomatitis. J Pediatr 1987;110:43–6.
[17] Feder HM. Cimetidine treatment for periodic fever associated with aphthous stomatitis, pharyngitis and cervical adenits. Pediatr Infect Dis J 1992;11:318–21.
[18] Abramson JS, Givner LB, Thompson JN. Possible role of tonsillectomy and adenoidectomy in children with recurrent fever and tonsillopharyngitis. Pediatr Infect Dis J 1989;8:119–20.
[19] Lekstrom-Himes J, Dale JK, Kingma DW, Diaz PS, Jaffe ES, Straus SE. Periodic illness associated with Epstein-Barr virus infection. Clin Infect Dis 1996;22:22–7.
[20] Ryan ME, Ferrigno K, O'Boyle T, Long SS. Periodic fever and skin lesions caused by disseminated *Mycobacterium chelonae* infection in an immunocompetent child. Pediatr Infect Dis J 1996;15:270–2.
[21] Thomas KT, Feder HM, Lawton AR, Edwards KM. Periodic fever syndrome in children. J Pediatr 1999;135:15–22.
[22] Padeh S, Brezniak N, Zemer D, et al. Periodic fever, aphthous stomatitis, pharyngitis, and adenopathy syndrome: clinical characteristics and outcome. J Pediatr 1999;135:98–102.
[23] Long SS. Syndrome of periodic fever, aphthous stomatitis, pharyngitis, and adenitis (PFAPA)—what it isn't. What is it? J Pediatr 1999;135:1–5.
[24] Hammond W, Price TH, Souze LM. Treatment of cyclic neutropenia with granulocytic colony stimulating factor. N Engl J Med 1989;320:1306–11.
[25] Horwitz M, Benson KF, Person RE, Aprikyan AG, Dale DC. Neutrophil elastase mutations define a 21-day biological clock in cyclic hematopoiesis. Nat Genet 1999;23:433–6.
[26] Aprikyan A, Liles WC, Chi EY, Jonas M, Dale DC. Impaired survival of bone marrow hematopoietic progenitor cells in cyclic neutropenia. Blood 2001;97:147–53.
[27] Dale DC, Bolyard A, Aprikyan A. Cyclic neutropenia. Semin Hematol 2002;39:89–94.
[28] Ben-Chetrit E, Levy M. Familial Mediterranean fever. Lancet 1998;351:659–64.
[29] Aksentijevich I, Torosyan Y, Samuels J, et al. Mutation and haplotype studies of familial Mediterranean fever reveal new ancestral relationships and evidence for a high carrier frequency with reduced penetrance in the Ashkenazi Jewish population. Am J Hum Gen 1999;64:949–62.

[30] McDermott MF. A common pathway in periodic fever syndromes. Trends Immunol 2004;25:457–60.
[31] Stehlik C, Reed JC. The PYRIN connection: novel players in innate immunity and inflammation. J Exp Med 2004;200:551–8.
[32] van der Meer JW, Vossen JM, Radl J, et al. Hyperimmunoglobulinemia D and periodic fever: a new syndrome. Lancet 1984;i:1087–90.
[33] Houten SM, Kuis W, Duran M, et al. Mutations in *MVK*, encoding mevalonate kinase, cause hyperimmunoglobulinemia D and periodic fever syndrome. Nat Genet 1999;22:175–7.
[34] Drenth JPH, Cuisset L, Grateau G, et al. Mutations in the gene encoding mevalonate kinase cause hyper-D and periodic fever syndrome. Nat Genet 1999;22:178–81.
[35] Simon A, Kremer HPH, Wevers RA, et al. Mevalonate kinase deficiency: evidence for a phenotypic continuum. Neurology 2004;62:994–7.
[36] Drenth JPH, Haagsma CJ, van der Meer JWM, and the International Hyper-IgD Study Group. Hyperimmunoglobulinemia D and periodic fever syndrome: the clinical spectrum in a series of 50 patients. Medicine 1994;73:133–44.
[37] Saulsbury FT. Hyperimmunoglobulinemia D and periodic fever syndrome (HIDS) in a child with normal serum IgD, but increased serum IgA concentration. J Pediatr 2003;143:127–9.
[38] Simon A, Drewe E, van der Meer JWM, et al. Simvastatin treatment for inflammatory attacks of the hyperimmunoglobulinemia D and periodic fever syndrome. Clin Pharmacol Ther 2004;75:476–83.
[39] Takada K, Aksentijevich I, Mahadevan V, Dean JA, Kelley RI, Kastner DL. Favorable preliminary experience with etanercept in two patients with hyperimmunoglobulinemia D and periodic fever syndrome. Arthritis Rheum 2003;48:2645–51.
[40] Obici L, Manno C, Muda AO, et al. First report of systemic reactive (AA) amyloidosis in a patient with the hyperimmunoglobulinemia D with periodic fever syndrome. Arthritis Rheum 2004;50:2966–9.
[41] Williamson LM, Hull D, Mehta R, et al. Familial Hibernian fever. QJM 1982;51:469–80.
[42] Dodé C, André M, Bienvenu T, et al. The enlarging clinical, genetic, and population spectrum of tumor necrosis factor receptor-associated periodic syndrome. Arthritis Rheum 2002;46: 2181–8.
[43] Mulley J, Saar K, Hewitt G, et al. Gene localization for an autosomal dominant familial periodic fever to 12p13. Am J Hum Genet 1998;62:884–9.
[44] McDermott MF, Aksentijevich I, Galon J, et al. Germline mutations in the extracellular domains of the 55 kDa TNF receptor, TNF-R1, define a family of dominantly inherited autoinflammatory syndromes. Cell 1999;97:133–44.
[45] Saulsbury FT, Wispelwey B. Tumor necrosis factor receptor associated periodic syndrome (TRAPS) in a young adult who had features of periodic fever, aphthous stomatitis, pharyngitis, adenitis (PFAPA) as a child. J Pediatr 2005;146:283–5.
[46] Long SS. TRAPS and PFAPA. J Pediatr 2005;146:2A.
[47] Hull KM, Wong K, Wood GM, et al. Monocytic fasciitis: a newly recognized clinical feature of tumor necrosis factor receptor dysfunction. Arthritis Rheum 2002;46:2189–94.
[48] Lamprecht P, Moosig F, Adam-Klages S, et al. Small vessel vasculitis and relapsing panniculitis in tumor necrosis factor receptor associated periodic syndrome (TRAPS). Ann Rheum Dis 2004;63:1518–20.
[49] Aganna E, Hammond L, Hawkins PN, et al. Heterogeneity among patients with tumor necrosis factor receptor-associated periodic syndrome phenotypes. Arthritis Rheum 2003;48:2632–44.
[50] Galon J, Aksentijevich I, McDermott MF, O'Shea JJ, Kastner DL. *TNFRS1A* mutations and autoinflammatory syndromes. Curr Opin Immunol 2000;12:479–86.

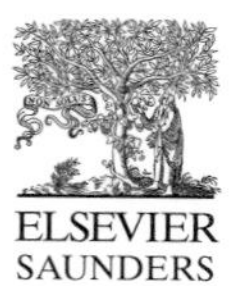

ELSEVIER
SAUNDERS

Pediatr Clin N Am 52 (2005) 837–867

PEDIATRIC CLINICS
OF NORTH AMERICA

Antiviral Therapies in Children: Has Their Time Arrived?

David W. Kimberlin, MD

Department of Pediatrics, Division of Pediatric Infectious Diseases, The University of Alabama at Birmingham, 1600 Seventh Avenue South, CHB 303, Birmingham, AL 35233, USA

Tremendous advances have occurred in recent decades in the development of safe and effective medications for the treatment of viral diseases. Until the last two to three decades, a central dogma of infectious diseases was that although antibiotics could target bacterial replication pathways effectively, similar success in the treatment of viral diseases was unlikely. Because viruses usurp host cell machinery for replication, it was assumed that attacking viruses inevitably would destroy normal cells. With the identification of virus-specific enzymes, however, safe targets for antiviral medications have been discovered. In general, antivirals exert their effects by interfering with attachment, entry, or uncoating of virus, thereby disabling their replication (Tables 1–3).

A total of 18 non-HIV antiviral agents and 17 HIV drugs currently are licensed by the US Food and Drug Administration (FDA). These antiviral agents are effective in the treatment or prevention of infections caused by herpes simplex virus (HSV), cytomegalovirus (CMV), varicella-zoster virus (VZV), HIV, respiratory syncytial virus (RSV), influenza A, influenza B, hepatitis B virus (HBV), hepatitis C virus (HCV), human papillomavirus (HPV), and lassa virus [1]. It is the clinician's responsibility to optimize the use of these powerful but sometimes

This work was supported under contract with the Virology Branch, Division of Microbiology and Infectious Diseases of the National Institute of Allergy and Infectious Diseases (NO1-AI-30025, NO1-AI -65306, NO1-AI -15113, NO1-AI-62554) and by grants from the General Clinical Research Center Program (M01-RR00032) and the State of Alabama.

E-mail address: dkimberlin@peds.uab.edu

doi:10.1016/j.pcl.2005.02.006 ***pediatric.theclinics.com***

Table 1
Antiviral choices for non-HIV clinical conditions

Virus	Clinical syndrome	Antiviral agent of choice	Alternative antiviral agents
Influenza A	Treatment	Rimantadine	Amantadine Oseltamivir (>1 year old)
	Prophylaxis	Rimantadine	Amantadine Oseltamivir (>1 year old) Zanamivir (>7 years old)
Influenza B	Treatment	Oseltamivir	Zanamivir (>7 years old)
Respiratory syncytial virus	Bronchiolitis or pneumonia in high-risk host	Ribavirin aerosol	
Cytomegalovirus	Retinitis in AIDS patients	Valganciclovir	Ganciclovir Cidofovir Foscarnet Ganciclovir ocular insert
	Pneumonitis, colitis; esophagitis in immunocompromised patients	Ganciclovir	Foscarnet Cidofovir Valganciclovir
Herpes simplex virus	Neonatal herpes	Acyclovir (IV)	
	HSV encephalitis	Acyclovir (IV)	
	HSV gingivostomatitis	Acyclovir (PO)	Acyclovir (IV)
	First episode genital infection	Acyclovir (PO)	Valaciclovir Famciclovir Acyclovir (IV) (severe disease)
	Recurrent genital herpes	Acyclovir (PO)	Valaciclovir Famciclovir
	Suppression of genital herpes	Acyclovir (PO)	Valaciclovir Famciclovir
	Whitlow	Acyclovir (PO)	
	Eczema herpeticum	Acyclovir (PO)	Acyclovir (IV) (severe disease)
	Mucocutaneous infection in immunocompromised host (mild)	Acyclovir (IV)	Acyclovir (PO) (if outpatient therapy acceptable)
	Mucocutaneous infection in immunocompromised host (moderate-to-severe)	Acyclovir (IV)	
	Prophylaxis in bone marrow transplant recipients	Acyclovir (IV)	Valaciclovir Famciclovir
	Acyclovir-resistant HSV	Foscarnet	Cidofovir
	Keratitis or keratoconjunctivitis	Trifluridine	Vidarabine
Varicella-zoster virus	Chickenpox, healthy child	Supportive care	Acyclovir (PO)
	Chickenpox, immunocompromised child	Acyclovir (IV)	
	Zoster (not ophthalmic branch of trigeminal nerve), healthy child	Supportive care	Acyclovir (PO)
	Zoster (ophthalmic branch of trigeminal nerve), healthy child	Acyclovir (IV)	
	Zoster, immunocompromised child	Acyclovir (IV)	Valaciclovir

Table 2
HIV drugs by class

Class of drug	Generic name	Brand name	Other names
Nucleoside reverse transcriptase inhibitors	Zidovudine	Retrovir	Azidothymidine, AZT, ZDV
	Didanosine	Videx	Dideoxyinosine, ddI
	Stavudine	Zerit	D4T
	Lamivudine	Epivir	3TC
	Abacavir	Ziagen	
	Emtricitabine	Emtriva	
Nonnucleoside reverse transcriptase inhibitors	Nevirapine	Viramune	
	Delavirdine	Rescriptor	
	Efavirenz	Sustiva	
Protease inhibitors	Saquinavir	Fortovase	
	Ritonavir	Norvir	
	Indinavir	Crixivan	
	Nelfinavir	Viracept	
	Amprenavir	Agenerase	
	Lopinavir-ritonavir	Kaletra	
	Atazanavir	Reyataz	
Fusion inhibitors	Enfuvirtide	Fuzeon	T20

toxic drugs. Although experience with their use is more limited in children than in adults, the future of antiviral therapeutics in pediatric patients is bright.

Antiviral agents used for treating herpesvirus infections

Antiviral therapy is established for the treatment and prevention of infections caused by four of the eight human herpesviruses (HHV) (HSV-1, HSV-2, VZV, and CMV). There are no agents of proven value for infections caused by Epstein-Barr virus (EBV), HHV-6, HHV-7, and HHV-8 (or Kaposi's sarcoma herpesvirus). All HHV are common causes of infection in children and adults. Disease is accentuated in high-risk, immunocompromised patients.

Nucleoside and nucleotide analogues

Acyclovir (acycloguanosine, Zovirax)

Commercially available since the 1980s, acyclovir remains in many regards the prototypic antiviral agent. The notable safety profile of acyclovir relates to its initial activation by the virus-encoded enzyme thymidine kinase (TK). Acyclovir is most active against HSV; activity against VZV also is substantial, but approximately 10-fold less. EBV is only moderately susceptible to acyclovir because EBV has minimal TK activity. Activity against CMV is poor because CMV does not have a unique TK, and CMV DNA polymerase is poorly inhibited by acyclovir triphosphate.

Table 3
Commonly used non-HIV drugs by class and mechanisms of action

Class	Nucleoside analogues	Nucleotide analogues	Inorganic phosphate analogues	Tricyclic amines	Neuraminidase inhibitors	Interferons
Mechanism of action	Monophosphorylated by viral enzyme, then triphosphorylated to active compound by cellular enzymes. Inhibits viral DNA polymerase	Diphosphorylated to active compound by cellular enzymes. Inhibits viral DNA polymerase	Noncompetitive inhibitor of viral DNA polymerase or HIV reverse transcriptase	Blocks M2 protein of influenza virus A, inhibiting initiation of viral replication	Inhibits influenza virus A and B neuraminidase, blocking release of progeny virus from infected cells	Induce production of more than two dozen effector proteins, leading to inhibition of viral penetration or uncoating, synthesis or methylation of mRNA, viral protein translation, or viral assembly and release
Examples	Acyclovir/valaciclovir Famciclovir/penciclovir Ganciclovir/valganciclovir	Cidofovir	Foscarnet	Amantadine Rimantadine	Oseltamivir Zanamivir	Interferon alfa Interferon beta Interferon gamma

Clinical utility. Acyclovir is effective in the treatment and suppression of genital herpes [2–12]. It also is effective in treating primary gingivostomatitis in pediatric patients [13], although it has only a modest effect in the treatment of recurrent herpes labialis [14–16]. Prophylactic acyclovir has been used to prevent reactivation of herpes labialis after exposure to UV radiation, facial surgery, or exposure to sun and wind while skiing [17–19]. Long-term suppressive therapy reduces the number of recurrences of oral infection in patients with histories of frequent recurrences [20]. Intravenous acyclovir improves morbidity and mortality in herpes simplex encephalitis [21,22] and in neonatal HSV disease [23–25]. Acyclovir also is indicated for the treatment of disseminated HSV infections in otherwise normal hosts, including pregnant women, and mucocutaneous HSV infections in immunocompromised hosts [26–29]. Topical therapy with acyclovir for HSV ocular infections is effective, but probably not superior to trifluridine [30]. Long-term suppressive therapy reduces the number of recurrences of ocular infection in patients with histories of frequent recurrences [31,32].

Persons at risk for developing severe varicella, such as patients with leukemia, should be treated early to prevent dissemination of VZV [33]. Treatment of immunologically normal children, adolescents, and adults with varicella using oral acyclovir produces only modest therapeutic benefit [34–36]. Treatment of patients with zoster with intravenous acyclovir results in more rapid clinical improvement [37–39]. Acute pain associated with zoster is diminished, although the frequency or severity of postherpetic neuralgia is not affected [39].

Antiviral resistance. Resistance of HSV to acyclovir has become an important clinical problem, especially in immunocompromised patients exposed to long-term therapy [40]. HSV resistance to acyclovir can result from mutations in either the viral TK gene or the viral DNA polymerase gene. Although these acyclovir-resistant isolates exhibit diminished virulence in animal models, in HIV-infected patients they can cause severe, progressive, debilitating mucosal disease and (rarely) visceral dissemination [41]. Although it is uncommon, genital herpes caused by acyclovir-resistant isolates also has been reported in immunocompetent hosts who usually have received long-term acyclovir therapy [42]. Acyclovir-resistant strains of VZV also occur, with mechanisms of resistance identical to those of HSV [43].

Pharmacokinetics and adverse effects. The oral bioavailability of acyclovir is poor, with only 15% to 30% of the oral formulation being absorbed. Acyclovir is widely distributed, with high concentrations attained in kidneys, lung, liver, heart, and skin vesicles; concentrations in the cerebrospinal fluid are about 50% of those in the plasma [44]. Acyclovir crosses the placenta and accumulates in breast milk. Dose modification is required in cases of renal insufficiency. Concomitant administration of probenicid prolongs acyclovir's half-life, whereas acyclovir can decrease the clearance and prolong the half-life of drugs such as methotrexate that are eliminated by active renal secretion.

Acyclovir is a safe, generally well-tolerated drug. Oral acyclovir sometimes causes mild gastrointestinal upset, rash, and headache. If it extravasates, intravenous acyclovir can cause severe inflammation, phlebitis, and sometimes a vesicular eruption leading to cutaneous necrosis at the injection site. If given by rapid intravenous infusion or to poorly hydrated patients or patients with preexisting renal compromise, intravenous acyclovir can cause reversible nephrotoxicity. This condition results from formation of acyclovir crystals precipitating in renal tubules and causing an obstructive nephropathy. The likelihood of renal toxicity of acyclovir is increased when administered with nephrotoxic drugs, such as cyclosporine or amphotericin B. Administration of acyclovir by the intravenous route occasionally is associated with rash, sweating, nausea, headache, hematuria, and hypotension. High doses of intravenous acyclovir in neonates and prolonged use of oral acyclovir after neonatal disease have been associated with neutropenia [45,46].

The most serious side effect of acyclovir is neurotoxicity, which usually occurs in subjects with compromised renal function who attain high serum concentrations of drug [47]. Neurotoxicity is manifest as lethargy, confusion, hallucinations, tremors, myoclonus, seizures, extrapyramidal signs, and changes in state of consciousness, developing within the first few days of initiating therapy. These signs and symptoms usually resolve spontaneously within several days of discontinuing acyclovir. Although acyclovir is mutagenic at high concentrations in some in vitro assays, it is not teratogenic in animals. Limited human data suggest that acyclovir use in pregnant women is not associated with congenital defects or other adverse pregnancy outcomes [48].

Valaciclovir (Valtrex)

Valaciclovir is the L-valyl ester of acyclovir that is converted rapidly to acyclovir after oral administration by first-pass metabolism in the liver [49]. It has a safety and efficacy profile similar to acyclovir, but offers potential pharmacokinetic advantages. Valaciclovir dosages in children are not established. A valaciclovir oral suspension has been formulated and is undergoing phase I evaluation in infants and children.

Clinical utility. Valaciclovir is effective for the treatment and suppression of genital herpes [2,5,50–53] and recurrent herpes labialis [54–56]. Valaciclovir also is approved for the treatment of herpes zoster [57].

Antiviral resistance. Because valaciclovir is metabolized to acyclovir in the bloodstream, antiviral resistance mechanisms are identical to those of acyclovir.

Pharmacokinetics and adverse effects. The bioavailability of valaciclovir exceeds 50%, which is three to five times greater than that of acyclovir [58]. The area under the drug concentration time curve approximates that seen after intravenous acyclovir.

The profiles of adverse effects and potential drug interactions observed with valaciclovir therapy are the same as those observed with acyclovir treatment. Manifestations resembling thrombotic microangiopathy have been described in patients with advanced HIV disease receiving very high doses of valaciclovir (8 g/d), but the multitude of other medications being administered to such patients makes the establishment of a causal relationship to valaciclovir difficult [59].

Cidofovir (Vistide, HPMPC)

Cidofovir was first approved for use in the United States for the therapy of AIDS-associated retinitis caused by CMV, and this remains the main indication for this antiviral agent. In addition to its excellent activity against CMV [60], cidofovir is active against HSV and VZV, including ganciclovir-resistant and foscarnet-resistant CMV isolates and acyclovir-resistant and foscarnet-resistant HSV isolates [61]. Cidofovir also has shown in vitro activity against EBV, HHV-6, HHV-8, polyomaviruses, adenovirus, HPV, and poxviruses.

Clinical utility. Cidofovir has been used successfully in the management of disease caused by acyclovir-resistant HSV isolates [62]. The primary use for cidofovir currently is for the management of CMV retinitis in patients with AIDS [63,64]. Aggressive intravenous prehydration and coadministration of probenecid are required with each cidofovir dose.

Antiviral resistance. Only a few cidofovir-resistant CMV isolates have been reported. Cidofovir-resistant CMV isolates generally remain sensitive to foscarnet [65,66], although a CMV mutant resistant to ganciclovir, foscarnet, and cidofovir has been reported [67].

Pharmacokinetics and adverse effects. Cidofovir is a novel acyclic phosphonate nucleotide analogue. When phosporylated to the active cidofovir diphosphate, it exhibits a 25-fold to 50-fold greater affinity for the viral DNA polymerase compared with the cellular DNA polymerase, selectively inhibiting viral replication [68]. Only 2% to 26% of cidofovir is absorbed after oral administration, requiring that cidofovir be administered intravenously in the clinical management of patients. The plasma half-life of cidofovir is 2.6 hours, but active intracellular metabolites of cidofovir have half-lives of 17 to 48 hours [69]. Although cidofovir is less potent in vitro against HSV than is acyclovir, the prolonged intracellular half-life increases its anti-HSV activity. Ninety percent of the drug is excreted in the urine, primarily by renal tubular secretion [70].

The principal adverse event associated with systemic administration of cidofovir is nephrotoxicity. Cidofovir concentrates in renal cells in amounts 100 times greater than in other tissues, producing severe proximal convoluted tubule nephrotoxicity when concomitant hydration and administration of probenicid are not employed [69,70]. Renal toxicity manifests as proteinuria and glycosuria. As a result of its potential for nephrotoxicity, cidofovir should not be administered concomitantly with other potentially nephrotoxic agents (eg, intravenous aminoglycosides [tobramycin, gentamicin, and amikacin], amphotericin B, foscarnet, intravenous pentamidine, vancomycin, and nonsteroidal anti-inflammatory drugs).

Other toxicities of cidofovir include neutropenia, ocular hypotony, and metabolic acidosis. Cidofovir is carcinogenic, is teratogenic, and causes hypospermia in animal studies. The safety and efficacy of cidofovir in children have not been studied. Because of the risk of long-term carcinogenicity and reproductive toxicity, the use of cidofovir in children warrants caution.

Famciclovir (Famvir) and penciclovir (Denavir)

Famciclovir is the oral prodrug of penciclovir. The spectrum of activity of penciclovir and famciclovir against herpesviruses is similar to that of acyclovir. In addition to HSV, penciclovir is active in vitro against VZV, EBV, and HBV.

Clinical utility. Famciclovir is effective in the treatment and suppression of genital herpes [71–73]. Topical penciclovir reduces time to healing and duration of pain in patients with recurrent herpes labialis [74,75]. Famciclovir also is effective in the treatment of herpes zoster [76].

Antiviral resistance. Because penciclovir, like acyclovir, must be activated by the viral encoded TK enzyme, TK-deficient viral strains are resistant to acyclovir and penciclovir. Strains of HSV whose resistance to acyclovir is conferred by alteration of the TK enzyme or by DNA polymerase mutations may remain sensitive to penciclovir [43].

Pharmacokinetics and adverse effects. Famciclovir is the inactive diacetyl ester prodrug of penciclovir, an acyclic nucleoside analogue. After oral ingestion and systemic absorption, famciclovir is rapidly deacetylated and oxidized to form the active parent drug penciclovir. The bioavailability of penciclovir after oral administration of famciclovir is about 70%. Penciclovir attains high intracellular concentrations and has a long intracellular half-life (7–20 hours). Although it is much less potent against herpesvirus DNA polymerase in vitro, it is clinically effective against these viruses. Dosage reduction of famciclovir is recommended for patients with compromised renal function [77].

Famciclovir is as well tolerated as acyclovir. Complaints of nausea, diarrhea, and headache occur at frequencies similar to those reported by placebo recipients. No clinically significant drug interactions have been reported to date. The safety and efficacy of famciclovir and topical penciclovir in children have not been established, although phase I studies of oral famciclovir are beginning. No liquid or suspension formulation exists currently.

Ganciclovir (Cytovene, DHPG)

Ganciclovir was the first antiviral available for the treatment and prevention of infections caused by CMV. Ganciclovir's greatest in vitro activity is against

CMV. It is also as active as acyclovir against HSV-1 and HSV-2 and almost as active against VZV.

Clinical utility. Ganciclovir is indicated for the treatment and prevention of life-threatening and sight-threatening CMV infections in immunocompromised patients [78–84]. Ganciclovir also is useful for prevention of CMV infections in high-risk immunocompromised subjects [85–92]. Ganciclovir has shown limited benefit in the treatment of neonates with congenital CMV infection [93].

Antiviral resistance. Ganciclovir resistance is most likely to occur in patients receiving long-term therapy. Antiviral resistance should be suspected when disease progression or continued recovery of virus occur despite ganciclovir therapy.

Pharmacokinetics and adverse effects. Oral bioavailability of ganciclovir is poor, with less than 10% of drug being absorbed after oral administration [94–96]. Concentrations of ganciclovir in the CNS range from 24% to 70% of the concentrations in the plasma, with brain concentrations of approximately 38% of plasma levels [97]. Dosage reduction, roughly proportional to the degree of reduction in creatinine clearance, is necessary in persons with impaired renal function [98,99].

Myelosuppression is the most common adverse effect of ganciclovir; dose-related neutropenia (<1000 white blood cells/mm^3) is the most consistent hematologic disturbance, with an incidence of about 40% of ganciclovir-treated patients [94]. Neutropenia is dose limiting in about 15% of subjects and is reversible on cessation of drug. Thrombocytopenia (<50,000 platelets/mm^3) occurs in approximately 20% of treated patients, whereas anemia occurs in about 2% of ganciclovir recipients.

In preclinical test systems, ganciclovir is mutagenic, carcinogenic, and teratogenic. Additionally, it causes irreversible reproductive toxicity in animal models. The use of ganciclovir in pediatric patients warrants caution because of this potential for long-term carcinogenicity and reproductive toxicity. Administration of ganciclovir to pediatric patients should be undertaken only after careful evaluation and only if the potential benefits of treatment outweigh the potential risks.

Valganciclovir (Valcyte)

Valganciclovir is an L-valine ester prodrug of ganciclovir and as such has the same mechanism of action, antiviral spectrum, and potential for development of resistance as ganciclovir [100]. Valganciclovir was approved by the FDA in 2001. Because it is well absorbed after oral administration, it may represent a favorable alternative to intravenously administered ganciclovir for the treatment and suppression of CMV infections in immunocompromised hosts.

Clinical utility. Valganciclovir has similar indications to ganciclovir. Based on limited controlled trials published to date, however, it currently is approved for the induction and maintenance therapy of CMV retinitis [101].

Pharmacokinetics and adverse effects. Valganciclovir is converted rapidly to ganciclovir, with a mean plasma half-life of about 30 minutes [102]. The absolute bioavailability of valganciclovir exceeds 60% and is enhanced by about 30% with concomitant administration of food [103]. The area under the curve of ganciclovir after oral administration of valganciclovir is one third to one half of that attained after intravenous administration of ganciclovir. Patients with impaired renal function require dosage reduction that is roughly proportional to their reduction in creatinine clearance [100]. Based on data from 370 subjects participating in clinical trials, the most common side effects associated with valganciclovir therapy include diarrhea (41%), nausea (30%), neutropenia (27%), anemia (26%), and headache (22%) [100].

Trifluridine (trifluorothymidine, Viroptic)

Trifluridine is a pyrimidine nucleoside active in vitro against HSV-1 and HSV-2 (including acyclovir-resistant strains), CMV, and certain adenoviruses [104]. Trifluridine is approved only for topical use in the management of primary keratoconjunctivitis and recurrent keratitis caused by HSV. It is more active than idoxuridine in HSV ocular infections [105] and is the treatment of choice for the topical treatment of HSV keratitis. Adverse effects include local discomfort, irritation, and edema and less commonly hypersensitivity reactions and superficial punctate or epithelial keratopathy. It is supplied as a 1% ophthalmic solution, 1 drop to be instilled in each eye up to nine times a day.

Vidarabine (ara-A, adenine arabinoside, Vira-A)

Licensed for use in the United States in 1977 as the first antiviral agent for use against herpesviruses, vidarabine occupies a special place in the historical development of antiviral compounds. Use of systemic vidarabine has been replaced by acyclovir, however, because of acyclovir's more favorable toxicity profile and greater ease of administration. Intravenous vidarabine has not been available in the United States since 1992, although a topical preparation remains on the market for the treatment of HSV keratitis. Although trifluridine is the antiviral agent of choice for the topical treatment of HSV keratitis, vidarabine is a suitable alternative in patients in whom trifluridine cannot be used [106–108]. Resistance to vidarabine is conferred by mutations in the viral DNA polymerase gene. Acyclovir-resistant clinical HSV isolates virtually always retain in vitro susceptibility to vidarabine [43].

Inorganic phosphate analogues

Foscarnet (PFA, Foscavir)

Foscarnet is the only antiherpes drug that is not a nucleoside or nucleotide analogue. Foscarnet inhibits all known human herpesviruses, including acyclovir-resistant HSV and VZV strains and most ganciclovir-resistant CMV isolates. It also is active against HIV. Rather than being a first-line drug, foscarnet is useful for the treatment of infections caused by resistant herpesviruses. The safety and efficacy of foscarnet in pediatric patients has not been established. Because of potential dental and bone toxicity, the administration of foscarnet to pediatric patients should be undertaken only after careful evaluation and only if the potential benefits for treatment outweigh the potential risks.

Clinical utility. Foscarnet is effective for therapy of life-threatening and sight-threatening CMV infections in immunocompromised patients [79,109–111]. Foscarnet also is effective in the therapy of CMV infections caused by ganciclovir-resistant strains of CMV [109] and has been used successfully in the management of disease caused by acyclovir-resistant HSV isolates [112,113].

Antiviral resistance. Foscarnet is active against most acyclovir-resistant HSV and VZV isolates and most ganciclovir-resistant CMV isolates [43,112,113]. Strains of CMV, HSV, and VZV with threefold to fivefold reduced sensitivity to foscarnet have been reported [67,114,115]. These isolates may respond to therapy with acyclovir [114] or cidofovir [115].

Pharmacokinetics and adverse effects. Foscarnet is poorly absorbed after oral administration, with a bioavailability of only about 20%, limiting foscarnet's delivery to the intravenous route. Data are limited regarding tissue distribution, but cerebrospinal fluid concentrations are about two thirds of those in serum. Eighty percent of an administered dose of foscarnet is eliminated unchanged in the urine; half-life is 48 hours. Dosage adjustments are necessary even in the presence of minimal degrees of renal dysfunction. The degree of dose reduction is proportional to reduction in creatinine clearance. There are no pharmacokinetic data for foscarnet in neonates.

The most common adverse effects of foscarnet are nephrotoxicity and metabolic derangements. Evidence of nephrotoxicity includes azotemia, proteinuria, acute tubular necrosis, crystalluria, and interstitial nephritis [116]. Serum creatinine concentrations increase in 50% of patients, usually during the second week of therapy. Renal function returns to normal within 2 to 4 weeks of discontinuing therapy in most affected patients. Metabolic disturbances associated with foscarnet therapy include symptomatic hypocalcemia and hypercalcemia and hypophosphatemia and hyperphosphatemia [94]. Hypocalcemia is due to direct chelation of ionized calcium by the drug, and patients can have paresthesias, tetany, seizures, and arrhythmias.

Concomitant use of amphotericin B, cyclosporine, gentamicin, and other nephrotoxic drugs increases the likelihood of renal dysfunction associated with foscarnet therapy. Coadministration of pentamidine increases the risk of hypocalcemia. Anemia and neutropenia are more common when patients also are receiving zidovudine. No drug-drug interactions are known to exist with the concomitant use of foscarnet and ganciclovir.

Antiviral agents used for treating respiratory virus infections

Infections of the respiratory tract of children are common and can result in significant morbidity, particularly in children with underlying pulmonary, cardiac, or immunologic abnormalities. Of the respiratory tract viral pathogens, licensed therapies currently exist for influenza A, influenza B, and RSV.

Tricyclic amines

Amantadine (Symmetrel) and rimantadine (Flumadine)

Amantadine and rimantadine are closely related antiviral agents that were approved for use in the United States in 1966 (amantadine) and 1993 (rimantadine). Amantadine and rimantadine are active only against influenza A viruses; rimantadine is 4-fold to 10-fold more active than amantadine [117]. Although these agents are useful for the prevention and treatment of infections caused by influenza A virus, vaccination against influenza is a more cost-effective means of reducing disease burden.

Clinical utility. Amantadine and rimantadine are useful for the prevention and treatment of infections caused by influenza type A virus in children and adults [118–122]. Drug therapy results in reduced duration of viral excretion, fever, and other systemic complaints. Compared with placebo, the duration of illness is shortened by about 1 day.

Antiviral resistance. Resistance to these drugs typically appears in the treated subject within 2 to 3 days of initiating therapy, and more than 25% of treated patients shed resistant strains by day 5 of treatment [123]. Although the clinical significance of isolating resistant strains from treated subjects is not clear, transmission of resistant strains to household contacts can occur, and failure of drug prophylaxis can result [123].

Pharmacokinetics and adverse effects. Amantadine and rimantadine are well absorbed after oral administration; food does not interfere with absorption of either drug [124,125]. Concentrations of both antivirals in nasal secretions exceed 50% of serum concentrations. Substantial dose adjustments of amantadine are necessary in persons with impaired renal function [126].

In general, side effects are less frequent and less severe with rimantadine. The most common complaints associated with the administration of both drugs are dose-related gastrointestinal and CNS symptoms [127]. Common gastrointestinal complaints include nausea, vomiting, and dyspepsia. Common CNS disturbances, evident in about 10% of amantadine and 2% of rimantadine recipients, include anxiety, depression, insomnia, difficulty in concentration, and confusion; hallucinations and seizures occur less often. Long-term amantadine therapy has been associated with vision loss, hypotension, urinary retention, peripheral edema, and congestive heart failure. In children, the incidence of side effects in rimantadine recipients is similar to that observed in placebo recipients [128].

Neuraminidase inhibitors

The biologic action of this class of antiviral agents results from inhibition of influenza neuraminidase. Because neuraminidase is required for optimal release of progeny virus from infected cells, inhibition of this enzyme decreases the spread of virus and the intensity of infection. Neuraminidase is a highly conserved enzyme in influenza viruses, and the neuraminidase inhibitors are active against all strains of influenza type A and influenza type B viruses.

Oseltamivir (Tamiflu)

Clinical utility. Oseltamivir is an oral antiviral medication that is effective in the prevention and treatment of infections caused by either influenza A or influenza B viruses in adults and children [123,129–133]. Duration of illness in adult and pediatric drug recipients is reduced by 1 to 1.5 days compared with duration of illness among placebo recipients [130–132]. Oseltamivir is licensed for use in children one year of age and older.

Antiviral resistance. A report indicates that the development of resistance occurs in about 18% of treated children during the course of therapy [134].

Pharmacokinetics and adverse effects. Oseltamivir is an ethyl ester prodrug, hydrolyzed by hepatic esterases to biologically active oseltamivir carboxylate. The oral bioavailability of oseltamivir is about 75%; coadministration with food does not affect absorption. More than 90% of oseltamivir is metabolized to oseltamivir carboxylate. The half-life of oseltamivir carboxylate is 6 to 10 hours; it is eliminated by glomerular filtration and tubular secretion [132]. Dose adjustment is recommended for patients with impaired renal function.

About 10% of patients treated with oseltamivir experience nausea without vomiting, and an additional 10% have nausea with vomiting. These side effects generally are mild and usually occur on the first 2 days of therapy. Insomnia and vertigo also occasionally occur in oseltamivir recipients.

Zanamivir (Relenza)

Clinical utility. Inhaled zanamivir is effective in the prevention and treatment of infections caused by either influenza A or influenza B viruses in adults and children [135–141]. On average, zanamivir-treated patients improve 1 to 2.5 days faster than placebo recipients [141].

Antiviral resistance. Decreased susceptibility to zanamivir has been described in an immunocompromised patient infected with influenza B [142].

Pharmacokinetics and adverse effects. Zanamivir is administered by oral inhalation because it has poor oral bioavailability. Less than 15% of an inhaled dose of zanamivir distributes to the airways and lungs; most is deposited in the oropharynx [143]. Nonetheless, high concentrations of drug in sputum exist for 6 hours after inhalation. About 10% of an inhaled dose of zanamivir is absorbed [143]. The plasma half-life of zanamivir ranges from 2.5 to 5 hours; drug is excreted unchanged in the urine. No adjustment in dosing is necessary for renal insufficiency because of the limited amount of systemically absorbed drug.

Zanamivir is well tolerated. A decline in pulmonary function and bronchospasm have been reported in some patients with underlying airway disease [144].

Nucleoside Analogues

Ribavirin (Virazole, Rebetron)

Ribavirin is available for inhaled use for the therapy of severe lower respiratory tract infection caused by RSV. It also is available as an oral and intravenous formulation for the therapy of hepatitis and lassa fever.

Clinical utility. Ribavirin aerosol is approved for the therapy of lower respiratory tract infections caused by RSV, but controversy exists over the circumstances under which its use is indicated in infants and children [27]. Intravenously administered ribavirin is effective in the prevention and management of life-threatening infections caused by Lassa fever and hemorrhagic fever with renal syndrome [145,146]. Although there are anecdotal reports of ribavirin therapy of other infections, including infections caused by influenza, parainfluenza, and measles virus, efficacy against these infections is not established. Ribavirin in combination with interferon alfa (Rebetron) is useful in the management of infections caused by HCV [147,148].

Pharmacokinetics and adverse effects. Ribavirin is active against a wide range of RNA and DNA viruses, including myxoviruses, paramyxoviruses, arenaviruses, bunyaviruses, herpesviruses, adenoviruses, poxviruses, and retroviruses [149]. Activity against RNA viruses is greater than activity against DNA viruses.

The aerosolized formulation of ribavirin (Virazole) and the oral formulation in combination with interferon alfa (Rebetron) are approved for use in the United States. Aerosolized delivery of ribavirin is accomplished with a small-particle aerosol generator (SPAG) that delivers a steady flow of small particles. The oral bioavailability of ribavirin is about 40%. Levels of ribavirin in cerebrospinal fluid are approximately 70% of plasma concentrations of drug [150].

Ribavirin is concentrated in red blood cells, and high concentrations of the drug are associated with reversible anemia [151]. Increases in serum bilirubin, iron, and uric acid also may result from systemic therapy.

Aerosolized ribavirin occasionally is associated with mild conjunctival irritation and rash. Transient wheezing may accompany therapy. When used in mechanically ventilated infants, unless careful attention is paid to modifying the circuitry and frequently changing in-line filters, ribavirin can precipitate, plugging the ventilator valves and tubing [152].

Significant teratogenic or embryocidal effects have been shown for ribavirin in all animal species in which adequate studies have been conducted. Concern exists for health care personnel caring for children receiving aerosolized ribavirin who may be exposed inadvertently to the drug. Only 1 of 29 health care workers evaluated in two studies in which drug was being administered to children by ventilator, oxygen tent, or oxygen hood had detectable drug in red blood cells, however, and none had drug detected in urine or serum samples [153,154].

Antiviral agents used for treating hepatitis viruses and papillomaviruses

Treatment of HBV and HCV has advanced rapidly over recent years. Although improvements in antiviral drugs for these viral diseases are still needed, the therapeutic options that exist today represent a significant advance compared with just a few years ago. Antiviral agents in use for the treatment of HBV and HCV include interferon (HBV and HCV), lamivudine (HBV), adefovir (HBV), and ribavirin (in combination with interferon) (HCV). A substantial challenge for treating infected pediatric patients is knowing when to initiate therapy. Study of existing drugs and molecules under development in the pediatric population is essential to define pediatric treatment algorithms more clearly.

HPV infections are among the most prevalent of sexually transmitted diseases, with 75% of women in the United States acquiring genital HPV infection at some point in their lives. HPV infections of the genital tract are of medical and public health concern because of their propensity to lead to the development of cervical cancer, and because they can be transmitted to the respiratory tract of a newborn child, resulting in juvenile-onset recurrent respiratory papillomatosis.

Interferons and pegylated interferons

Interferons are a family of nonspecific regulatory proteins associated with a variety of antiviral, antiproliferative, and immunomodulating activities [27, 155]. There are two major types of interferons. Type 1 (α and β) interferons are secreted by all nucleated cells after viral infection; interferon-α is predominantly produced by virus-infected leukocytes, and interferon-β is produced by fibroblasts. Type II interferon (γ) is the product of antigen-stimulated or mitogen-stimulated lymphocytes. Interferons do not have direct antiviral activity, but rather exert their antiviral effects by inducing production of more than two dozen effector proteins in exposed cells. Antiviral activity also can be facilitated by the complex interactions between interferons and other components of the immune system, resulting in modification of host response to infection [27,156]. Interferons are active against a broad range of viruses, although, in general, they are more active against RNA viruses than DNA viruses.

Clinical utility

Interferon alfa therapy is effective in the management of HBV [157] and HCV [158,159] infections. The combination of oral ribavirin with interferon alfa (Rebetron) improves the efficacy of interferon alfa [147,148,160]. Data suggest that the combination of pegylated (long-acting) interferon plus ribavirin produces additional significant improvements in the rate of sustained virologic response compared with nonpegylated interferon plus ribavirin [161]. Interferon alfa also is recommended for the therapy of recalcitrant anogenital warts caused by papillomaviruses [162]. Therapy may be administered directly into lesions or systemically. The most commonly accepted adjuvant therapy for juvenile-onset recurrent respiratory papillomatosis is the systemic administration of interferon alfa-2a [163–167].

Pharmacokinetics and adverse effects

More than 80% of interferon alfa is absorbed after intramuscular or subcutaneous injection; plasma levels peak at 4 to 8 hours [168]. Although the plasma half-life is only 2 to 4 hours, antiviral activity peaks at about 24 hours, slowly decreasing over the next 6 days [169]. Negligible plasma levels of interferon beta are detected after intramuscular or subcutaneous injection; concentrations of interferon gamma vary. Low concentrations of interferon are detectable in body tissues and fluid, and negligible amounts are excreted in the urine [168].

At interferon doses at and greater than 1 to 2 million IU, most persons develop an influenza-like illness, with fever, chills, headache, myalgia, arthralgia, and gastrointestinal disturbances [170]. These symptoms typically appear during the first week of therapy and remit with continued therapy, rarely necessitating therapy discontinuation or dosage modification. The major therapy-limiting toxicities of systemically administered interferon are neuropsychiatric complications and bone marrow suppression [171]. About 10% to 20% of interferon recipients develop neuropsychiatric problems. Neutropenia and thrombocytopenia are the most common signs of bone marrow suppression [172].

Because interferon interferes with the function of the hepatic cytochrome P-450 enzymes, it can increase significantly the half-life of drugs metabolized by these enzymes, such as theophylline. Interferon also increases the bone marrow suppression of myelotoxic drugs, such as zidovudine.

Nucleoside and nucleotide analogues

Ribavirin (Rebetron)

Oral ribavirin has been coadministrated with either interferon alfa or pegylated interferon for the treatment of HCV infections in adults. Current therapeutic regimens in adults result in long-term improvement of disease in approximately onethird of adults treated. No consensus exists, however, on the treatment of children with chronic HCV infection. Efficacy using interferon plus ribavirin is greatest for non–type 1 genotypes. Type 1 genotypes are encountered most frequently in the United States.

Adefovir (Hepsera)

Adefovir is an inhibitor of HBV viral replication. It also has in vitro activity against HIV, although it has not been shown to suppress HIV RNA in patients.

Clinical utility. Adefovir is indicated for the treatment of chronic HBV in adults with evidence of active viral replication and either evidence of persistent elevations in serum aminotransferases or histologically active disease [173]. The optimal duration of adefovir treatment and the relationship between treatment response and long-term outcomes, such as hepatocellular carcinoma or decompensated cirrhosis, are not known.

Antiviral resistance. To date, mutations within the HBV DNA polymerase that confer resistance to adefovir have not been identified in clinical trials.

Pharmacokinetics and adverse effects. Adefovir is an acyclic nucleoside analogue of AMP. It is administered as a diester prodrug and is converted rapidly to the active drug after ingestion. It is active against HBV. Oral bioavailability of adefovir is approximately 60%. Adefovir concentrations are not affected by administration with food. Persons with moderately or severely impaired renal function or persons on hemodialysis require adefovir dosage modification. Pharmacokinetic studies have not been performed in children.

Severe acute exacerbation of hepatitis has been reported in patients who have discontinued anti-HBV therapy, including adefovir therapy. Patients at risk of or having underlying renal dysfunction may experience nephrotoxicity associated with adefovir administration. Lactic acidosis and severe hepatomegaly with steatosis have been reported with the use of nucleoside analogues alone or in combination with other antiretrovirals.

Nucleoside reverse transcriptase inhibitors

Lamivudine (Epivir, 3TC)

Lamivudine inhibits the reverse transcriptase of HIV and HBV and is discussed is more detail in the section on HIV. Lamivudine has been used for the treatment of chronic HBV infection in children and adults [174–176].

Lamivudine-resistant HBV mutants occur in one third of subjects by the end of 1 year of therapy and in two thirds by the end of 4 years of treatment [174]. Lamivudine resistance usually is manifest clinically as breakthrough infection, defined as reappearance of HBV DNA in serum after its initial disappearance. Most patients continue to have lower serum HBV DNA and alanine aminotransferase levels compared with pretreatment levels, perhaps as a result of decreased fitness of the lamivudine-resistant mutants.

Antiviral agents used for treating HIV

Therapeutic agents for the treatment of HIV infection in children have increased rapidly. Four classes of compounds currently are licensed for administration to patients with HIV infection: nucleoside reverse transcriptase inhibitors (NRTIs), non-nucleoside reverse transcriptase inhibitors (NNRTIs), protease inhibitors, and, most recently, fusion inhibitors. Therapeutic trials in children support the value of combination therapies, particularly the inclusion of protease inhibitors, when viral load is high and CD4 cell counts are low. Noncompliance with the medical regimen is a frequent and often limiting occurrence in pediatric HIV patients. As with adults, adverse events, such as alterations in lipid metabolism, insulin-refractory diabetes, and metabolic acidosis, all are problematic for children. Because of the large number of antiretroviral medications and their similarities within classes, summaries are provided here by class, with brief reports on individual drugs following.

Nucleoside reverse transcriptase inhibitors

NRTIs are the cornerstone of most highly active antiretroviral treatment regimens. NRTIs are phosphorylated intracellularly, with thymidine analogues (zidovudine or stavudine) being preferentially phosphorylated in activated cells, whereas lamivudine and didanosine are preferentially phosphorylated in resting cells [177]. Optimal use of NRTIs combines a thymidine analogue with lamivudine or didanosine such that both cell types are included. Zidovudine and stavudine should not be administered together, however, because they compete for the same activating enzymes and are clinically antagonistic [178]. Abacavir is a newer agent and the first guanosine-derived NRTI. With the exception of zidovudine and abacavir, the NRTIs are primarily renally eliminated as unchanged parent drug. As a result, drug-drug interactions are much less common with this class of agents.

Zidovudine (azidothymidine, AZT, ZDV, Retrovir)

Zidovudine is indicated for the treatment of HIV infections in children and for prevention of perinatal (mother-to-infant) transmission. It was the first compound licensed for the treatment of AIDS and remains a key medication in treatment paradigms, being used in combination with lamivudine and with

NNRTIs and protease inhibitors. Neonates unable to receive oral dosing may be treated intravenously with zidovudine. Currently, zidovudine is used most frequently in fixed combination with lamivudine (Combivir).

Didanosine (dideoxyinosine, ddI, Videx)

Didanosine is used in the treatment of HIV infection of children and adults, usually in combination with either zidovudine or stavudine. In adults, administration is recommended 1 hour before or 2 hours after meals. This dosing constraint may not be an issue in children because absorption does not seem to be altered substantially by food. An enteric-coated formulation of didanosine (ddI EC) has been developed for once-daily dosing. Because the drug is cleared by the kidney, dose reduction is required in cases of renal insufficiency. Adverse reactions after didanosine administration to children include pancreatitis, peripheral neuropathy, altered hepatic function, and myalgia and, less frequently than zidovudine, leukopenia, anemia, and thrombocytopenia.

Stavudine (d4T, Zerit)

Stavudine often is used in combination with lamivudine or didanosine and with either a NNRTI or protease inhibitor.

Lamivudine (Epivir, 3TC)

Lamivudine is used frequently with zidovudine in the form of Combivir. Lamivudine also is used frequently for the treatment of HIV in combination with stavudine, a NNRTI, or a protease inhibitor. HIV resistance to lamivudine appears rapidly with monotherapy. Combination therapy with zidovudine prolongs the time to the appearance of zidovudine resistance.

Abacavir (Ziagen)

Abacavir often is used in combination with lamivudine and zidovudine and with either a NNRTI or protease inhibitor. Fatal hypersensitivity reactions have been associated with abacavir use. Anyone developing signs or symptoms of hypersensitivity, including fever, skin rash, fatigue, nausea, vomiting, diarrhea, or abdominal pain, should discontinue abacavir immediately. Abacavir *should not* be restarted after a hypersensitivity reaction because more severe symptoms recur within hours and may include life-threatening hypotension and death.

Emtricitabine (Emtriva)

Emtricitabine is a synthetic nucleoside analogue of cytosine that is indicated, in combination with other antiretroviral agents such as didanosine and efavirenz, for the treatment of HIV-1-infected adults.

Non-nucleoside reverse transcriptase inhibitors

NNRTIs have been of considerable interest in the development of simplified highly active antiretroviral treatment regimens because the pharmacokinetic profiles for some of these drugs allow once-daily or twice-daily administration. NNRTIs also inhibit HIV reverse transcriptase, but do not require intracellular activation. The three NNRTIs currently available are hepatically metabolized by cytochrome P-450 enzymes. As a result, significant drug-drug interactions can occur. Efavirenz and nevirapine induce CYP3A4, whereas delavirdine is the only NNRTI that inhibits CYP3A4, causing concentrations of concomitant drugs metabolized by the same pathway to be increased. Because hepatic enzyme activity is depressed during the postnatal period, significant alterations in the disposition of this class of drugs may occur. Data on the pharmacokinetics of NNRTIs in children are limited. Immature enzymatic activity in newborns is evident by the decreased elimination of nevirapine in this group of patients.

Nevirapine (Viramune)

Nevirapine is a NNRTI that is structurally similar to the benzodiazepines. Because of the rapid and invariable appearance of resistance, it is not used as monotherapy. The potency of nevirapine ensures its utility in combination therapy, however, particularly in three-drug regimens. The major side effect of nevirapine is the development of a rash. The most severe form of rash is a Stevens-Johnson syndrome, requiring discontinuation of therapy. The frequency and severity of rash can be diminished by starting treatment at a lower dose (usually 50% of the maintenance dose and escalating to full therapy after approximately 4 weeks).

Delavirdine (Rescriptor)

Delavirdine is used frequently as combination therapy with two NRTIs, such as zidovudine and didanosine, with or without a protease inhibitor. Dosing recommendations for delavirdine in pediatric patients are not available, and there is no commercially available liquid formulation. Delavirdine has a myriad of drug interactions. Drugs that decrease delavirdine levels include antacids, phenytoin, phenobarbital, carbamazepine, rifabutin (with concomitant increase in rifabutin levels), rifampin, clarithromycin (with concomitant increase in clarithromycin levels), H_2 inhibitors (eg, cimetidine, ranitidine), and nelfinavir. Delavirdine increases concentrations of saquinavir, nelfinavir, and indinavir when given in combination.

Efavirenz (Sustiva)

Efavirenz frequently is used in combination with two or more NRTIs, with or without a protease inhibitor. Efavirenz has produced numerous birth defects in animal models and is contraindicated in pregnancy. This contraindication has potential implications for its use in adolescent females, in whom consistent contraceptive use may be unreliable.

Protease inhibitors

Protease inhibitors represent a major advance in the treatment of HIV infection. The HIV protease enzyme is responsible for post-translational cleavage of polyproteins into smaller, more functional proteins. Protease inhibitors block this enzyme, leading to the production of immature noninfectious virions [179,180]. Protease inhibitors are large, lipophilic organic bases that also are metabolized by cytochrome P-450 enzymes and have the potential for significant drug-drug interactions. Although the pharmacokinetics of protease inhibitors have been evaluated in older children, it is imperative that pharmacokinetic data are determined in younger children because the activity of cytochrome P-450 enzymes vary with age.

Saquinavir (Fortovase)

Saquinavir is used in combination therapy with NRTIs or NNRTIs. Because of poor oral bioavailability, saquinavir is not the protease inhibitor of choice in the management of HIV infections. Its use in combination with ritonavir is potentially beneficial, however. Saquinavir is metabolized by the cytochrome P-450 enzyme system; ritonavir and nelfinavir increase the plasma levels of saquinavir, a fact that has been used in the development of combination protease inhibitor therapies. Because saquinavir concentrations are substantially diminished by efavirenz, the two drugs should not be used together. Pediatric doses for saquinavir have not been established.

Ritonavir (Norvir)

Ritonavir is a peptide-like inhibitor of HIV proteases that is used in combination with NRTIs or NNRTIs. Adverse reactions associated with ritonavir therapy include nausea, vomiting, anorexia, and taste perversion. Ritonavir should be taken with meals to reduce the taste and nausea-inducing effects. Ritonavir syrup can be mixed with a variety of products, particularly products with high fat content, to improve taste. Ritonavir increases levels of saquinavir, and as such low doses of ritonavir sometimes are used in combination with saquinavir to achieve higher saquinavir concentrations.

Indinavir (Crixivan)

Indinavir is administered with NRTIs or NNRTIs. Administration of indinavir should be accompanied by a light snack and not with antacids or didanosine. Adverse reactions associated with indinavir therapy include nephrolithiasis, hematuria, and occasionally hyperbilirubinemia.

Nelfinavir (Viracept)

Nelfinavir is given in combination with NRTIs or NNRTIs. Adverse events associated with nelfinavir administration include diarrhea, rash, leukopenia, and neutropenia.

Amprenavir (Agenerase)

Amprenavir has exhibited synergistic anti-HIV-1 activity in vitro in combination with abacavir, zidovudine, didanosine, or saquinavir and additive anti-HIV-1 activity in combination with indinavir, nelfinavir, and ritonavir. In vivo correlations for these combinations have not been studied adequately to ensure that they also occur. When using this protease inhibitor in pediatric patients, the quantity of propylene glycol in the product precludes its use in children younger than 4 years old.

Lopinavir/Ritonavir (Kaletra)

Lopinavir-ritonavir combination is a new inhibitor of HIV protease. The addition of ritonavir enhances the concentrations of lopinavir that can be achieved after oral administration. It is given in combination with NRTIs or NNRTIs. Because of its ritonavir component, lopinavir-ritonavir liquid has a poorly tolerated taste.

Atazanavir (Reyataz)

Atazanavir is an azapeptide inhibitor of HIV-1 protease that is used in combination with other antiretroviral agents, such as two NRTIs, for the treatment of HIV-1 infection. The drug interaction list associated with atazanavir is extensive, necessitating careful review and consideration before initiating HIV treatment with this compound. Coadministration of atazanavir is *contraindicated* with drugs that are highly dependent on CYP3A for clearance and for which elevated plasma concentrations are associated with serious or life-threatening events; these drugs are midazolam, triazolam, dihydroergotamine, ergotamine, ergonovine, methylergonovine, cisapride, and pimozide. Other drugs that *should not* be used with atazanavir include rifampin, irinotecan, bepridil, lovastatin, simvastatin, indinavir, proton-pump inhibitors, and St. John's wort (*Hypericum perforatum*). Atazanavir has been shown to prolong the P-R interval on the electrocardiogram in a concentration-dependent and dose-dependent fashion in some patients. Most patients taking atazanavir experience asymptomatic elevations in indirect (unconjugated) bilirubin related to inhibition of UDP-glucuronosyl transferase. This hyperbilirubinemia is reversible on discontinuation of atazanavir. Because of the risk of kernicterus, atazanavir should not be administered to pediatric patients younger than age 3 months.

Fusion inhibitors

A promising new class of compounds that has received FDA approval is the fusion inhibitors. This class interferes with the entry of HIV-1 into cells through the inhibition of viral fusion to cell membranes. Of this new class, only enfuvirtide is commercially available currently.

Enfuvirtide (T20, Fuzeon)

Enfuvirtide interferes with the entry of HIV-1 into cells by inhibiting fusion of viral and cellular membranes. In combination with other antiretroviral agents, it is indicated for the treatment of HIV-1 infection in treatment-experienced patients with evidence of HIV-1 replication despite ongoing antiretroviral therapy. Enfuvirtide exhibits additive to synergistic effects in cell culture assays when combined with individual members of various antiretroviral classes, including zidovudine, lamivudine, nelfinavir, indinavir, and efavirenz.

Summary

The pace of discovery and development of new antiviral agents has increased dramatically since the 1980s. Antiviral drugs are currently available for the treatment of herpesvirus infections (HSV, VZV, CMV), respiratory virus infections (influenza A, influenza B, RSV), hepatitis virus infections (HBV, HCV), HPV infections, and HIV infections. The safety profiles of the various antiviral agents vary from drug to drug, necessitating a thorough understanding of each antiviral agent being used. Two factors that can limit the utility of antiviral drugs are toxicity and the development of antiviral resistance. The development of resistance is not a frequent issue among immunocompetent patients. Resistance most commonly develops in immunocompromised persons receiving antiviral treatment for prolonged periods.

References

[1] Keating MR. Antiviral agents. Mayo Clin Proc 1992;67:160–78.

[2] Centers for Disease Control and Prevention. Sexually transmitted diseases treatment guidelines 2002. MMWR Morb Mortal Wkly Rep 2002;51(RR-6):12–7.

[3] Bryson YJ, Dillon M, Lovett M, et al. Treatment of first episodes of genital herpes simplex virus infection with oral acyclovir: a randomized double-blind controlled trial in normal subjects. N Engl J Med 1983;308:916–21.

[4] Mertz GJ, Critchlow CW, Benedetti J, et al. Double-blind placebo-controlled trial of oral acyclovir in first-episode genital herpes simplex virus infection. JAMA 1984;252:1147–51.

[5] Tyring SK, Douglas Jr JM, Corey L, Spruance SL, Esmann J, The Valaciclovir International Study Group. A randomized, placebo-controlled comparison of oral valacyclovir and acyclovir in immunocompetent patients with recurrent genital herpes infections. Arch Dermatol 1998; 134:185–91.

[6] Douglas JM, Critchlow C, Benedetti J, et al. A double-blind study of oral acyclovir for suppression of recurrences of genital herpes simplex virus infection. N Engl J Med 1984; 310:1551–6.

[7] Mindel A, Faherty A, Carney O, Patou G, Freris M, Williams P. Dosage and safety of long-term suppressive acyclovir therapy for recurrent genital herpes. Lancet 1988;1:926–8.

[8] Mertz GJ, Jones CC, Mills J, et al. Long-term acyclovir suppression of frequently recurring genital herpes simplex virus infection: a multicenter double-blind trial. JAMA 1988;260: 201–6.

[9] Straus SE, Takiff HE, Seidlin M, et al. Suppression of frequently recurring genital herpes: a placebo-controlled double-blind trial of oral acyclovir. N Engl J Med 1984;310:1545–50.
[10] Mertz GJ, Eron L, Kaufman R, et al. Prolonged continuous versus intermittent oral acyclovir treatment in normal adults with frequently recurring genital herpes simplex virus infection. Am J Med 1988;85:14–9.
[11] Wald A, Corey L, Cone R, Hobson A, Davis G, Zeh J. Frequent genital herpes simplex virus 2 shedding in immunocompetent women: effect of acyclovir treatment. J Clin Invest 1997;99: 1092–7.
[12] Wald A, Zeh J, Barnum G, Davis LG, Corey L. Suppression of subclinical shedding of herpes simplex virus type 2 with acyclovir. Ann Intern Med 1996;124:8–15.
[13] Aoki FY, Law BJ, Hammond GW, et al. Acyclovir (ACV) suspension for treatment of acute herpes simplex virus (HSV) gingivostomatitis in children: a placebo (PL) controlled, double blind trial. Presented at 33rd Interscience Conference on Antimicrobial Agents and Chemotherapy. New Orleans. Abstract #1530. October 17–20, 1993.
[14] Raborn GW, McGaw WT, Grace M, Percy J. Treatment of herpes labialis with acyclovir: review of three clinical trials. Am J Med 1988;85:39–42.
[15] Raborn GW, McGaw WT, Grace M, Tyrrell LD, Samuels SM. Oral acyclovir and herpes labialis: a randomized, double-blind, placebo-controlled study. J Am Dent Assoc 1987;115:38–42.
[16] Spruance SL, Stewart JC, Rowe NH, McKeough MB, Wenerstrom G, Freeman DJ. Treatment of recurrent herpes simplex labialis with oral acyclovir. J Infect Dis 1990;161:185–90.
[17] Spruance SL, Hamill ML, Hoge WS, Davis LG, Mills J. Acyclovir prevents reactivation of herpes simplex labialis in skiers. JAMA 1988;260:1597–9.
[18] Gold D, Corey L. Acyclovir prophylaxis for herpes simplex virus infection. Antimicrob Agents Chemother 1987;31:361–7.
[19] Spruance SL, Freeman DJ, Stewart JC, et al. The natural history of ultraviolet radiation-induced herpes simplex labialis and response to therapy with peroral and topical formulations of acyclovir. J Infect Dis 1991;163:728–34.
[20] Rooney JF, Straus SE, Mannix ML, et al. Oral acyclovir to suppress frequently recurrent herpes labialis: a double-blind, placebo-controlled trial. Ann Intern Med 1993;118:268–72.
[21] Whitley RJ, Alford CA, Hirsch MS, et al. Vidarabine versus acyclovir therapy in herpes simplex encephalitis. N Engl J Med 1986;314:144–9.
[22] Skoldenberg B, Forsgren M, Alestig K, et al. Acyclovir versus vidarabine in herpes simplex encephalitis: randomised multicentre study in consecutive Swedish patients. Lancet 1984;2: 707–11.
[23] Kimberlin DW, Lin CY, Jacobs RF, et al. Safety and efficacy of high-dose intravenous acyclovir in the management of neonatal herpes simplex virus infections. Pediatrics 2001;108:230–8.
[24] American Academy of Pediatrics. Herpes simplex. In: Pickering LK, editor. Red Book: 2003 report of the Committee on Infectious Diseases. 26th edition. Elk Grove Village (IL): American Academy of Pediatrics; 2003. p. 344–53.
[25] Whitley RJ, Nahmias AJ, Soong SJ, Galasso GG, Fleming CL, Alford CA. Vidarabine therapy of neonatal herpes simplex virus infection. Pediatrics 1980;66:495–501.
[26] Wade JC, Newton B, McLaren C, Flournoy N, Keeney RE, Meyers JD. Intravenous acyclovir to treat mucocutaneous herpes simplex virus infection after marrow transplantation: a double-blind trial. Ann Intern Med 1982;96:265–9.
[27] Kimberlin DW, Prober CG. Antiviral agents. In: Long SS, Pickering LK, Prober CG, editors. Principles and practice of pediatric infectious diseases. 2nd edition. Philadelphia: Churchill Livingstone; 2003. p. 1527–47.
[28] Meyers JD, Wade JC, Mitchell CD, et al. Multicenter collaborative trial of intravenous acyclovir for treatment of mucocutaneous herpes simplex virus infection in the immunocompromised host. Am J Med 1982;73:229–35.
[29] Shepp DH, Newton BA, Dandliker PS, Flournoy N, Meyers JD. Oral acyclovir therapy for mucocutaneous herpes simplex virus infections in immunocompromised marrow transplant recipients. Ann Intern Med 1985;102:783–5.
[30] Hovding G. A comparison between acyclovir and trifluorothymidine ophthalmic ointment in

the treatment of epithelial dendritic keratitis: a double blind, randomized parallel group trial. Acta Ophthalmol (Copenh) 1989;67:51–4.

[31] Herpetic Eye Disease Study Group. Acyclovir for the prevention of recurrent herpes simplex virus eye disease. N Engl J Med 1998;339:300–6.

[32] Herpetic Eye Disease Study Group. Oral acyclovir for herpes simplex virus eye disease: effect on prevention of epithelial keratitis and stromal keratitis. Arch Ophthalmol 2000;118: 1030–6.

[33] Whitley RJ. Therapeutic approaches to varicella-zoster virus infections. J Infect Dis 1992; 166:S51–7.

[34] Dunkle LM, Arvin AM, Whitley RJ, et al. A controlled trial of acyclovir for chickenpox in normal children. N Engl J Med 1991;325:1539–44.

[35] Balfour Jr HH, Rotbart HA, Feldman S, et al. Acyclovir treatment of varicella in otherwise healthy adolescents. J Pediatr 1992;120:627–33.

[36] Wallace MR, Bowler WA, Murray NB, Brodine SK, Oldfield 3rd EC. Treatment of adult varicella with oral acyclovir: a randomized, placebo-controlled trial. Ann Intern Med 1992; 117:358–63.

[37] Whitley RJ, Straus SE. Therapy for varicella-zoster virus infections: where do we stand? Infect Dis Clin Pract 1993;2:100–8.

[38] McGill J, MacDonald DR, Fall C, McKendrick GD, Copplestone A. Intravenous acyclovir in acute herpes zoster infection. J Infect 1983;6:157–61.

[39] Wood MJ, Ogan PH, McKendrick MW, Care CD, McGill JI, Webb EM. Efficacy of oral acyclovir treatment of acute herpes zoster. Am J Med 1988;85:79–83.

[40] Englund JA, Zimmerman ME, Swierkosz EM, Goodman JL, Scholl DR, Balfour Jr HH. Herpes simplex virus resistant to acyclovir: a study in a tertiary care center. Ann Intern Med 1990;112:416–22.

[41] Gateley A, Gander RM, Johnson PC, Kit S, Otsuka H, Kohl S. Herpes simplex virus type 2 meningoencephalitis resistant to acyclovir in a patient with AIDS. J Infect Dis 1990;161: 711–5.

[42] Kost RG, Hill EL, Tigges M, Straus SE. Brief report: recurrent acyclovir-resistant genital herpes in an immunocompetent patient. N Engl J Med 1993;329:1777–82.

[43] Kimberlin DW, Coen DM, Biron KK, et al. Molecular mechanisms of antiviral resistance. Antiviral Res 1995;26:369–401.

[44] Wagstaff AJ, Faulds D, Goa KL. Aciclovir: a reappraisal of its antiviral activity, pharmacokinetic properties and therapeutic efficacy. Drugs 1994;47:153–205.

[45] Kimberlin D, Powell D, Gruber W, et al. Administration of oral acyclovir suppressive therapy after neonatal herpes simplex virus disease limited to the skin, eyes and mouth: results of a phase I/II trial. Pediatr Infect Dis J 1996;15:247–54.

[46] Kimberlin DW, Lin CY, Jacobs RF, et al. Natural history of neonatal herpes simplex virus infections in the acyclovir era. Pediatrics 2001;108:223–9.

[47] Revankar SG, Applegate AL, Markovitz DM. Delirium associated with acyclovir treatment in a patient with renal failure. Clin Infect Dis 1995;21:435–6.

[48] Stone KM, Reiff-Eldridge R, White AD, et al. Pregnancy outcomes following systemic prenatal acyclovir exposure: conclusions from the International Acyclovir Pregnancy Registry, 1984–1999. Birth Defects Res 2004;70:201–7.

[49] Jacobson MA. Valaciclovir (BW256U87): the L-valyl ester of acyclovir. J Med Virol 1993; (Suppl 1):150–3.

[50] Fife KH, Barbarash RA, Rudolph T, Degregorio B, Roth R, The Valaciclovir International Herpes Simplex Virus Study Group. Valaciclovir versus acyclovir in the treatment of first-episode genital herpes infection: results of an international, multicenter, double-blind, randomized clinical trial. Sex Transm Dis 1997;24:481–6.

[51] Spruance SL, Tyring SK, DeGregorio B, Miller C, Beutner K, The Valaciclovir HSV Study Group. A large-scale, placebo-controlled, dose-ranging trial of peroral valaciclovir for episodic treatment of recurrent herpes genitalis. Arch Intern Med 1996;156:1729–35.

[52] Leone PA, Trottier S, Miller JM. Valacyclovir for episodic treatment of genital herpes:

a shorter 3-day treatment course compared with 5-day treatment. Clin Infect Dis 2002;34: 958–62.

[53] Reitano M, Tyring S, Lang W, et al. Valaciclovir for the suppression of recurrent genital herpes simplex virus infection: a large-scale dose range-finding study. J Infect Dis 1998;178:603–10.

[54] Spruance SL, Jones TM, Blatter MM, et al. High-dose, short-duration, early valacyclovir therapy for episodic treatment of cold sores: results of two randomized, placebo-controlled, multicenter studies. Antimicrob Agents Chemother 2003;47:1072–80.

[55] Baker D, Eisen D. Valacyclovir for prevention of recurrent herpes labialis: 2 double-blind, placebo-controlled studies. Cutis 2003;71:239–42.

[56] Baker DA, Deeter RG, Redder K, Phillips JA. Valacyclovir effective for suppression of recurrent HSV-1 herpes labialis. Presented at 40th Interscience Conference on Antimicrobial Agents and Chemotherapy. Toronto, Ontario, Canada. Abstract #464. September 17–20, 2000.

[57] Beutner KR, Friedman DJ, Forszpaniak C, Andersen PL, Wood MJ. Valaciclovir compared with acyclovir for improved therapy for herpes zoster in immunocompetent adults. Antimicrob Agents Chemother 1995;39:1546–53.

[58] Soul-Lawton J, Seaber E, On N, Wootton R, Rolan P, Posner J. Absolute bioavailability and metabolic disposition of valaciclovir, the L-valyl ester of acyclovir, following oral administration to humans. Antimicrob Agents Chemother 1995;39:2759–64.

[59] Bell WR, Chulay JD, Feinberg JE. Manifestations resembling thrombotic microangiopathy in patients with advanced human immunodeficiency virus (HIV) disease in a cytomegalovirus prophylaxis trial (ACTG 204). Medicine 1997;76:369–80.

[60] Andrei G, Snoeck R, Schols D, Goubau P, Desmyter J, De Clercq E. Comparative activity of selected antiviral compounds against clinical isolates of human cytomegalovirus. Eur J Clin Microbiol Infect Dis 1991;10:1026–33.

[61] Safrin S, Cherrington J, Jaffe HS. Cidofovir: review of current and potential clinical uses. Adv Exp Med Biol 1999;458:111–20.

[62] Lalezari JP, Drew WL, Glutzer E, et al. Treatment with intravenous (S)-1-[3-hydroxy-2-(phosphonylmethoxy)propyl]-cytosine of acyclovir-resistant mucocutaneous infection with herpes simplex virus in a patient with AIDS. J Infect Dis 1994;170:570–2.

[63] Studies of Ocular Complications of AIDS Research Group in collaboration with the AIDS Clinical Trials Group. Parenteral cidofovir for cytomegalovirus retinitis in patients with AIDS: the HPMPC peripheral cytomegalovirus retinitis trial: a randomized, controlled trial. Ann Intern Med 1997;126:264–74.

[64] Lalezari JP, Stagg RJ, Kuppermann BD, et al. Intravenous cidofovir for peripheral cytomegalovirus retinitis in patients with AIDS: a randomized, controlled trial. Ann Intern Med 1997;126:257–63.

[65] Lurain NS, Spafford LE, Thompson KD. Mutation in the UL97 open reading frame of human cytomegalovirus strains resistant to ganciclovir. J Virol 1994;68:4427–31.

[66] Lurain NS, Thompson KD, Holmes EW, Read GS. Point mutations in the DNA polymerase gene of human cytomegalovirus that result in resistance to antiviral agents. J Virol 1992;66: 7146–52.

[67] Kimberlin DW, Crumpacker CS, Straus SE, et al. Antiviral resistance in clinical practice. Antiviral Res 1995;26:423–38.

[68] Ho HT, Woods KL, Bronson JJ, De Boeck H, Martin JC, Hitchcock MJ. Intracellular metabolism of the antiherpes agent (S)-1-[3-hydroxy-2-(phosphonylmethoxy)propyl]cytosine. Mol Pharmacol 1992;41:197–202.

[69] Cundy KC, Petty BG, Flaherty J, et al. Clinical pharmacokinetics of cidofovir in human immunodeficiency virus-infected patients. Antimicrob Agents Chemother 1995;39:1247–52.

[70] Lalezari JP, Drew WL, Glutzer E, et al. (S)-1-[3-hydroxy-2-(phosphonylmethoxy)propyl] cytosine (cidofovir): results of a phase I/II study of a novel antiviral nucleotide analogue. J Infect Dis 1995;171:788–96.

[71] Sacks SL, Aoki FY, Diaz-Mitoma F, Sellors J, Shafran SD, The Canadian Famciclovir Study Group. Patient-initiated, twice-daily oral famciclovir for early recurrent genital herpes: a randomized, double-blind multicenter trial. JAMA 1996;276:44–9.

[72] Diaz-Mitoma F, Sibbald RG, Shafran SD, Boon R, Saltzman RL, The Collaborative Famciclovir Genital Herpes Research Group. Oral famciclovir for the suppression of recurrent genital herpes: a randomized controlled trial. JAMA 1998;280:887–92.

[73] Mertz GJ, Loveless MO, Levin MJ, et al. Oral famciclovir for suppression of recurrent genital herpes simplex virus infection in women: a multicenter, double-blind, placebo-controlled trial. Arch Intern Med 1997;157:343–9.

[74] Boon R, Goodman JJ, Martinez J, Marks GL, Gamble M, Welch C. Penciclovir cream for the treatment of sunlight-induced herpes simplex labialis: a randomized, double-blind, placebo-controlled trial. Penciclovir Cream Herpes Labialis Study Group. Clin Ther 2000;22: 76–90.

[75] Spruance SL, Rea TL, Thoming C, Tucker R, Saltzman R, Boon R. Penciclovir cream for the treatment of herpes simplex labialis: a randomized, multicenter, double-blind, placebo-controlled trial. Topical Penciclovir Collaborative Study Group. JAMA 1997;277:1374–9.

[76] Tyring S, Barbarash RA, Nahlik JE, et al. Famciclovir for the treatment of acute herpes zoster: effects on acute disease and postherpetic neuralgia: a randomized, double-blind, placebo-controlled trial. Ann Intern Med 1995;123:89–96.

[77] Boike SC, Pue MA, Freed MI, et al. Pharmacokinetics of famciclovir in subjects with varying degrees of renal impairment. Clin Pharmacol Ther 1994;55:418–26.

[78] Drew WL. Cytomegalovirus infection in patients with AIDS. Clin Infect Dis 1992;14:608–15.

[79] Dieterich DT, Poles MA, Lew EA, et al. Concurrent use of ganciclovir and foscarnet to treat cytomegalovirus infection in AIDS patients. J Infect Dis 1993;167:1184–8.

[80] Anduze-Faris BM, Fillet AM, Gozlan J, et al. Induction and maintenance therapy of cytomegalovirus central nervous system infection in HIV-infected patients. AIDS 2000;14: 517–24.

[81] Dieterich DT, Kotler DP, Busch DF, et al. Ganciclovir treatment of cytomegalovirus colitis in AIDS: a randomized, double-blind, placebo-controlled multicenter study. J Infect Dis 1993; 167:278–82.

[82] Reed EC, Wolford JL, Kopecky KJ, et al. Ganciclovir for the treatment of cytomegalovirus gastroenteritis in bone marrow transplant patients: a randomized, placebo-controlled trial. Ann Intern Med 1990;112:505–10.

[83] Reed EC, Bowden RA, Dandliker PS, Lilleby KE, Meyers JD. Treatment of cytomegalovirus pneumonia with ganciclovir and intravenous cytomegalovirus immunoglobulin in patients with bone marrow transplants. Ann Intern Med 1988;109:783–8.

[84] Emanuel D, Cunningham I, Jules-Elysee K, et al. Cytomegalovirus pneumonia after bone marrow transplantation successfully treated with the combination of ganciclovir and high-dose intravenous immune globulin. Ann Intern Med 1988;109:777–82.

[85] Rayes N, Oettle H, Schmidt CA, et al. Preemptive therapy in CMV-antigen positive patients after liver transplantation–a prospective trial. Ann Transplant 1999;4:12–7.

[86] Kelly J, Hurley D, Raghu G. Comparison of the efficacy and cost effectiveness of pre-emptive therapy as directed by CMV antigenemia and prophylaxis with ganciclovir in lung transplant recipients. J Heart Lung Transplant 2000;19:355–9.

[87] Mori T, Okamoto S, Matsuoka S, et al. Risk-adapted pre-emptive therapy for cytomegalovirus disease in patients undergoing allogeneic bone marrow transplantation. Bone Marrow Transplant 2000;25:765–9.

[88] Reddy V, Hao Y, Lipton J, et al. Management of allogeneic bone marrow transplant recipients at risk for cytomegalovirus disease using a surveillance bronchoscopy and prolonged pre-emptive ganciclovir therapy. J Clin Virol 1999;13:149–59.

[89] Egan JJ, Lomax J, Barber L, et al. Preemptive treatment for the prevention of cytomegalovirus disease: in lung and heart transplant recipients. Transplantation 1998;65:747–52.

[90] Duncan SR, Paradis IL, Dauber JH, Yousem SA, Hardesty RL, Griffith BP. Ganciclovir prophylaxis for cytomegalovirus infections in pulmonary allograft recipients. Am Rev Respir Dis 1992;146:1213–5.

[91] Merigan TC, Renlund DG, Keay S, et al. A controlled trial of ganciclovir to prevent cytomegalovirus disease after heart transplantation. N Engl J Med 1992;326:1182–6.

[92] Seu P, Winston DJ, Holt CD, Kaldas F, Busuttil RW. Long-term ganciclovir prophylaxis for successful prevention of primary cytomegalovirus (CMV) disease in CMV-seronegative liver transplant recipients with CMV-seropositive donors. Transplantation 1997;64:1614–7.
[93] Kimberlin DW, Lin CY, Sanchez PJ, et al. Effect of ganciclovir therapy on hearing in symptomatic congenital cytomegalovirus disease involving the central nervous system: a randomized, controlled trial. J Pediatr 2003;143:16–25.
[94] Markham A, Faulds D. Ganciclovir: an update of its therapeutic use in cytomegalovirus infection. Drugs 1994;48:455–84.
[95] Frenkel LM, Capparelli EV, Dankner WM, et al. Oral ganciclovir in children: pharmacokinetics, safety, tolerance, and antiviral effects. J Infect Dis 2000;182:1616–24.
[96] Jacobson MA, de Miranda P, Cederberg DM, et al. Human pharmacokinetics and tolerance of oral ganciclovir. Antimicrob Agents Chemother 1987;31:1251–4.
[97] Fletcher C, Sawchuk R, Chinnock B, de Miranda P, Balfour Jr HH. Human pharmacokinetics of the antiviral drug DHPG. Clin Pharmacol Ther 1986;40:281–6.
[98] Swan SK, Munar MY, Wigger MA, Bennett WM. Pharmacokinetics of ganciclovir in a patient undergoing hemodialysis. Am J Kidney Dis 1991;17:69–72.
[99] Spector SA, Hsia K, Wolf D, Shinkai M, Smith I. Molecular detection of human cytomegalovirus and determination of genotypic ganciclovir resistance in clinical specimens. Clin Infect Dis 1995;21:S170–3.
[100] Cocohoba JM, McNicholl IR. Valganciclovir: an advance in cytomegalovirus therapeutics. Ann Pharmacother 2002;36:1075–9.
[101] Martin DF, Sierra-Madero J, Walmsley S, et al. A controlled trial of valganciclovir as induction therapy for cytomegalovirus retinitis. N Engl J Med 2002;346:1119–26.
[102] Jung D, Dorr A. Single-dose pharmacokinetics of valganciclovir in HIV- and CMV-seropositive subjects. J Clin Pharmacol 1999;39:800–4.
[103] Brown F, Banken L, Saywell K, Arum I. Pharmacokinetics of valganciclovir and ganciclovir following multiple oral dosages of valganciclovir in HIV- and CMV-seropositive volunteers. Clin Pharmacokinet 1999;37:167–76.
[104] Carmine AA, Brogden RN, Heel RC, Speight TM, Avery GS. Trifluridine: a review of its antiviral activity and therapeutic use in the topical treatment of viral eye infections. Drugs 1982;23:329–53.
[105] Pavan-Langston D. Major ocular viral infections. In: Galasso GJ, Whitley RJ, Merigan TC, editors. Antiviral agents and viral diseases of man. 3rd edition. New York: Raven Press; 1990. p. 183–233.
[106] Hyndiuk RA, Hull DS, Schultz RO, Chin GN. Adenine arabinoside in idoxuridine unresponsive and intolerant herpetic keratitis. Am J Ophthalmol 1975;79:655–8.
[107] Pavan-Langston D, Dohlman CH. A double blind clinical study of adenine arabinoside therapy of viral keratoconjunctivitis. Am J Ophthalmol 1972;74:81–8.
[108] Coster DJ, McKinnon JR, McGill JI, Jones BR, Fraunfelder FT. Clinical evaluation of adenine arabinoside and trifluorothymidine in the treatment of corneal ulcers caused by herpes simplex virus. J Infect Dis 1976;133:A173.
[109] Jacobson MA, Drew WL, Feinberg J, et al. Foscarnet therapy for ganciclovir-resistant cytomegalovirus retinitis in patients with AIDS. J Infect Dis 1991;163:1348–51.
[110] Nelson MR, Connolly GM, Hawkins DA, Gazzard BG. Foscarnet in the treatment of cytomegalovirus infection of the esophagus and colon in patients with the acquired immune deficiency syndrome. Am J Gastroenterol 1991;86:876–81.
[111] Youle M, Chanas A, Gazzard B. Treatment of acquired immune deficiency syndrome (AIDS)-related pneumonitis with foscarnet: a double-blind placebo controlled study. J Infect 1990;20: 41–50.
[112] Safrin S, Berger TG, Gilson I, et al. Foscarnet therapy in five patients with AIDS and acyclovir-resistant varicella-zoster virus infection. Ann Intern Med 1991;115:19–21.
[113] Safrin S, Crumpacker C, Chatis P, et al. A controlled trial comparing foscarnet with vidarabine for acyclovir-resistant mucocutaneous herpes simplex in the acquired immunodeficiency syndrome. N Engl J Med 1991;325:551–5.

[114] Safrin S, Kemmerly S, Plotkin B, et al. Foscarnet-resistant herpes simplex virus infection in patients with AIDS. J Infect Dis 1994;169:193–6.
[115] Snoeck R, Andrei G, Gerard M, et al. Successful treatment of progressive mucocutaneous infection due to acyclovir- and foscarnet-resistant herpes simplex virus with (S)-1-(3-hydroxy-2-phosphonylmethoxypropyl)cytosine (HPMPC). Clin Infect Dis 1994;18:570–8.
[116] Studies of Ocular Complications of AIDS Research Group in collaboration with the AIDS Clinical Trials Group. Mortality in patients with the acquired immunodeficiency syndrome treated with either foscarnet or ganciclovir for cytomegalovirus retinitis. N Engl J Med 1992;326:213–20.
[117] Valette M, Allard JP, Aymard M, Millet V. Susceptibilities to rimantadine of influenza A/H1N1 and A/H3N2 viruses isolated during the epidemics of 1988 to 1989 and 1989 to 1990. Antimicrob Agents Chemother 1993;37:2239–40.
[118] Couch RB. Prevention and treatment of influenza. N Engl J Med 2000;343:1778–87.
[119] Douglas Jr RG. Prophylaxis and treatment of influenza. N Engl J Med 1990;322:443–50.
[120] Hall CB, Dolin R, Gala CL, et al. Children with influenza A infection: treatment with rimantadine. Pediatrics 1987;80:275–82.
[121] Van Voris LP, Newell PM. Antivirals for the chemoprophylaxis and treatment of influenza. Semin Respir Infect 1992;7:61–70.
[122] Demicheli V, Jefferson T, Rivetti D, Deeks J. Prevention and early treatment of influenza in healthy adults. Vaccine 2000;18:957–1030.
[123] Hayden FG, Couch RB. Clinical and epidemiologic importance of influenza A viruses resistant to amantadine and rimantadine. Rev Med Virol 1992;2:89–96.
[124] Aoki FY, Sitar DS. Clinical pharmacokinetics of amantadine hydrochloride. Clin Pharmacokinet 1988;14:35–51.
[125] Capparelli EV, Stevens RC, Chow MS, Izard M, Wills RJ. Rimantadine pharmacokinetics in healthy subjects and patients with end-stage renal failure. Clin Pharmacol Ther 1988;43:536–41.
[126] Horadam VW, Sharp JG, Smilack JD, et al. Pharmacokinetics of amantadine hydrochloride in subjects with normal and impaired renal function. Ann Intern Med 1981;94:454–8.
[127] Dolin R, Reichman RC, Madore HP, Maynard R, Linton PN, Webber-Jones J. A controlled trial of amantadine and rimantadine in the prophylaxis of influenza A infection. N Engl J Med 1982;307:580–4.
[128] Clover RD, Crawford SA, Abell TD, Ramsey Jr CN, Glezen WP, Couch RB. Effectiveness of rimantadine prophylaxis of children within families. Am J Dis Child 1986;140:706–9.
[129] Munoz FM, Galasso GJ, Gwaltney Jr JM, et al. Current research on influenza and other respiratory viruses: II international symposium. Antiviral Res 2000;46:91–124.
[130] Treanor JJ, Hayden FG, Vrooman PS, et al. Efficacy and safety of the oral neuraminidase inhibitor oseltamivir in treating acute influenza: a randomized controlled trial. US Oral Neuraminidase Study Group. JAMA 2000;283:1016–24.
[131] Nicholson KG, Aoki FY, Osterhaus AD, et al. Efficacy and safety of oseltamivir in treatment of acute influenza: a randomised controlled trial. Neuraminidase Inhibitor Flu Treatment Investigator Group. Lancet 2000;355:1845–50.
[132] Wood ND, Aitken M, Sharp S, Evison H. Tolerability and pharmacokinetics of the influenza neuraminidase inhibitor Ro-64–0802 (GS4071) following oral administration of the prodrug Ro-64–0796 (GS4104) to healthy male volunteers. Presented at 37th Interscience Conference on Antimicrobial Agents and Chemotherapy (ICAAC). Toronto. Abstract #A-123. September 28–October 1, 1997.
[133] Whitley RJ, Hayden FG, Reisinger KS, et al. Oral oseltamivir treatment of influenza in children. Pediatr Infect Dis J 2001;20:127–33.
[134] Kiso M, Mitamura K, Sakai-Tagawa Y, et al. Resistant influenza A viruses in children treated with oseltamivir: descriptive study. Lancet 2004;364:759–65.
[135] Monto AS, Robinson DP, Herlocher ML, Hinson Jr JM, Elliott MJ, Crisp A. Zanamivir in the prevention of influenza among healthy adults: a randomized controlled trial. JAMA 1999;282:31–5.

[136] Kaiser L, Henry D, Flack NP, Keene O, Hayden FG. Short-term treatment with zanamivir to prevent influenza: results of a placebo-controlled study. Clin Infect Dis 2000;30:587–9.

[137] Hayden FG, Gubareva LV, Monto AS, et al. Inhaled zanamivir for the prevention of influenza in families. Zanamivir Family Study Group. N Engl J Med 2000;343:1282–9.

[138] Makela MJ, Pauksens K, Rostila T, et al. Clinical efficacy and safety of the orally inhaled neuraminidase inhibitor zanamivir in the treatment of influenza: a randomized, double-blind, placebo-controlled European study. J Infect 2000;40:42–8.

[139] MIST (Management of Influenza in the Southern Hemisphere Trialists) Study Group. Randomised trial of efficacy and safety of inhaled zanamivir in treatment of influenza A and B virus infections. Lancet 1998;352:1877–81.

[140] Hedrick JA, Barzilai A, Behre U, et al. Zanamivir for treatment of symptomatic influenza A and B infection in children five to twelve years of age: a randomized controlled trial. Pediatr Infect Dis J 2000;19:410–7.

[141] Gubareva LV, Kaiser L, Hayden FG. Influenza virus neuraminidase inhibitors. Lancet 2000; 355:827–35.

[142] Gubareva LV, Matrosovich MN, Brenner MK, Bethell RC, Webster RG. Evidence for zanamivir resistance in an immunocompromised child infected with influenza B virus. J Infect Dis 1998;178:1257–62.

[143] Cass LM, Brown J, Pickford M, et al. Pharmacoscintigraphic evaluation of lung deposition of inhaled zanamivir in healthy volunteers. Clin Pharmacokinet 1999;1:21–31.

[144] Cass LM, Gunawardena KA, Macmahon MM, Bye A. Pulmonary function and airway responsiveness in mild to moderate asthmatics given repeated inhaled doses of zanamivir. Respir Med 2000;94:166–73.

[145] McCormick JB, King IJ, Webb PA, et al. Lassa fever: effective therapy with ribavirin. N Engl J Med 1986;314:20–6.

[146] Holmes GP, McCormick JB, Trock SC, et al. Lassa fever in the United States: investigation of a case and new guidelines for management. N Engl J Med 1990;323:1120–3.

[147] Poynard T, Marcellin P, Lee SS, et al. Randomised trial of interferon alpha2b plus ribavirin for 48 weeks or for 24 weeks versus interferon alpha2b plus placebo for 48 weeks for treatment of chronic infection with hepatitis C virus. International Hepatitis Interventional Therapy Group (IHIT). Lancet 1998;352:1426–32.

[148] McHutchison JG, Gordon SC, Schiff ER, et al. Interferon alfa-2b alone or in combination with ribavirin as initial treatment for chronic hepatitis C. Hepatitis Interventional Therapy Group. N Engl J Med 1998;339:1485–92.

[149] Huggins JW. Prospects for treatment of viral hemorrhagic fevers with ribavirin, a broad-spectrum antiviral drug. Rev Infect Dis 1989;11(Suppl):S750–61.

[150] Connor E, Morrison S, Lane J, Oleske J, Sonke RL, Connor J. Safety, tolerance, and pharmacokinetics of systemic ribavirin in children with human immunodeficiency virus infection. Antimicrob Agents Chemother 1993;37:532–9.

[151] Laskin OL, Longstreth JA, Hart CC, et al. Ribavirin disposition in high-risk patients for acquired immunodeficiency syndrome. Clin Pharmacol Ther 1987;41:546–55.

[152] Frankel LR, Wilson CW, Demers RR, et al. A technique for the administration of ribavirin to mechanically ventilated infants with severe respiratory syncytial virus infection. Crit Care Med 1987;15:1051–4.

[153] Centers for Disease Control and Prevention. Assessing exposures of health-care personnel to aerosols of ribavirin—California. MMWR Morb Mortal Wkly Rep 1988;37:560–3.

[154] Rodriguez WJ, Bui RH, Connor JD, et al. Environmental exposure of primary care personnel to ribavirin aerosol when supervising treatment of infants with respiratory syncytial virus infections. Antimicrob Agents Chemother 1987;31:1143–6.

[155] Borden EC, Fall LA. Interferons: biochemical, cell growth, inhibitory, and immunological effects. Prog Hematol 1981;350:1–64.

[156] Baron S, Coppenhaver DH, Dianzani F, et al. Introduction to the interferon system. In: Baron S, editor. Interferon: principles and medical applications. Galveston (TX): University of Texas Medical Branch; 1992. p. 1–15.

[157] Hirschman SZ. Current therapeutic approaches to viral hepatitis. Clin Infect Dis 1995;20: 741–3.

[158] Davis GL, Balart LA, Schiff ER, et al. Treatment of chronic hepatitis C with recombinant interferon alfa: a multicenter randomized, controlled trial. Hepatitis Interventional Therapy Group. N Engl J Med 1989;321:1501–6.

[159] Hagiwara H, Hayashi N, Mita E, et al. Detection of hepatitis C virus RNA in serum of patients with chronic hepatitis C treated with interferon-alpha. Hepatology 1992;15:37–41.

[160] Davis GL, Esteban-Mur R, Rustgi V, et al. Interferon alfa-2b alone or in combination with ribavirin for the treatment of relapse of chronic hepatitis C. International Hepatitis Interventional Therapy Group. N Engl J Med 1998;339:1493–9.

[161] Fried MW, Shiffman ML, Reddy KR, et al. Peginterferon alfa-2a plus ribavirin for chronic hepatitis C virus infection. N Engl J Med 2002;347:975–82.

[162] Eron LJ, Judson F, Tucker S, et al. Interferon therapy for condylomata acuminata. N Engl J Med 1986;315:1059–64.

[163] Healy GB, Gelber RD, Trowbridge AL, Grundfast KM, Ruben RJ, Price KN. Treatment of recurrent respiratory papillomatosis with human leukocyte interferon: results of a multicenter randomized clinical trial. N Engl J Med 1988;319:401–7.

[164] Leventhal BG, Kashima HK, Mounts P, et al. Long-term response of recurrent respiratory papillomatosis to treatment with lymphoblastoid interferon alfa-N1. N Engl J Med 1991;325: 613–7.

[165] Haglund S, Lundquist PG, Cantell K, Strander H. Interferon therapy in juvenile laryngeal papillomatosis. Arch Otolaryngol 1981;107:327–32.

[166] Steinberg BM, Gallagher T, Stoler M, Abramson AL. Persistence and expression of human papillomavirus during interferon therapy. Arch Otolaryngol Head Neck Surg 1988;114:27–32.

[167] Schuurman AM, Van Den Broek P. Results of treatment with alpha-interferon in adult-onset laryngeal papillomatosis. Clin Otolaryngol Allergy Sci 1986;11:447–53.

[168] Wills RJ. Clinical pharmacokinetics of interferons. Clin Pharmacokinet 1990;19:390–9.

[169] Barouki FM, Witter FR, Griffin DE, et al. Time course of interferon levels, antiviral state, 2′,5′-oligoadenylate synthetase and side effects in healthy men. J Interferon Res 1987;7:29–39.

[170] Renault PF, Hoofnagle JH. Side effects of alpha interferon. Semin Liver Dis 1989;9:273–7.

[171] McDonald EM, Mann AH, Thomas HC. Interferons as mediators of psychiatric morbidity. Lancet 1987;2:1175–8.

[172] CASL Hepatitis Consensus Group. Treatment of chronic viral hepatitis with alpha interferon: a consensus conference report. Can J Infect Dis 1994;5:107–12.

[173] Marcellin P, Chang TT, Lim SG, et al. Adefovir dipivoxil for the treatment of hepatitis B e antigen-positive chronic hepatitis B. N Engl J Med 2003;348:808–16.

[174] Dienstag JL, Schiff ER, Wright TL, et al. Lamivudine as initial treatment for chronic hepatitis B in the United States. N Engl J Med 1999;341:1256–63.

[175] Lai CL, Chien RN, Leung NW, et al. A one-year trial of lamivudine for chronic hepatitis B. Asia Hepatitis Lamivudine Study Group. N Engl J Med 1998;339:61–8.

[176] Hartman C, Berkowitz D, Shouval D, et al. Lamivudine treatment for chronic hepatitis B infection in children unresponsive to interferon. Pediatr Infect Dis J 2003;22:224–9.

[177] Gao WY, Shirasaka T, Johns DG, Broder S, Mitsuya H. Differential phosphorylation of azidothymidine, dideoxycytidine, and dideoxyinosine in resting and activated peripheral blood mononuclear cells. J Clin Invest 1993;91:2326–33.

[178] Havlir DV, Tierney C, Friedland GH, et al. In vivo antagonism with zidovudine plus stavudine combination therapy. J Infect Dis 2000;182:321–5.

[179] Debouck C. The HIV-1 protease as a therapeutic target for AIDS. AIDS Res Hum Retroviruses 1992;8:153–64.

[180] Kohl NE, Emini EA, Schleif WA, et al. Active human immunodeficiency virus protease is required for viral infectivity. Proc Natl Acad Sci U S A 1988;85:4686–90.

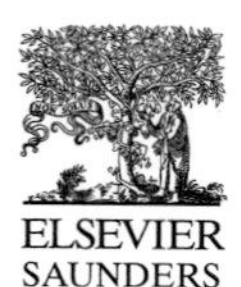

ELSEVIER
SAUNDERS

PEDIATRIC CLINICS
OF NORTH AMERICA

Pediatr Clin N Am 52 (2005) 869–894

Guidelines for the Selection of Antibacterial Therapy in Children

Alice L. Pong, MD, John S. Bradley, MD*

Children's Hospital and Health Center, 3020 Children's Way, MC 5041, San Diego, CA 92123, USA

Selection of appropriate anti-infective therapy can be challenging to the pediatrician. It is not sufficient to know the likely pathogens causing the infection and which antibiotics have been successful in the past. It also is necessary to know prevalent antibiotic resistance patterns and the effect that treatment might have on promoting the development of resistance in the specific patient being treated and in the general population. The evolution of penicillin-nonsusceptible *Streptococcus pneumoniae,* the increase in community-acquired methicillin-resistant *Staphylococcus aureus* (CA-MRSA), and the emergence of multidrug-resistant gram-negative pathogens are examples of how the susceptibility patterns of commonly treated bacteria can change. These changes might alter options for effective therapy dramatically.

Determining the appropriate dose of antibiotics for children also can be difficult. Clinical studies evaluating antimicrobial pharmacokinetics in neonates (from extremely low birth weight to full term), infants, and children are few in number compared with studies performed in adults. Doses often are extrapolated from data derived from adults. Adverse event profiles also are based in large part on studies performed in preclinical animal toxicology models or in clinical trials conducted in older subjects. The clinical relevance of understanding how effectively antibiotics inhibit or kill pathogens at the site of infection, termed *pharmacodynamics,* has been integrated only recently into clinical investigations conducted in adults [1]. Similar studies in children to validate these concepts do not exist. This article reviews factors important in the selection of antimicrobial agents in infants and children. Recommendations for antibiotic therapy for a wide range of infections occurring in children are provided.

* Corresponding author.
E-mail address: jbradley@chsd.org (J.S. Bradley).

0031-3955/05/$ – see front matter
doi:10.1016/j.pcl.2005.02.008

pediatric.theclinics.com

Factors affecting antibiotic selection

When choosing an antibacterial agent, the following factors are the most important to consider.

- *Microbiology.* What are the most common organisms causing the infection? What are the local antibiotic susceptibility patterns? Are resistance mechanisms likely already present in the pathogens; will additional mechanisms become apparent on exposure to the antibiotic?
- *Pharmacodynamics.* Would treatment with the agent result in the type of exposure known to optimize the desired biologic effect on the pathogens?
- *Pharmacokinetics.* Based on the expected absorption, metabolism, elimination, and distribution of the drug to the site of infection, what is the ideal route and dose of drug to prescribe?
- *Monte Carlo simulation* [2]. In the specific population being treated for any given tissue sites of infection and for any given pathogens, what risk of treatment failure is acceptable?
- *Host.* What host factors might affect drug selection and dosing?
- *Antibiotic adverse reactions.* Are there potential side effects that might affect the relative risks and benefits of therapy? What toxicities should be anticipated, either directly or as a result of drug-drug interactions?

Microbiology

Most infections occur as a result of disruption in host defenses (physical or immunologic) in combination with virulence factors of the bacteria. Highly virulent organisms cause disease in healthy and immunocompromised hosts, whereas low-virulence organisms usually are pathogenic only in immunocompromised hosts. In general, most organisms that cause community-acquired infections are part of the child's normal bacterial flora, resulting from exposure to other children in the community. Skin and soft tissue infections are caused most commonly by *S. aureus* or beta-hemolytic streptococci, whereas upper and lower respiratory tract infections are caused commonly by *S. pneumoniae* and nontypable *Haemophilus influenzae*. Resistance to antibiotics can occur with any organism. Local epidemiologic data are key to assessing the prevalent patterns of resistance in a community.

The susceptibility of a specific pathogen to a specific antibiotic can be measured in the microbiology laboratory by defining the lowest concentration of the antibiotic that can inhibit the growth of the pathogen, the *minimum inhibitory concentration* (MIC). Not all isolates of a single pathogen, such as *Escherichia coli,* have exactly the same MIC for a given antibiotic. Although some isolates might remain completely susceptible to an antibiotic, such as ampicillin, a variety of different antibiotic resistance mechanisms involving ampicillin and other antibiotics might exist in other *E. coli* isolates. This variation in susceptibility gives rise to the concept of a distribution of MICs for specific bacteria infecting a population of children from a defined region over a specified period. This concept of susceptibility distribution has been shown in isolates of pneumococcus with respect to susceptibility to penicillin. The distribution of MICs has been shown to vary by site of isolation of the pneumococcus (middle ear fluid, blood, or cerebrospinal fluid) and by region of the United States [3]. In an ongoing national surveillance project of pneumococcal resistance in children, organisms isolated in Houston, Texas, have tended to be more resistant than organisms isolated in Pittsburgh, Pennsylvania. Organisms isolated in middle ear fluid from children with otitis media on average have been more resistant than organisms isolated from cerebrospinal fluid [4,5].

This observed distribution of susceptibilities in bacterial pathogens is often more apparent in hospitals and long-term care settings, where resistance patterns vary and are notably dependent on the institution. Local clinical laboratory data and hospital antibiograms are helpful in directing empirical therapy. For individual patient care, obtaining bacterial cultures from the site of infection to identify the organism and determine specific antibiotic susceptibility is essential for selecting successful therapy and minimizing the overuse of antibiotics. Hospital-associated infections (eg, wounds, urinary tract infections, ventilator-associated pneumonia) can be particularly difficult to treat because variability in the types of bacteria isolated and in their susceptibility patterns is extensive. For the management of serious infections, a strategy based on susceptibility testing of the isolated pathogen is the standard of care.

Patterns of resistance change over time. Over 5 years there has been an increase in CA-MRSA [6–8]. In contrast to hospital-acquired MRSA (HA-MRSA), which has been a challenge for adult and pediatric providers for many years, these community-acquired strains frequently are found in otherwise healthy children. The usual predisposing factors for MRSA, including antibiotic exposure and prior hospitalization, often are not present in children infected by CA-MRSA. In contrast to HA-MRSA, the community-acquired strains often retain susceptibility to non–β-lactam antibiotics, such as clindamycin, trimethoprim-sulfamethoxazole, and the macrolides. Resistance to methicillin and the other β-lactam antibiotics is based on an alteration in a specific transpeptidase, penicillin-binding protein 2a, which is conferred by the *mecA* gene. The alteration in protein structure of this transpeptidase is the same one as that seen in HA-MRSA. The differences in susceptibility between HA-MRSA and CA-MRSA can be explained, however, by the antibiotic resistance cassette in which the *mecA* gene is found.

Many strains of CA-MRSA contain a much smaller cassette (SCCmec IV) composed of resistance genes only for the β-lactam antibiotics [9–11]. There is evidence that some of these community-acquired strains have evolved from community-acquired methicillin-susceptible strains of *S. aureus* and not from HA-MRSA [12]. Evolving patterns of resistance underscore the need to obtain cultures and antibiotic susceptibilities, especially when the patient does not respond clinically to antibiotic therapy previously believed to be effective. Mecha-

Table 1
Examples of pediatric bacterial pathogens with emergence of antibiotic resistance, mechanism of resistance, and relevance to patient care

Organism	Mechanism of resistance	Clinical implication
Streptococcus pneumoniae	Alteration in the binding site of the antibiotic to one or more transpeptidases (penicillin binding proteins)	Relative resistance to β-lactam agents (penicillins and cephalosporins)
	Alteration in the ribosomal binding site of antibiotics	Resistance to macrolide agents
	Efflux pump to expel an antibiotic from the cytoplasm	Relative resistance to macrolide agents
Staphylococcus aureus	Alteration in the binding site of a specific transpeptidase (mec A)	Resistance to all β-lactams
	Alteration at ribosomal binding site	Resistance to macrolides and clindamycin
	Efflux pump to expel antibiotics from the cytoplasm	Relative resistance to macrolides
Escherichia coli, Klebsiella	β-lactamases with activity extended beyond ampicillin (extended-spectrum β-lactamases)	Resistance to cefotaxime, ceftriaxone, and ceftazidime
Enterobacter, Serratia, and some other Enterobacteriaceae	Chromosomal β-lactamases that are deregulated and hyperproduced (ampC)	Resistance to cefotaxime, ceftriaxone, and ceftazidime
Pseudomonas aeruginosa	Multiple β-lactamases each with activity against different β-lactam antibiotics	Resistance to multiple β-lactam agents, including ceftazidime
	Cell wall porin protein–deficient bacteria	Carbapenem resistance
	Multiple efflux pumps to expel antibiotics from the cytoplasm	Resistance to β-lactams, fluoroquinolones, others

Data from references [23–25].

nisms of antibiotic resistance in pediatric bacterial pathogens and their resulting clinical implications are outlined in Table 1.

Pharmacodynamics

Pharmacodynamics is recognized as an important concept in predicting the microbiologic and clinical success of antibiotic treatment. Depending on the class of antibiotic and the particular pathogen in question, the ability of the antibiotic to inhibit or kill an organism over minutes to hours might be quite different. In general, antibiotic effect is related directly to either the concentration attained at the site of infection or the time during which an effective concentration of the antibiotic is present at the site of infection. For some antibiotics, such as aminoglycosides and fluoroquinolones [1,13,14], higher concentrations and greater drug exposure result in more rapid killing. Drug exposure is related to the total area under the curve, depicted by plotting serum drug concentrations from the time of administration to the time of elimination (Fig. 1). For β-lactams, optimal activity is related to time during which the antibiotic concentration remains above the MIC at the site of infection over a dosing interval, or the "percent-time-above-MIC." Inhibitory activity can be optimized by achieving antibiotic concentrations at the site of infection for a duration that is greater than 40% of the dosing interval (eg, for 4.8 hours out of every 12 hours for antibiotics that are administered every 12 hours) for some antibiotic-pathogen combinations. For these interactions, having greater antibiotic concentrations at the site of infection would not achieve a greater inhibitory effect. In addition to the time-above-MIC effect, the macrolides, clindamycin, vancomycin, and linezolid all exhibit a postantibiotic effect, with organisms requiring substantial time to begin regrowth after exposure to the antibiotic [14].

Pharmacokinetics

Dosing guidelines usually are based on information obtained from clinical trials conducted on a few relatively normal, healthy children. For many antibiotics, dosing guidelines have been extrapolated from studies conducted in adults. The absorption, concentration profile, distribution, metabolism, and excretion of an antibiotic in a sick child who might have compromised organ function might not be predicted accurately from existing literature. Patient-to-patient variability in pharmacokinetics must be anticipated. Selecting the most appropriate antibiotic dose when switching from intravenous to oral therapy depends most on the absorption characteristics of the oral agent. In general, most antibiotics when given parenterally result in higher, more reproducible serum concentrations than when given orally (see Fig. 1). Most β-lactam antibiotics administered orally have fair bioavailability; serum concentrations usually are approximately 5% to 10% of those obtained when β-lactam antibiotics are given parenterally [15]. Quinolones and the oxazolidinone antibiotic, linezolid, have excellent bioavailability, however, with serum concentrations and antibiotic exposure after an oral dose being close to that found after an intravenous dose [16–18].

Compliance is not an issue with parenteral treatment, although an indwelling catheter is needed, and complications with the catheters and administration devices might occur. Oral therapy is associated with fewer serious complications. Absorption, compliance, and the palatability of the drug present a different set of problems with oral therapy, however.

Data are limited regarding the specific concentrations of antibiotics in many tissues and organs. It is predictable, however, that antibiotic concentrations would be different in various body compartments, and that the elimination half-lives of antibiotics at each of these sites would vary. There are limitations to predicting the effectiveness of therapy based on general pharmacokinetic principles. When data are available, pharmacokinetic/pharmacodynamic modeling is informative. Antibiotic therapy of otitis media provides an example of how differences in

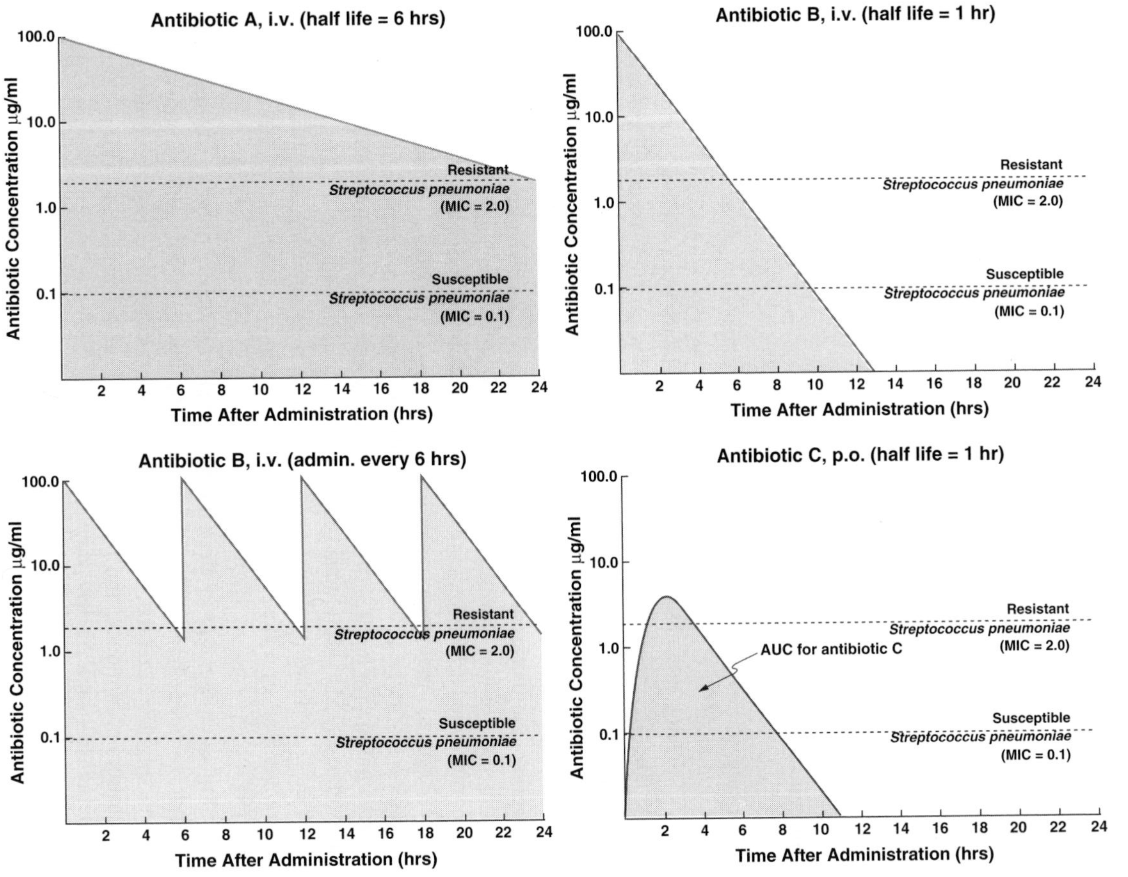
Antibiotic A, i.v. (half life = 6 hrs)
Antibiotic B, i.v. (half life = 1 hr)
Antibiotic B, i.v. (admin. every 6 hrs)
Antibiotic C, p.o. (half life = 1 hr)
Antibiotic Concentration µg/ml
100.0
10.0
1.0
0.1
Time After Administration (hrs)
2 4 6 8 10 12 14 16 18 20 22 24
Resistant
Streptococcus pneumoniae
(MIC = 2.0)
Susceptible
Streptococcus pneumoniae
(MIC = 0.1)
AUC for antibiotic C

antibiotic exposure between the bloodstream and the site of infection affect dosing recommendations. Middle ear fluid concentrations of ceftriaxone are known to approximate the concentrations in serum, with documented peak concentrations in middle ear fluid of 80 μg/mL [19]. Although ceftriaxone has an elimination half-life of 4 to 6 hours in the serum, its measured elimination half-life in middle ear fluid is closer to 24 hours [19]. Concentrations of ceftriaxone in middle ear fluid remain well above the MIC for most strains of *S. pneumoniae* and non-typable *H. influenzae* for at least 72 hours after a single dose. With validation of clinical and microbiologic efficacy of a single dose of ceftriaxone for otitis media in prospective clinical trials, the US Food and Drug Administration approved this dosing regimen for otitis media.

In the population of children to be treated for a particular infection, one can estimate the antibiotic exposure in infected tissues achieved at a specific antibiotic dose. By combining information on antibiotic exposure with information on the range of antibiotic susceptibilities of the pathogens causing the infection, one can estimate the percent of children who would be cured of their infections at a specific antibiotic dosage.

Monte Carlo simulation

When an antibiotic is prescribed, the clinician should be able to predict the likelihood that a certain dose would cure the infection. The acceptable level of certainty with the prediction varies according to the clinical circumstances. An anticipated cure rate of 80% to 90% might be acceptable in the management of a nonserious infection, such as cystitis caused by *E. coli* in a healthy child. In contrast, this would not be an acceptable cure rate for a child with leukemia hospitalized with neutropenia and pneumonia caused by *Pseudomonas aeruginosa*. The therapy in these two situations would be dramatically different; the dose of the appropriate antibiotic necessary to achieve the desired "target attainment" in both children can be predicted by Monte Carlo simulation [2]. This simulation is performed using a computer program that considers the distributions of MICs of a selected antibiotic against the probable pathogens (*E. coli* or *Pseudomonas* in the examples here), the expected range of antibiotic concentrations at the site of infection for various antibiotic dosages, and knowledge of the pharmacodynamic characteristics of the antibiotic that determine the type of antibiotic exposure required. The computer simulates the distributions of MICs and pharmacokinetics in a population of children with characteristics approxi-

Fig. 1. The area under the curve *(shaded area)* for different antibiotics. The area under the curve provides a measure of antibiotic exposure to bacterial pathogens. The greatest exposure comes with antibiotics that have a long serum half-life and are administered parenterally *(upper left panel, antibiotic A)*. The lowest exposure occurs with oral administration *(lower right panel, antibiotic C)*. Dosing of antibiotic B once a day *(upper right panel)* provides far less exposure than dosing the same antibiotic every 6 hours *(lower left panel)*. (© John S. Bradley, MD.)

Table 2
Antimicrobial therapy for common infections seen in children*

Clinical diagnosis	Usual pathogen(s)	Therapy	Comments
Skin and soft tissue infections			
Note: Community-acquired methicillin-resistant *Staphylococcus aureus* (CA-MRSA) is now prevalent (representing >20% of all isolates) in many areas. Penicillins and cephalosporins are not active against these strains. Vancomycin is active against virtually all strains and should be used for all life-threatening and severe infections. Clindamycin, TMP-SMZ and linezolid are potentially active and can be used for mild-to-moderate infections			
Oxacillin, methicillin, and nafcillin are all highly active against methicillin-susceptible *Staphylococcus aureus* (MSSA) and are considered roughly equivalent in efficacy. Cefazolin, although less active in vitro than the antistaphylococcal penicillins, is therapeutically equivalent in mild-to-moderate infections, can be given less frequently, and is better tolerated than the penicillins			
Bites, animal and human	*Pasteurella multocida* (animal), *Eikenella corrodens* (human), *Staphylococcus* spp. and *Streptococcus* spp	Augmentin 45 mg/kg/d (amoxicillin component) PO div q8h (amoxicillin:clavulanate ratio of 7:1) × 5–7 d; for hospitalized patients, use ticarcillin/clavulanate, 200 mg ticarcillin/kg/d div q6h *or* ampicillin and clindamycin	Consider rabies prophylaxis for animal bites; consider tetanus prophylaxis; human bites often have mixed aerobes and anaerobes with a very high rate of infection (do not close open wounds)
Impetigo	*S. aureus* (methicillin-susceptible or methicillin-resistant), group A strep (*S. pyogenes*)	Mupirocin topically to lesions tid; *or* (for extensive lesions) cephalexin 50–75 mg/kg/d PO div tid	Cleanse infected area with soap and water; bathe daily. For CA-MRSA: clindamycin, TMP/SMZ, or linezolid
Lymphadenitis	*S. aureus* (MSSA or MRSA), group A strep	Empiric IV therapy: oxacillin 150 mg/kg/d IV div q6h *or* cefazolin 100 mg/kg/d IV div q8h initially; for possible CA-MRSA: clindamycin 30 mg/kg/d IV div q8h or vancomycin 40 mg/kg/d IV q8h	Oral therapy for MSSA: cephalexin *or* dicloxacillin. For CA-MRSA: clindamycin, TMP/SMZ, or linezolid
Myositis, suppurative (synonyms: tropical myositis, pyomyositis)	*S. aureus*	Oxacillin 150 mg/kg/d IV div q6h *or* cefazolin 100 mg/kg/d IV div q8h 14–21 d; alternatives: vancomycin *or* clindamycin	Surgical drainage or excision when needed; for severe infections, add gentamicin for synergy. For CA-MRSA: clindamycin, TMP/SMZ, or linezolid

Necrotizing fasciitis	*S. aureus*, group A strep, mixed aerobic/ anaerobic, or staphylococcal, depending on the location of infection, age of the child	Penicillin G 200,000–250,000 U/kg/d div q6h *and* clindamycin 40 mg/kg/d div q8h; *add* cefotaxime to the above regimen *or* use meropenem or imipenem as single drug therapy if gram-negative aerobic bacilli suspected	Aggressive, emergent debridement; consider IVIG to bind bacterial toxins for life-threatening disease; if *S. aureus* is isolated, use oxacillin or cefazolin rather than clindamycin, unless MRSA
Pyoderma, abscesses, cervical lymphadenitis	*S. aureus*, group A strep	Cephalexin 50–75 mg/kg/d PO div tid; *or* dicloxacillin (as above); × 5–10 d	Incision and drainage when indicated; oxacillin or cefazolin IV or vancomycin for serious infections. For oral therapy for CA-MRSA: clindamycin, TMP-SMZ, or linezolid
Cellulitis, periorbital (Preseptal infection)			
Associated with entry site lesion on skin	*S. aureus*, group A strep	Oxacillin 150 mg/kg/d IV div q6h *or* cefazolin 100 mg/kg/d IV div q8h; for regions with high prevalence of CA-MRSA: clindamycin 40 mg/kg/d IV div q8h *or* vancomycin 40 mg/kg/d div q8h; × 10–14 d	Oral antistaphylococcal antibiotic for less severe infection, or for convalescent therapy after the infection has clearly responded to IV therapy
Bacteremia	*S. pneumoniae* (pneumoccus) or *H. influenzae* type b in unimmunized children	Cefuroxime or cefotaxime 100–150 mg/kg/d IV, IM div q8h; *or* ceftriaxone 50 mg/kg/d once daily × 10–14 d	R/O meningitis
Associated with sinusitis (more commonly presenting as nontender edema, not cellulitis); rarely sinus pathogens may erode anteriorly into soft tissue		As for sinusitis: initially cefuroxime or cefotaxime 100–150 mg/kg/d IV, IM div q8h; *or* ceftriaxone 50 mg/kg/d once daily 5–7 d, followed by oral antibiotics to complete 21 d	For oral antibiotic therapy, see Otitis media and Sinusitis

(continued on next page)

Table 2 (*continued*)

Clinical diagnosis	Usual pathogen(s)	Therapy	Comments
Skin and soft tissue infections			
Cellulitis, orbital (Postseptal infection)		Cefotaxime 150 mg/kg/d div q8h or ceftriaxone 50 mg/kg/d once daily; *and* antistaphylococcal therapy (oxacillin 150 mg/kg/d IV div q6h or cefazolin 100 mg/kg/d IV div q8h; *or* for CA-MRSA, consider vancomycin 40 mg/kg/d div q8h or clindamycin 40 mg/kg/d IV div q8h) × 10–14 d	Usually secondary to sinus infection: staphylococcal or respiratory tract flora; surgical drainage of pus, if present by CT scan in orbit or subperiosteal tissue
Bone and joint infections			
Osteomyelitis			
Infants and children, acute infection	*S. aureus*, group A strep, rarely *Kingella*	As above: for communities with over 5–10% MRSA, start empirical therapy with clindamycin 40 mg/kg/d IV div q8h *or* vancomycin 40 mg/kg/d IV div q8h; otherwise start oxacillin 150 mg/kg/d IV div q6h *or* cefazolin 100 mg/kg/d IV div q8h Transition to oral therapy may be considered with cephalexin 100 mg/kg/d div q6–8h or dicloxacillin 100 mg/kg/d div q6h for MSSA once clinical improvement is documented and compliance ensured. Total therapy (IV plus PO) for 4–6 wk	In children with open fractures secondary to trauma, consider adding ceftazidime for extended aerobic gram-negative activity (pending culture results). Oral therapy alternatives for CA-MRSA include clindamycin, TMP/SMZ, and linezolid

Osteomyelitis of the foot (osteochondritis after a puncture wound)	*Pseudomonas aeruginosa*	Ceftazidime 150 mg/kg/d IV, IM div q8h *or* ticarcillin 200–300 mg/kg/d IV div q6h; *and* tobramycin 67.5 mg/kg/d IM, IV div q8h; *or* cefepime 150 mg/kg/d IV, div q8h; *or* meropenem 60 mg/kg/d IV, div q8h; × 10 d	Thorough surgical debridement required (second drainage procedure needed in at least 20% of children). For convalescent therapy after clinical resolution, consider ciprofloxacin 30 mg/kg/d PO, div bid
Arthritis, bacterial			
Infants	*S. aureus*, group A strep; consider pneumococcus and *H. influenzae* type b in unimmunized children	For isolates documented to be MSSA: oxacillin 150 mg/kg/d IV div q6h *or* cefazolin 100 mg/kg/d IV div q8h × 21 d; empirical therapy in communities with 5–10% MRSA: clindamycin 40 mg/kg/d IV div q8h *or* vancomycin 40 mg/kg/d div q8h. As for osteomyelitis, transition to oral therapy may be considered once clinically improved	For penicillin-susceptible pneumococci or group A strep: penicillin G 200,000 U/kg/d IV div q6h × 14 d or longer; for penicillin-nonsusceptible pneumococci, ceftriaxone 50–75 mg/kg/d IV, IM, once daily, *or* cefotaxime 100–150 mg/kg/d IV, IM div q8h
Children	*S. aureus*, group A strep	For MSSA isolates: oxacillin 150 mg/kg/d IV div q6h *or* cefazolin 100 mg/kg/d IV div q8h. Total therapy (IV plus PO) for 3 wk; empirical therapy for suspected MRSA as above: clindamycin 40 mg/kg/d IV div q8h *or* vancomycin 40 mg/kg/d IV div q8h. As for osteomyelitis, transition to oral therapy may be considered once clinically improved	Pneumococcus is unusual past infancy. Oral therapy alternatives for CA-MRSA include clindamycin, TMP/SMZ, and linezolid

(continued on next page)

Table 2 (*continued*)

Clinical diagnosis	Usual pathogen(s)	Therapy	Comments
Ear and sinus infections			
External otitis, bacterial	*P. aeruginosa, S.aureus*	Antibiotic solution delivered to wick inserted into canal: neomycin/polymyxin B or fluoroquinolone (ciprofloxacin or ofloxacin); with hydrocortisone	Optimal therapy not well studied; cleaning canal of detritus important
Otitis media, acute			
Note on acute otitis media: Several antibiotic regimens are effective for acute otitis media. High-dose amoxicillin (80–90 mg/kg/d) is considered the most effective oral agent against *S. pneumoniae*. Other drugs active against β-lactamase-producing *H. influenzae* and penicillin-resistant *S. pneumoniae* should be considered for amoxicillin failures or relapses. The physician should consider advantages and disadvantages regarding antibacterial spectrum, palatability of suspensions, and cost. Some physicians observe the child >2 years for 72 h in milder cases before starting antibiotic therapy, watching for spontaneous resolution (often noted with *Moraxella* and *Haemophilus*). Although prophylaxis is only rarely indicated in an attempt to limit antibiotic exposure, amoxicillin or other antibiotics can be used in one half the therapeutic dose once or twice daily to prevent infections.			
Otitis media, acute			
Infants and children	Pneumococcus, nontypable *H. influenzae, Moraxella* most common	Usual therapy: amoxicillin 90 mg/kg/d PO bid; failures caused by either β-lactamase–producing *Haemophilus* or penicillin-resistant pneumococcus The following offer better activity than amoxicillin against β-lactamase–positive *Haemophilus* and *Moraxella*: amoxicillin/clavulanate (Augmentin), cefdinir, cefprozil, cefpodoxime, cefuroxime, azithromycin, clarithromycin, erythromycin-sulfisoxazole PO, *or* ceftriaxone 50 mg/kg/d IM q24h × 1–3 doses It is difficult to achieve better activity	High-dose amoxicillin (90 mg/kg/d) should be used for empirical therapy in most regions of the world, given the high prevalence of penicillin-nonsusceptible pneumococci causing otitis. The high serum and middle ear fluid concentrations achieved with 45 mg/kg/dose of amoxicillin, combined with its long middle ear fluid half-life, allow for a therapeutic antibiotic exposure to pathogens in the middle ear with only twice-daily dosing of amoxicillin; Augmentin ES-600 combines high-dose amoxicillin (90 mg/kg/d) with clavulanate. For failure with a second treatment course, tympanocentesis differentiates persisting infxn from resolving inflammation

		against penicillin-resistant pneumococci with oral therapy than with high-dose amoxicillin; options include ceftriaxone 50 mg/kg/d IM q24h × 1–3 doses, *or* a macrolide-class antibiotic (azithromycin, clarithromycin, or erythromycin-sulfisoxazole); caution: 40% of penicillin-resistant pneumococci are also macrolide-resistant, *or* clindamycin (not active against *H. influenzae* or *M. catarrhalis*)	
Sinusitis, acute	Nontypable *H. influenzae*, pneumococcus, other streptococci, *Moraxella*	Same antibiotic therapy as for acute otitis media, but 14–21 d may be needed. Prolonged therapy may be necessary while mucosal swelling resolves and ventilation of sinus is restored	Little prospective data exist on bid therapy with high-dose amoxacillin (90 mg/kg/d) in sinus infections, but this dosing regimen should be as effective as in otitis. Sinus irrigations for severe disease or failure to respond
Oropharyngeal infections			
Dental abscess	Oral aerobic and anaerobic flora	Clindamycin 30 mg/kg/d PO, IV, IM div q6–8h *or* penicillin G 100,000–200,000 U/kg/d IV div q6h	Usually oral aerobes and anaerobes; tooth extraction may be necessary
Epiglottitis (aryepiglottitis, supraglottitis)	*H. influenzae* type b; consider *S. aureus* in immunized children	Cefuroxime 100–150 mg/kg/d IV, IM div q8h *or* cefotaxime 150 mg/kg/d IV div q8h or ceftriaxone 50 mg/kg/d IV, IM q24h × 7–10 d	Provide airway. For staphylococcia, consider oxacillin 150 mg/kg/d IV div q6h *or* cefazolin 100 mg/kg/d IV div q8h *or* vancomycin 40 mg/kg/d IV div q8h
Peritonsillar cellulitis or abscess	Group A strep with mixed oral flora	Clindamycin 30 mg/kg/d PO, IV, IM div q8h *and* cefotaxime 150 mg/kg/d IV div q8h	Consider incision and drainage for abscess. Alternatives: meropenem or imipenem; piperacillin/tazobactam

(continued on next page)

Table 2 (*continued*)

Clinical diagnosis	Usual pathogen(s)	Therapy	Comments
Oropharyngeal infections			
Pharyngitis	Group A strep	Penicillin V 50–75 mg/kg/d PO div bid or tid, or amoxicillin 50–75 mg/kg/d div bid or tid 10 d *or* benzathine penicillin 25,000 U/kg IM (max 1.2 million U) as a single dose; erythromycin for penicillin-allergic patients	For the uncommon failures, or frequent relapses, amoxicillin/clavulanate, cephalosporins, or clindamycin may be more effective
Retropharyngeal or lateral pharyngeal cellulitis or abscess	Mixed aerobic and anaerobic oral flora	Clindamycin 30 mg/kg/d PO, IV, IM div q8h *and* cefotaxime 150 mg/kg/d IV div q8h or ceftriaxone 50 mg/kg/d IV q24h	Consider incision and drainage; possible airway compromise, mediastinitis Alternatives: meropenem or imipenem
Tracheitis, bacterial	*S. aureus* (consider CA-MRSA), group A strep, pneumococcus, *H. influenzae,* type b	Vancomycin 40 mg/kg/d IV div q8h, or oxacillin 150 mg/kg/d IV div q6h or cefazolin 100 mg/kg/d IV div q8h *and* cefotaxime 150 mg/kg/d div q8h or ceftriaxone 50 mg/kg/d q24h	May represent bacterial superinfection of viral laryngotracheobronchitis
Lower respiratory tract infections			
Abscess, lung - primary (severe, necrotizing)	Pneumococcus, *S. aureus* (consider CA-MRSA), group A strep	Empirical therapy with ceftriaxone 50–75 mg/kg/d q24h or cefotaxime 150 mg/kg/d div q8h *and* vancomycin 40 mg/kg/d IV div q8h × 14–21 d or longer	Bronchoscopy necessary if abscess fails to drain; surgical excision rarely necessary For MSSA: oxacillin 150 mg/kg/d IV div q6h or cefazolin 100 mg/kg/d IV div q8h; or for CA-MRSA: clindamycin 30–40 mg/kg/d IV div q8h
Pertussis		Erythromycin (estolate may be preferable) 40 mg/kg/d PO div qid × 14 d; limited clinical data suggest that azithromycin (10 mg/kg/d × 5 d) or clarithromycin (15 mg/kg/d × 14 d) may be used as alternatives	Hospitalize young infants; avoid mist therapy; avoid cough suppressants; Isolate for the first 5 d of therapy; Provide macrolide prophylaxis to family members

Pneumonia, aspiration	Polymicrobial infection with oral aerobes and anaerobes	Clindamycin 30–40 mg/kg/d PO, IM, IV div q8h *or* meropenem 60 mg/kg/d IV div q8h if additional gram-negative aerobic coverage is needed; × ≥10 d	Alternatives: imipenem IV or piperacillin/tazobactam IV or ticarcillin/clavulanate IV
Pneumonia: lobar or segmental consolidation			Consider *H. influenzae* type b in unimmunized child
Community-acquired	Pneumococcus (even if immunized), group A strep, and *S. aureus* more likely in younger infants; *Mycoplasma pneumoniae* and other atypical agents may cause lobar pneumonia in school-age children and adolescents	Empirical therapy for hospitalized children: cefuroxime 150 mg/kg/d IV, IM div q8h, *or* ceftriaxone 50 mg/kg/d IV, IM q24h, *or* cefotaxime 150 mg/kg/d div q8h; × 10–14 days; for suspect mycoplasma and other atypical pneumonia pathogens, *add* a macrolide (erythromycin IV or PO, azithromycin IV or PO, clarithromycin PO) Empirical oral outpatient therapy for less severe illness: amoxicillin 80–90 mg/kg/d PO div q8h; for atypical pneumonia, *add* agents as above	Change to PO after improvement (decreased fever, no oxygen needed); Alternative IV agents include clindamycin for susceptible strains of staphylococcus and pneumococcus. Oral therapy for bacterial pathogens may also be successful with: amoxicillin/clavulanate, cefdinir, cefprozil, cefpodoxime or cefuroxime.
	Pneumococcal, penicillin-susceptible	Penicillin G 150,000 U/kg/d IV div q4–6h × 10 d	Change to PO penicillin V 50–75 mg/kg/d div qid to tid after improvement
	Pneumococcal, penicillin-resistant	Ceftriaxone 50 mg/kg/d q24h, or cefotaxime 150 mg/kg/d div q8h for 10–14 d	Addition of vancomycin has *not* been required for eradication of penicillin-resistant strains causing lobar or bronchopneumonia
With empyema	Same pathogens as for community- acquired pneumonia; consider CA-MRSA	Empirical therapy: ceftriaxone 50–75 mg/kg/d q24h or cefotaxime 150 mg/kg/d div q8h *and* vancomycin 40 mg/kg/d IV div q8h × 10–14 d	Initial therapy based on Gram stain of empyema fluid; typically clinical improvement is slow, with persisting but decreasing "spiking" fever for 2–3 wk; for susceptible strains of staph, use β-lactam therapy; for susceptible CA-MRSA: clindamycin

(continued on next page)

Table 2 (*continued*)

Clinical diagnosis	Usual pathogen(s)	Therapy	Comments
Lower respiratory tract infections			
Pneumonia: lobar or segmental consolidation			
With empyema	Group A strep	Penicillin G 150,000 U/kg/d IV div q4–6h × 10 d	Closed chest tube drainage of purulent fluid; change to PO penicillin V 50–75 mg/kg/day, div qid to tid, or amoxicillin 75 mg/kg/d div tid after clinical improvement
	Pneumococcal	(See above, Pneumonia: Lobar or segmental consolidation)	Definitive therapy is based on susceptibility of strain
	S. aureus (consider CA-MRSA)	Vancomycin 40 mg/kg/d div q8h. For susceptible strains of MSSA: oxacillin or cefazolin. For susceptible strains of MRSA: clindamycin × ≥21 d	Closed chest tube drainage of empyema; consider adding gentamicin for synergy; may benefit from video-assisted thoracoscopic drainage
Pneumonia, nosocomial	*P. aeruginosa,* gram-negative enteric bacilli *(Enterobacter, Klebsiella, Serratia, E. coli), Acinetobacter, Stenotrophomonas* and gram-positive organisms including MRSA and *enterococcus*, including vancomycin-resistant strains (VRE)	Should be institution-specific, based on hospital's nosocomial pathogens and their susceptibilities. Commonly used regimens include meropenem 60 mg/kg/d div q8h *or* piperacillin/tazobactam 240–300 mg/kg/d div q6–8h, *or* cefepime 150 mg/kg/d div q8h; with/without gentamicin 6–7.5 mg/kg/d div q8h; *and* vancomycin 40 mg/kg/d div q8h	Pathogens that cause hospital-acquired pneumonia often have multidrug resistance. Cultures are critical. Empirical therapy is often based on prior colonization and hospital epidemiology

Other bacterial pneumonias of established etiology			
	Chlamydia pneumoniae (TWAR), *C. psittaci*, or *C. trachomatis*	A macrolide *or* doxycycline (patients >7 y); ampicillin for *C. trachomatis*	
Legionnaires' disease	*Legionella pneumophila*	A macrolide and rifampin	
	M. pneumoniae	A macrolide or doxcycline	
Heart infections			
Endocarditis	Regimens not well defined in children; consider vancomycin *and* gentamicin for echocardiogram-positive endocarditis, pending culture results; combination provides bactericidal activity against most strains of streptococci, enterococci, and staphylococci (including MRSA)		
	Viridans streptococcus	Fully susceptible to penicillin: penicillin G 200,000 U/kg/d IV div q4–6h × 30 d; *or* penicillin G *and* gentamicin 6–7.5 mg/kg/d IM, IV div q8h × 14 d; *or* ceftriaxone 50 mg/kg/d IV, IM q24h 30 d	Tolerant to penicillin: penicillin G 200,000–300,000 U/kg/d IV div q4–6h *and* gentamicin 6–7.5 mg/kg/d IM, IV div q8h; *or* vancomycin 40–60 mg/kg/d IV div q8h; × 4–6 wk Follow echocardiogram for resolution of vegetation
	Enterococcus	Ampicillin 200 mg/kg/d IV, IM div q6h *and* gentamicin 6–7.5 mg/kg/d IV div q8h; *or* vancomycin 40 mg/kg/d IV div q8h *and* gentamicin 6–7.5 mg/kg/d IV div q8h; × 4–6 wk	Combined treatment used for synergistic bactericidal activity. Use susceptibility results to guide therapy
	S. aureus (consider community-acquired or hospital-acquired MRSA), *S. epidermidis*	Vancomycin 40 mg/kg/d IV div q8h. For susceptible strains: nafcillin or oxacillin 150 mg/kg/d IV div q6h; × 6 wk; *add* gentamicin or rifampin for slow clinical or microbiologic response (at least for the first 2 wk of therapy)	Surgery may be necessary in acute phase; avoid cephalosporins because of conflicting data on efficacy. Consider continuing therapy at end of 6 wk if vegetations persist on echocardiogram. Consult an infectious disease specialist for prosthetic valve endocarditis

(continued on next page)

Table 2 (*continued*)

Clinical diagnosis	Usual pathogen(s)	Therapy	Comments
Heart infections			
Endocarditis	Pneumococcus, gonococcus, group A strep	Penicillin G 150,000 U/kg/d IV div q4–6h × 30 d; alternatives: ceftriaxone or vancomycin	Ceftriaxone for gonococcus until susceptibilities known
Gastrointestinal infections			
Colitis, antibiotic-associated	*Clostridium difficile* toxin	Metronidazole 30 mg/kg/d PO div qid *or* vancomycin 40 mg/kg/d PO div qid × 7 d	Vancomycin PO may cause emergence of vancomycin-resistant enterococci in gut
Gastritis, peptic ulcer disease	*Helicobacter pylori*	Clarithromycin 7.5 mg/kg/dose 2–3 times each day *and* amoxicillin 40 mg/kg/dose (max 1 g) PO bid *and* omeprazole 0.6–0.7 mg/kg/dose PO qd 2 wk, followed by omeprazole alone × 2 wk	Most data from studies in adults; other regimens include bismuth, metronidazole, or other proton-pump inhibitors
Gastroenteritis	*Aeromonas*	TMP/SMZ as for shigellosis	Possible alternatives based on in vitro susceptibilities: fluoroquinolones, cefotaxime/ceftriaxone, cefepime
	Campylobacter jejuni	Erythromycin 40 mg/kg/d PO div qid × 5 d or azithromycin 10 mg/kg/d × 3 d	Alternatives: doxycycline and ciprofloxacin
Cholera	*Vibrio cholerae*	Doxycycline 4 mg/kg/d (max 200 mg/d) PO div bid	Ciprofloxacin; TMP/SMZ (if susceptible)
	Escherichia coli—a Note on E. coli and diarrheal disease: Antibiotic susceptibility of *E. coli* varies considerably from region to region in the world. For mild-to-moderate disease, TMP/SMX may be started as initial therapy. For severe disease, oral second- and third-generation cephalosporins (cefixime, cefuroxime, cefaclor, cefprozil, ceftibuten, cefdinir, cefpodoxime) may be used. Cultures and antibiotic susceptibility testing are recommended for significant disease		
Enterotoxigenic (traveler's diarrhea)	*E. coli* (ST or LT toxin producing)	TMP/SMZ or cefixime 8 mg/kg/d PO qd × 5–7 d	Most illnesses brief and self-limited; alternative (for adults): ciprofloxacin

Enterohemorrhagic	O157:H7; STEC (shiga toxin-producing *E. coli*); associated with hemolytic-uremic syndrome	Controversy on whether treatment results in more or less toxin-mediated renal damage. Withhold therapy, if possible; otherwise for severe infection, therapy as for enterotoxigenic strains	Injury to colonic mucosa may lead to invasive bacterial colitis
Salmonellosis			
Nontyphoid strains	*Salmonella*	Usually none for self-limited diarrhea. For persisting symptomatic infection: cefixime as for shigellosis; *or* for susceptible strains: amoxicillin 50 mg/kg/d PO div tid; *or* TMP/SMZ (8 mg/kg/d of TMP component) PO div bid; × 5–7 d	For severe colitis, a septic clinical picture, bacteremia, or compromised hosts: treat with ceftriaxone IV, IM
Typhoid fever	*S. typhi*	Ceftriaxone 50 mg/kg/d IV, IM q24h, or cefotaxime 150 mg/kg/d IV div q8h; ciprofloxacin 30 mg/kg/d IV, PO div bid; *or* azithromycin 12 mg/kg on day 1, followed by 6 mg/kg daily × 4 d	Ciprofloxacin or azithromycin for ceftriaxone-resistant strains; watch for relapse if ceftriaxone used
Shigellosis	*Shigella*	Cefixime 8 mg/kg/d PO qd; *or* azithromycin 12 mg/kg PO on day 1, followed by 6 mg/kg daily × 4 d; *or* ciprofloxacin 30 mg/kg/d PO div bid; *or* for susceptible strains: TMP/SMZ (8 mg/kg/d of TMP component) PO div bid; × 5 d	Ampicillin (not amoxicillin) when *Shigella* susceptible Avoid antiperistaltic drugs Treat to decrease communicability, even if symptoms resolving
	Yersinia enterocolitica	Antimicrobial therapy probably not of value for mild disease in normal hosts. Cefotaxime IV for TMP-SMZ IV for severe infection.	May mimic appendicitis. Limited clinical data exist on oral therapy; ciprofloxacin for adults
Perirectal abscess	*S. aureus*, enteric gram-negative bacilli, anaerobes	Clindamycin 30–40 mg/kg/d IV div q8h *and* gentamicin, cefotaxime, or ceftriaxone	*S. aureus* common, but may be mixed with coliforms, anaerobes; surgical drainage

(continued on next page)

Table 2 (*continued*)

Clinical diagnosis	Usual pathogen(s)	Therapy	Comments
Gastrointestinal infections			
Peritonitis			
Primary	Pneumococcus	Ceftriaxone 50 mg/kg/d q24h or cefotaxime 150 mg/kg/d div q8h; if penicillin-susceptible, penicillin G 150,000 U/kg/d IV div q6h; × 7–10 d	Other antibiotics according to culture and susceptibility tests
Secondary to bowel perforation or appendicitis	Enteric gram-negative bacilli, *Bacteroides, Enterococcus*	Meropenem 60 mg/kg/d IV div q8h or imipenem 60 mg/kg/d IV div q6h; *or* clindamycin 30 mg/kg/d IV, IM div q8h *and* ampicillin 150 mg/kg/d div q8h and gentamicin 6–7.5 mg/kg/d IV, IM div q8h; × ≥10 d	Many other regimens claimed to be effective for intra-abdominal infection based on limited data. No published data on oral convalescent therapy
Secondary to peritoneal dialysis	Check culture	Antibiotic added to dialysate in concentrations approximating those attained in serum for systemic disease (eg, 8 g/mL for gentamicin; 50 g/mL for vancomycin)	Selection of antibiotic based on organism isolated from peritoneal fluid; systemic antibiotics if there is accompanying bacteremia
Urinary tract infections			
Note: Antibiotic susceptibility profiles of *E. coli* vary considerably. For mild-to-moderate disease, TMP/SMZ may be started as initial therapy. For severe disease, obtain cultures and begin oral second- and third-generation cephalosporins (cefuroxime, cefaclor, cefprozil, cefixime, ceftibuten, cefdinir, cefpodoxime). Antibiotic susceptibility testing helps direct therapy			
Acute cystitis	*E. coli* most common; also caused by *Klebsiella*, other enteric gram-negative bacilli	TMP/SMZ (8 mg/kg/d of TMP component) PO div bid for mild-to-moderate disease, *or* cefixime 8 mg/kg/d PO qd OR (for patients >18 yr) ciprofloxacin 500 mg PO bid × 7–10 d	Alternative: amoxicillin 30 mg/kg/d PO div tid if susceptible. Follow-up culture after 36–48 h treatment if still symptomatic. Ceftibuten should be equivalent to cefixime in treatment of urinary tract infection

Acute pyelonephritis	See Acute cystitis	Ceftriaxone 50 mg/kg/d IV, IM q24h *or* gentamicin 5–6 mg/kg/d IV, IM div q8h or given as a single dose q24h; switch to oral therapy after clinical response. If organisms resistant to amoxicillin and TMP/SMZ, an oral second- or third-generation cephalosporin should be effective; × 10 d total therapy	Parenteral therapy if sepsis suspected; If bacteremia documented, and infant is <2–3 mo of age, R/O meningitis and treat 14 d IV or IM
Prophylaxis for recurrent UTI		TMP/SMZ (2 mg/kg TMP component) PO qd OR nitrofurantoin 1–2 mg/kg PO qd at bedtime	Prophylaxis for patients with reflux or frequent infections; resistance eventually develops to any antibiotic used
CNS infections			
Abscess, brain	Respiratory tract flora, skin flora, or bowel flora, depending on the pathogenesis of infection in a particular child	Until etiology established: meropenem 120 mg/kg/d div q8h; *or* nafcillin 150–200 mg/kg/d IV div q6h *and* cefotaxime 200–300 mg/kg/d IV div q6h or ceftriaxone 100 mg/kg/d IV div q24h *and* metronidazole 30 mg/kg/d IV, div q8h; × 7–10 d after successful drainage; longer therapy if no surgery (3–6 wk)	Surgery; anaerobes common. If CA-MRSA suspected *based* on skin lesions or other foci of staphylococci, *add* vancomycin pending culture results. If secondary to chronic otitis, use cefepime or meropenem for anti-*Pseudomonas* activity. Follow abscess size with CT scans
Meningitis, bacterial			

Notes

-Iinitial empirical therapy for suspected pneumococcal meningitis should be with vancomycin *plus* cefotaxime or ceftriaxone until susceptibility test results are available

-Dexamethasone (0.6 mg/kg/d IV div q6h × 2 d) as an adjunct to antibiotic therapy decreases hearing deficits and possibly other neurologic sequelae in *Haemophilus* meningitis and possibly other types. The first dose of dexamethasone preferably is given before or concurrent with the first dose of atibiotic. There is probably no benefit if given >1 h after the antibiotic is given

(continued on next page)

Table 2 (*continued*)

Clinical diagnosis	Usual pathogen(s)	Therapy	Comments
CNS infections			
Empirical therapy		Cefotaxime 200–300 mg/kg/d IV div q6h *or* ceftriaxone 100 mg/kg/d IV div q24h. *Add* vancomycin 60 mg/kg/d IV div q8h if Gram stain suggests pneumococcus	Alternative: meropenem 120 mg/kg/d IV div q8h
	H. influenzae type b	Cefotaxime 200–300 mg/kg/d IV div q6h *or* ceftriaxone 100 mg/kg/d IV div q1224h; 10 d	Alternative: ampicillin 200–400 mg/kg/d IV div q6h (for β-lactamase–negative strains) *or* chloramphenicol 100 mg/kg/d IV div q6h
	Pneumococcus (*S. pneumoniae*)	When pneumococcus is suspected on culture, *add* vancomycin 60 mg/kg/d IV div q8h until susceptibility results are known. For penicillin-susceptible and cephalosporin-susceptible strains: penicillin G 250,000 U/kg/d IV div q4–6h, *or* ceftriaxone 100 mg/kg/d IV div q24h or cefotaxime 200–300 mg/kg/d IV div q6h; × 10 d; for penicillin-resistant pneumococci: continue the combination of vancomycin and ceftriaxone IV	Some pneumococci may be resistant to penicillin, but susceptible to cefotaxime and ceftriaxone and may be treated with these antibiotics alone
	Meningococcus (*Neisseria meningitis*)	Penicillin G 250,000 U/kg/d IV div q4h × 7 d; *or* ceftriaxone 100 mg/kg/d IV div q24h, *or* cefotaxime 200 mg/kg/d IV div q6h	Rare strains are resistant to penicillin; meningococcal prophylaxis: rifampin 10 mg/kg PO, q12h × 4 doses *or* ceftriaxone 125–250 mg IM once *or* ciproflaxin 500 mg PO once (adults)

Miscellaneous systemic infections			
Bacteremia	Meningococcus; if unimmunized, pneumococcus and *H. influenzae* type b	Ceftriaxone 50 mg/kg/d IM, IV q24h, *or* cefotaxime 150 mg/kg/d IV, div q8h; Until afebrile 24 h (usually 2–5 d), then convalescent oral therapy	R/O meningitis, other focal infection; oral convalescent therapy (amoxicillin 75–100 mg/ kg/d PO div tid) to complete 7 d (meningococcus) to 10 d (pneumococcus, *Haemophilus*)
Cat-scratch disease	*Bartonella henselae*	Supportive (aspiration of pus); azithromycin 12 mg/kg/d PO qd × 5 d shortens the duration of adenopathy	Aminoglycosides, rifampin, TMP/SMZ, ciprofloxacin, cefotaxime also may be effective. Azithromycin dose is that used for group A strep pharyngitis
Lyme disease	*Borrelia burgdorferi*	Early localized or early disseminated disease: doxycycline (patients >7 y) 4 mg/kg/d (max 200 mg/d) PO div bid *or* amoxicillin 50 mg/kg/d (max 1.5 g/d) PO div tid × 14–21 d Arthritis (no CNS infection): oral therapy as outlined above, for 28 d Bell's palsy: treat with oral therapy (doxycycline) × 21–28 d Neuroborreliosis: ceftriaxone IV, *or* cefotaxime IV *or* penicillin G IV × 14–21 d	Neurologic evaluation, including lumbar puncture, if there is clinical suspicion of CNS involvement; children who have persistent or recurrent joint swelling after recommended courses should repeat treatment with another 4-wk course of oral antibiotics or with a 2- to 4-wk course of ceftriaxone IV; guidelines available at http://www.journals.uchicago.edu/IDSA/guidelines/

Abbreviation: TMP/SMZ, trimethoprim/sulfamethoxazole.

* This table should be considered a rough guideline for the "usual" patient. Dosages recommended are for patients without renal or hepatic failure. Duration of treatment should be individualized. The periods recommended are based on common practice and general experience. Critical evaluations of duration of therapy have been carried out in only a few diseases. In general, a longer duration of therapy should be used (1) for tissues in which antibiotic concentrations may not be high (eg, abscess, bone), (2) when the organisms are less susceptible to antibiotic therapy, (3) when a relapse of infection is unacceptable (eg, CNS infections), or (4) when the host is immuno compromised in some way.

mating those of the child being treated. The simulation provides the physician with the percent of children who achieve a cure at each dose of antibiotic under consideration.

Although these simulations are now an integral part of drug development within the pharmaceutical industry, the US Food and Drug Administration, and the National Institutes of Health, these computer simulations are not yet available in most hospitals or clinics to help the clinicians on the frontlines. Experts involved in making recommendations for antibiotic therapy for infected children have access to published or presented data on Monte Carlo simulations, however, for an ever-increasing number of different antibiotic treatment regimens for many different pathogens causing specific infections.

Host

Host factors, such as patient age and underlying disease, are important considerations in selecting appropriate antibiotic therapy for suspected bacterial infections. Host factors influence the types of bacteria likely to be pathogenic and the anticipated pharmacokinetics and side-effect profiles of different antibiotics. Neonates, especially preterm infants, have immature immunity and disruption of their mucosal and skin barriers by the use of ventilators and deep indwelling catheters. Antibiotic dosing is complicated by pharmacokinetic profiles distinct from the pharmacokinetic profiles of older children. Because of a larger total body water content and higher proportion of extracellular fluid, neonates typically have a larger volume of distribution for certain antibiotics compared with older infants and children. Newborns also have impaired renal function, especially during the first few weeks of life [20–22]. The mg/kg doses for certain antibiotics in these neonates might need to be greater to compensate for the larger volume of distribution and given less frequently to compensate for delayed renal excretion.

Antibiotic adverse reactions

Safety is a major consideration in selection of an appropriate antibiotic for children. All antibiotics have potential side effects, and it is important for the clinician to be aware of how these might affect the patient. Each class of antibiotics has associated risks, and different antibiotics within the same class often have different rates of adverse events. The β-lactams have proved to be among the safest antibiotics for children. Macrolides, aminoglycosides, glycopeptides, sulfonamides, and quinolones all have documented toxicities; some of these antibiotics also have the potential to interfere with drug metabolism of other, concurrently prescribed medications.

Summary

Understanding of the microbiology of infectious pathogens and their mechanisms of resistance has grown tremendously in the past decades. Technologic advances have enabled clinicians to establish the genetic basis for many bacterial resistance phenotypes. The challenge continues: to choose safe and effective antimicrobial agents that are administered to children in a way that maximizes clinical and microbiologic cure, while minimizing adverse drug effects and the development of antibiotic resistance. Table 2 gives examples of infections commonly seen in children and what antibiotics are believed to be reasonable therapy based on the principles discussed in this article [22].

References

[1] Drusano GL. Antimicrobial pharmacodynamics: critical interactions of 'bug and drug.' Nat Rev Microbiol 2004;2:289–300.

[2] Bradley JS, Dudley MN, Drusano GL. Predicting efficacy of antiinfectives with pharmacodynamics and Monte Carlo simulation. Pediatr Infect Dis J 2003;22:982–92.

[3] Centers for Disease Control and Prevention. Geographic variation in penicillin resistance in *Streptococcus pneumoniae*—selected sites, United States, 1997. MMWR Morb Mortal Wkly Rep 1999;48:656–61.

[4] Kaplan SL, Mason Jr EO, Barson WJ, et al. Three-year multicenter surveillance of systemic pneumococcal infections in children. Pediatrics 1998;102:538–45.

[5] Mason Jr EO, Kaplan SL, Lamberth LB, Tillman J. Increased rate of isolation of penicillin-resistant *Streptococcus pneumoniae* in a children's hospital and in vitro susceptibilities to antibiotics of potential therapeutic use. Antimicrob Agents Chemother 1992;36:1703–7.

[6] Salgado CD, Farr BM, Calfee DP. Community-acquired methicillin-resistant *Staphylococcus aureus*: a meta-analysis of prevalence and risk factors. Clin Infect Dis 2003;36:131–9.

[7] Frank AL, Marcinak JF, Mangat PD, Schreckenberger PC. Community-acquired and clindamycin-susceptible methicillin-resistant *Staphylococcus aureus* in children. Pediatr Infect Dis J 1999; 18:993–1000.

[8] Dufour P, Gillet Y, Bes M, et al. Community-acquired methicillin-resistant *Staphylococcus aureus* infections in France: emergence of a single clone that produces Panton-Valentine leukocidin. Clin Infect Dis 2002;35:819–24.

[9] Livermore DM. Antibiotic resistance in staphylococci. Int J Antimicrob Agents 2000;16:S3–10.

[10] Ma XX, Ito T, Tiensasitorn C, et al. Novel type of staphylococcal cassette chromosome mec identified in community-acquired methicillin-resistant *Staphylococcus aureus* strains. Antimicrob Agents Chemother 2002;46:1147–52.

[11] Daum RS, Ito T, Hiramatsu K, et al. A novel methicillin-resistance cassette in community-acquired methicillin resistant *Staphylococcus aureus* isolates of diverse genetic backgrounds. J Infect Dis 2002;186:1344–7.

[12] Charlebois ED, Perdreau-Remington F, Kreiswirth B, et al. Origins of community strains of methicillin-resistant *Staphylococcus aureus*. Clin Infect Dis 2004;39:47–54.

[13] Craig WA. Pharmacokinetic/pharmacodynamic parameters: rational for antibacterial dosing of mice and men. Clin Infect Dis 1998;26:1–12.

[14] Craig WA. Basic pharmacodynamics of antibacterials with clinical applications to the use of beta-lactams, glycopeptides, and linezolid. Infect Dis Clin North Am 2003;17:479–501.

[15] McEvoy GK, editor. AHFS Drug Information 2003. Bethesda (MD): American Society of Health-System Pharmacists; 2003.

[16] Furlanut M, Brollo L, Lugatti E, et al. Pharmacokinetic aspects of levofloxacin 500 mg once

daily during sequential intravenous/oral therapy in patients with lower respiratory tract infections. J Antimicrob Chemother 2003;51:101–6.

[17] Saravolatz LD, Leggett J. Gatifloxacin, gemifloxacin, and moxifloxacin: the role of 2 newer fluoroquinolones. Clin Infect Dis 2003;37:1210–5.

[18] Stalker DJ, Jungbluth GL, Hopkins NK, Batts DH. Pharmacokinetics and tolerance of single- and multiple-dose oral or intravenous linezolid, an oxazolidinone antibiotic, in healthy volunteers. J Antimicrob Chemother 2003;51:1239–46.

[19] Gudnason T, Gudbrandsson F, Barsanti F, Kristinsson KG. Penetration of ceftriaxone into the middle ear fluid of children. Pediatr Infect Dis J 1998;17:258–60.

[20] Aperia A, Broberger O, Broberger U, Herin P, Zetterstrom R. Postnatal development of renal function in pre-term and full-term infants. Acta Paediatr Scand 1981;70:183–7.

[21] Capparelli EV, Lane JR, Romanowski GL, et al. The influences of renal function and maturation on vancomycin elimination in newborns and infants. J Clin Pharmacol 2001;41:927–34.

[22] Bradley JS, Nelson JD, editors. Nelson's pocket book of pediatric antimicrobial therapy. 16th edition. Buenos Aires, Argentina: Acindes; 2005 [in press].

[23] Pong A, Bradley JS. Clinical challenges of nosocomial infections caused by antibiotic-resistant pathogens in pediatrics. Semin Pediatr Infect Dis 2004;15:21–9.

[24] Bush K. New beta-lactamases in gram-negative bacteria: diversity and impact on the selection of antimicrobial therapy. Clin Infect Dis 2001;32:1085–9 [Epub].

[25] Widdowson CA, Klugman KP. Molecular mechanisms of resistance to commonly used non-betalactam drugs in *Streptococcus pneumoniae*. Semin Respir Infect 1999;14:255–68.

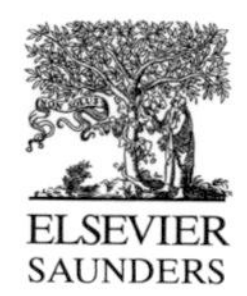

ELSEVIER
SAUNDERS

Pediatr Clin N Am 52 (2005) 895–915

PEDIATRIC CLINICS
OF NORTH AMERICA

Antifungal Agents in Children

William J. Steinbach, MD[a,b,*]

[a]*Department of Pediatrics, Division of Pediatric Infectious Diseases, Box 3499, Duke University Medical Center, Durham, NC 27710, USA*
[b]*Department of Molecular Genetics and Microbiology, Duke University Medical Center, Durham, NC 27710, USA*

Fungal pathogens are an increasingly recognized complication of organ transplantation and the ever more potent chemotherapeutic regimens for childhood malignancies. There has been a recent surge in the development of antifungals, including new formulations of older drugs and the discovery of a class of agents with a novel target. More recent studies have expanded knowledge on how to optimize the utility of these new agents. Because of the paucity of pediatric data, however, many recommendations for use of antifungals in children are derived from experience in adult patients.

This article provides a brief overview of the current state of systemic antifungal therapy. Currently licensed drugs, including amphotericin B and its lipid derivates; 5-fluorocytosine; the azoles, including fluconazole, itraconazole, and voriconazole; and a representative of the new class of echinocandin agents, caspofungin, are discussed. Newer second-generation azoles (posaconazole and ravuconazole) and echinocandins (micafungin and anidulafungin) that are likely to be licensed in the United States in the next few years also are addressed. The

* Department of Pediatrics, Division of Pediatric Infectious Diseases, Box 3499, Duke University Medical Center, Durham, NC 27710.

E-mail address: stein022@mc.duke.edu

doi:10.1016/j.pcl.2005.02.009

pediatric.theclinics.com

Table 1
Spectrum of activity of selected antifungal agents

Antifungal	Important clinical uses
Amphotericin B	*Blastomyces dermatitidis*, *Coccidioides immitis*, *Cryptococcus neoformans*, *Histoplasma capsulatum*, *Paracoccidioides brasiliensis*, *Sporotrix schenckii,* most *Candida* species, *Aspergillus,* Zygomycetes (*not: Candida lusitaniae, Scedosporium, Fusarium, Trichosporon*)
5-Fluorocytosine	Only in combination therapy for *Candida, C. neoformans*, dematiaceous molds
Fluconazole	Most *Candida, C. neoformans, B. dermatitidis, H. capsulatum, C. immitis, P. brasiliensis* (*not: Candida krusei, Candida glabrata, Aspergillus*)
Itraconazole	*Candida, Aspergillus, B. dermatitidis, H. capsulatum, C. immitis, P. brasiliensis*
Voriconazole	*Candida, Aspergillus, Fusarium, B. dermatitidis, H. capsulatum, C. immitis, Malassezia* species, *Scedosporium*, dematiaceous molds (*not*: Zygomycetes; *caution*: *C. glabrata*)
Caspofungin	*Candida, Aspergillus* (*not: C. neoformans, Fusarium*, Zygomycetes)

antifungal spectra of each agent are presented on Table 1, and recommended dosages are summarized on Table 2.

Polyenes: amphotericin B

Mechanism of action

The oldest antifungal class is the polyene macrolides, amphotericin B and nystatin. Since its initial approval for use in 1958, amphotericin B deoxycholate remains the "gold standard" for the therapy of many invasive fungal infections and the comparative agent for all newer antifungal agents. Amphotericin B binds to ergosterol, the major sterol found in fungal cytoplasmic membranes, creating transmembrane channels resulting in an increased permeability to monovalent cations. Fungicidal activity is believed to be caused by leakage of essential nutrients from the fungal cell.

Pharmacology and toxicities

The fungicidal activity of amphotericin B is concentration-dependent, increasing directly with the amount of drug attained at the site of infection. Amphotericin B also has a prolonged postantifungal effect. That is, antifungal activity persists even after the concentration of drug declines to less than the amount needed to kill the fungus. These pharmacodynamic characteristics suggest that a single daily dose of amphotericin B would be effective [1]. Although there is a relationship between total dose administered and tissue concentrations [2], there is no conclusive clinical evidence that doses greater than 1 mg/kg/d

Table 2
Preferred pediatric dosing of approved systemic antifungal agents

Drug class	Antifungal drug	Preferred adult dosing	Preferred pediatric dosing	Pedatric dosing comments
Polyene	Amphotericin B deoxycholate (Fungizone)	1–1.5 mg/kg/d	1–1.5 mg/kg/d	Children generally can tolerate higher doses than adults
	Amphotericin B lipid complex (Abelcet)	5 mg/kg/d*	5 mg/kg/d	
	Amphotericin B colloidal dispersion (Amphocil; Amphotec)	5 mg/kg/d*	5 mg/kg/d	
	Liposomal amphotericin B (AmBisome)	5 mg/kg/d*	5 mg/kg/d	
Pyrimidine analogue	5-Fluorocytosine (Ancobon)	150 mg/kg/d divided q6h	150 mg/kg/d divided q6h	Use caution with large oral volume for neonates
Triazole	Fluconazole (Diflucan)	100–800 mg/d; 3–6 mg/kg/d	6–12 mg/kg/d	Dose higher in children due to shorter half-life; neonates require further special dosing
	Itraconazole (Sporanox)	200–400 mg/d	2.5–5 mg/kg/dose bid	Dosing BID preferred in children
	Voriconazole (VFend)	Load: 6 mg/kg/dose bid × 1 d Maintenance: 3–4 mg/kg/dose bid	Load: 6 mg/kg/dose bid × 1 d Maintenance: 4–8 mg/kg/dose BID†	Linear pharmacokinetics in children; exact pediatric dose not yet determined, but believed to be greater than adult dosing
Echinocandin	Caspofungin (Cancidas)	Load: 70 mg qd × 1 d Maintenance: 50 mg qd	Load: 70 mg/m^2 QD × 1 d Maintenance: 50 mg/m^2 qd	Dosing for hepatic insufficiency in children is 35 mg/m^2 qd, similar to the adult decrease to 35 mg qd

* Abelcet is officially recommended at 5 mg/kg/d; Amphocil, at 3–5 mg/kg/d; and AmBisome, at 1–5 mg/kg/d. Most clinical data have been obtained with the use of these preparations at 5 mg/kg/d, and most clinicians use and prefer this higher dosing.

† Suggested dosing by the author; exact pediatric dosing for voriconazole not yet determined.

of amphotericin B deoxycholate are necessary for successful therapy [3,4]. Cerebrospinal fluid (CSF) concentrations are only 2% to 4% of serum concentrations [5], so this agent is a poor choice as monotherapy for the treatment of meningitis.

In addition to fungal ergosterol, amphotericin B binds to cholesterol in human cell membranes, likely accounting for its toxicity [6]. Lipid formulations of amphotericin B generally are better tolerated than the conventional deoxycholate preparation, perhaps because the lipid stabilizes the drug in a self-associated state so that it cannot interact with the cholesterol of human cellular membranes [7,8]. The reduced nephrotoxicity of lipid formulations also may result from their preferential binding to serum high-density lipoproteins. High-density lipoprotein–bound amphotericin B seems to be released to the kidney more slowly, or to a lesser degree, than conventional amphotericin B that is bound to low-density lipoproteins [9].

Three lipid-associated formulations of amphotercin B offer the advantage of an increased daily dose of the parent drug, better delivery to the primary reticuloendothelial organs (lungs, liver, spleen) [10,11], and reduced toxicity. The US Food and Drug Administration (FDA) approved amphotericin B lipid complex (ABLC, Abelcet) in December 1995, amphotericin B colloidal dispersion (ABCD, Amphocil, Amphotec) in December 1996, and liposomal amphotericin B (L-amphotericin B, AmBisome) in August 1997 [12]. It is postulated that activated monocytes/macrophages take up drug-laden lipid formulations and transport them to the site of infection, where phospholipases release free drug [12,13]. A multicenter maximum tolerated dose study of L-amphotericin B using doses of 7.5 to 15 mg/kg/d found a nonlinear plasma pharmacokinetic profile with a maximal concentration at 10 mg/kg/d and no demonstrable dose-limiting nephrotoxicity or infusion-related toxicity [14].

Amphotericin B nephrotoxicity is generally less severe in infants and children than in adults, likely resulting from the more rapid clearance of the drug in children. Reduced nephrotoxicity with a lipid formulation has been reported in adults and has been observed in children [15,16] and neonates [17]. A pharmacokinetic study of L-amphotericin B conducted in 39 children ranging in age from 1 to 17 years observed no dose-related trends in adverse events and a maximally tolerated dose of 10 mg/kg/d (Gilead Sciences, data on file). These results are similar to the results in studies conducted in adults [14]. A 56-center prospective study evaluated the safety and efficacy of L-amphotericin B administered to 260 adults, 242 children (<15 years old), and 43 infants (<2 months old) [18]. In general, the infants and children tolerated the largest doses of L-amphotericin B administered for the longest time (median 16 days) [18].

Clinical experience and pediatric data

The optimal duration of amphotericin B therapy is unknown, but likely depends on underlying disease, extent of fungal infection, resolution of neutropenia, degree of immunosuppression, and graft function after transplantation. No specific total dose of amphotericin B currently is recommended; rather, a standard approach is to initiate therapy with 1 mg/kg/d, reducing the dose if toxicity develops [19]. No data indicate that any of the amphotericin B lipid formulations are more effective than conventional amphotericin B [10,12,20–22]. A study of 56 infants with candidiasis, including 52 preterm infants, showed no differences in mortality or time to resolution of candidemia between neonates receiving conventional amphotericin B ($n = 34$), L-amphotericin B ($n = 6$), or ABCD ($n = 16$) [23]. The decision to prescribe a lipid formulation of amphotericin B should be based on the potential of reducing nephrotoxicity or infusion-related toxicity rather than anticipated therapeutic benefit.

In noncomparative studies, ABLC has been found to be an effective antifungal agent in children. In an open-label pediatric trial, complete or partial therapeutic response was observed in 70% (38 of 54) of patients, including 56% (14 of 25) of patients with aspergillosis and 81% (22 of 27) of patients with candidiasis [16]. A retrospective study of 46 children treated with ABLC reported an overall response rate of 83% (38 of 46), including 78% (18 of 23) against aspergillosis and 89% (17 of 19) against candidiasis [24].

Few published data exist on the use of lipid formulations of amphotericin B in neonates. One study that included 40 preterm neonates (mean birth weight 1090 g, mean gestational age 28.4 weeks) noted that L-amphotericin B was associated with clinical resolution in greater than 70% of patients with candidiasis [25]; other uncontrolled studies have confirmed the high response rates. In three other studies, 21 of 21, 35 of 37, and 20 of 24 neonates with candidiasis cleared their infections [26–28].

Pyrimidine analogues: 5-Fluorocytosine

Mechanism of action

5-Fluorocytosine (5-FC, Ancoban) is a fluorinated analogue of cytosine that has antimycotic activity resulting from the rapid conversion of 5-FC into 5-fluorouracil (5-FU) within susceptible fungal cells [29,30]. 5-FU inhibits fungal protein synthesis after incorporation into fungal RNA in place of uridylic acid or through inhibition of thymidylate synthetase, inhibiting fungal DNA synthesis [30]. 5-FC has little inherent antimold activity [31], and most reports detail clinical failure with monotherapy against yeast infections [32]. Antifungal resistance develops quickly to 5-FC monotherapy, so the drug should be used only in combination with other agents. 5-FC is thought to enhance the antifungal activity of amphotericin B, especially in anatomic sites where amphotericin B penetration is poor, such as CSF, heart valves, and the vitreal body [3]. One explanation for the synergism detected with amphotericin B plus 5-FC is that the membrane-permeabilizing effects of low concentrations of amphotericin B facilitate penetration of 5-FC to the cell interior [33].

Pharmacology and toxicities

5-FC is well absorbed after oral administration [30]. 5-FC distributes widely, attaining therapeutic concentrations in most body sites, such as the CSF, vitreous and peritoneal fluids, and inflamed joints, because it is small and highly water soluble and not bound by serum proteins to a great extent [30]. It is often technically difficult to treat neonates with 5-FC because of the large volume necessitated by using the oral formulation and the lack of an intravenous formulation available in the United States.

5-FC toxicity seems to be due to its conversion to 5-FU, with reports of 5-FU concentrations being in the range found after chemotherapeutic doses [34]. 5-FC may exacerbate myelosuppression in patients with neutropenia, and trough serum concentrations of 100 μg/mL or greater are associated with bone marrow aplasia. 5-FC serum concentrations should be monitored, and levels should be maintained at approximately 40 to 80 μg/mL. In a review of a multicenter trial of 194 patients who received amphotericin B plus 5-FC for cryptococcal meningitis, hematologic toxicity appeared in the first 2 weeks of therapy in 56% of patients and in the first 4 weeks of therapy in 87% [35].

Clinical experience and pediatric data

A pivotal trial showed that the combination of amphotericin B plus 5-FC was more effective than amphotericin B alone in the treatment of cryptococcal meningitis [36]. A subsequent multicenter study of 194 patients with cryptococcal meningitis concluded that 4 weeks of amphotericin B plus 5-FC was adequate for immunocompetent patients without neurologic complications, such as hydrocephalus. In immunocompromised patients, 6 weeks of combination therapy resulted in fewer relapses [37]. Amphotericin B combined with 5-FC currently is recommended as initial therapy for cryptococcal meningitis [38]. These two agents also are suggested for use in patients with candidal meningitis [39].

Data regarding the use of 5-FC in children are limited. One review of 17 cases of candidal meningitis that included 11 patients younger than 12 months old noted improvement in 15 patients treated with amphotericin B and 5-FC [40].

Azoles

Mechanism of action

The azole antifungals are heterocyclic synthetic compounds that inhibit the fungal lanosterol 14α-demethylase, which catalyzes a late step in ergosterol biosynthesis. The drugs block demethylation of the C-14 of lanosterol, leading to substitution of methylated sterols in the fungal cell membrane and depletion of ergosterol. The result is an accumulation of precursors leading to abnormalities in fungal membrane permeability, membrane-bound enzyme activity, and a lack of coordination of chitin synthesis [41,42].

Fluconazole

Pharmacology and toxicities

Fluconazole (Diflucan) is a triazole that was approved by the FDA for treatment of cryptococcosis and *Candida* infections in 1990. Fluconazole's activity is concentration-independent; it does not increase when the maximal fungistatic concentration is attained [43]. Fluconazole is available as either an oral or an intravenous form, and oral fluconazole is approximately 90% bioavailable. Unchanged drug is cleared predominantly by the kidneys; metabolism accounts for only a minor proportion of fluconazole clearance [44]. Drug concentrations in CSF and vitreous humor are approximately 80% of the concentrations found in blood [45]. Fluconazole passes into tissues and fluids rapidly, probably as a result of its relatively low lipophilicity and limited binding to plasma proteins. Concentrations of fluconazole are 10-fold to 20-fold higher in the urine than in the blood, and it is particularly appropriate for the therapy of fungal urinary tract infections.

The pharmacokinetics of fluconazole differ between adults and children. A review of five separate fluconazole pharmacokinetic studies that included 101 infants and children ranging in age from 2 weeks to 16 years [44] showed that fluconazole clearance is more rapid in children than adults. The mean plasma half-life was approximately 20 hours in children compared with 30 hours in adults. To achieve comparable drug exposure, the daily fluconazole dose needs to be approximately doubled for children older than 3 months to 6 to 12 mg/kg/d.

The volume of distribution of fluconazole is greater and more variable in neonates than in infants and children. There is also a slow elimination of fluconazole, however, with a mean half-life of 88.6 hours at birth, decreasing to approximately 55 hours by 2 weeks of age. Neonates should be treated with a higher dose of fluconazole to compensate for their increased volume of distribution, but the frequency of dosing needs to be decreased because of their slow elimination. Specifically, during the first 2 weeks of life, fluconazole should be dosed every 72 hours; this dosing interval can be reduced to 48 hours during the next 2 weeks of life [44]. The pharmacologic consequence of such a long half-life is that patients require at least 8 days to reach steady state [46].

Side effects of fluconazole are uncommon. In one study of 24 immunocompromised children, elevated transaminases were observed in only 2 children [47]. Another review of 562 children confirmed that pediatric results mirror the excellent safety profile seen in adults. The most common side effects were gastrointestinal upset (vomiting, diarrhea, nausea) (7.7%) or skin rash (1.2%) [48].

Clinical experience and pediatric data

In one clinical trial of 206 nonneutropenic adult patients with invasive candidiasis, the rate of successful therapy with 0.5 to 0.6 mg/kg/d of amphotericin B (79%) was similar to that with 400 mg/d of fluconazole (70%) [49]. Another multicenter trial of 219 mostly nonneutropenic adult patients with invasive candidiasis found that patients treated with a combination of fluconazole and amphotercin B ($n = 112$) showed no difference in the 30-day time to failure compared with patients treated with fluconazole alone ($n = 107$) [50]. Although a secondary analysis suggested that combination therapy was superior in efficacy to fluconazole alone, the difference in favorable outcome was small (69% versus 56%). A definitive conclusion regarding the benefit of this combination therapy to treat candidiasis is unproven.

Clinical and mycologic response was observed in 97% of 40 neonates and infants treated with fluconazole. These children had been nonresponsive or intolerant to standard antifungal therapy [51]. In another report, 80% of 40 neonates with invasive candidiasis were treated successfully with 6 mg/kg/d of fluconazole. Although three of these patients relapsed, they ultimately were cured with an increased dose of fluconazole (10 mg/kg/d) [52]. Finally, a prospective randomized study that compared fluconazole with amphotericin B in 24 infants with candidemia noted a survival benefit among infants treated with fluconazole (67%) compared with infants who received amphotericin B (55%) [53].

Fluconazole also has been evaluated for antifungal prophylaxis. Randomized, placebo-controlled clinical trials have shown that the prophylactic use of fluconazole after allogeneic bone marrow transplantation results in lower rates of candidal infection and graft-versus-host disease [54]. Studies conducted in adult stem cell transplant recipients observed that 200 mg/d of prophylactic fluconazole is as effective as 400 mg/d [55,56]. One concern with this patient population continues to be the lack of anti-*Aspergillus* activity with fluconazole. A prospective, placebo-controlled, randomized, double-blind evaluation of prophylactic fluconazole has been conducted in 100 low-birth-weight (<1000 g) infants. Six weeks of fluconazole therapy resulted in a statistically significant reduction in the incidence of fungal colonization (22% versus 60%) and a decrease in the development of invasive fungal infection (0% versus 20%) [57].

Itraconazole

Itraconazole (Sporanox) is fungicidal and has been available for clinical use since 1990 [58]. Limitations of itraconazole include lack of a parenteral formulation, erratic oral absorption in high-risk patients, and frequent drug interactions.

Pharmacology and toxicities

Itraconazole has a high volume of distribution and accumulates in tissues [42]. It is not reliably absorbed from the gastrointestinal tract and has high protein binding [1]. H_2 receptor antagonists may result in decreased drug absorption, whereas acidic beverages, such as colas or cranberry juice, may enhance absorption [59]. Administration of the capsular formulation with food increases absorption, but the oral suspension is better absorbed on an empty stomach [5].

Elimination of itraconazole is primarily hepatic; there is no need for dosage adjustment in the presence of renal function impairment [42].

Serum concentrations of itraconazole are much lower in children than in adults after administration of the oral solution. This is especially true in children younger than 5 years old [60–62]. Children usually need twice-daily dosing, whereas once-daily dosing is appropriate for adults.

Itraconazole is well tolerated. Nausea and vomiting occur in about 10% of subjects, and elevated transaminases occur in 5% [63]. Rare cases of cardiomyopathy have been reported in adults, but no cases have been described in children. Itraconzole is a potent inhibitor of the cytochrome CYP3A4 enzyme and can result in important drug interactions. Prior or concurrent use of rifampin, phenytoin, carbamazepime, and phenobarbital should be avoided, and concomitant use with cyclophosphamide should be discouraged [64]. Any drug handled by this cytochrome pathway with normally low bioavailability, extensive first-pass metabolism, or a narrow therapeutic window may be especially vulnerable [65].

Clinical experience and pediatric data

Itraconazole is currently more appealing as a prophylactic rather than a therapeutic agent. It may be superior to fluconazole for this purpose. In one large randomized, controlled trial conducted in 445 patients with hematologic malignancy, itraconazole oral solution prevented more fungal infections than fluconazole suspension. Specifically, six proven fungal infections, including four fatal cases, occurred in the fluconazole recipients compared with one nonfatal case of candidiasis in the itraconazole recipients [66]. Additionally, although there were no cases of invasive aspergillosis in the patients receiving itraconazole, four cases of aspergillosis were diagnosed among patients receiving fluconazole. Itraconazole and fluconazole prophylaxis had similar prophylactic efficacy in a trial conduced in liver transplant recipients [67]. Itraconazole also has been shown to be an effective prophylactic agent in patients infected with HIV. A double-blind, placebo-controlled trial conducted in 63 patients with HIV infection in Thailand showed a reduction in fungal infections from 16.7% in the placebo recipients to 1.6% in patients taking itraconazole [68].

There are no pivotal studies of itraconazole prophylaxis in children, and the few children enrolled in the larger prophylaxis studies were not analyzed separately. A phase I study in 26 HIV-infected children showed the cyclodextrin itraconazole solution was well tolerated and efficacious against oropharyngeal candidiasis, including responses in all patients with fluconazole-resistant isolates [62].

Voriconazole

Voriconazole (VFend) is a second-generation triazole and a synthetic derivative of fluconazole. Voriconazole combines the broad spectrum of antifungal activity of itraconazole with the increased bioavailability of fluconazole. It is fungicidal against *Aspergillus* and fungistatic against *Candida* species [58, 69–71].

Pharmacology and toxicities

Voriconazole metabolism is nonlinear in adults with an approximately threefold increase in the area under the concentration-time curve after a 33% increase in dosage. In contrast, elimination of voriconazole seems to be linear in children after doses of 3 mg/kg and 4 mg/kg every 12 hours [72].

Children require higher doses of voriconazole than adults to attain similar serum concentrations over time. Based on limited pharmacokinetic analyses, it seems that a pediatric dosage of 11 mg/kg administered every 12 hours is approximately bioequivalent to an adult dosage of 4 mg/kg given every 12 hours [72]. The correct pediatric dosage is unknown, but seems to be much higher than the dosage for adult patients. Using voriconazole at recommended doses for adults may lead to clinical failures in children.

After nearly complete oral absorption, voriconazole is extensively metabolized by the liver. As a result of a point mutation in the gene encoding CYP2C19, some people are poor metabolizers, and some are extensive metabolizers [73]. About 5% to 7% of whites and 20% of non-Indian Asians have a deficiency in expressing this enzyme. As a result, voriconazole levels are fourfold greater in these subjects than in homozygous subjects who metabolize the drug more extensively [74,75].

Voriconazole's main side effects include reversible dose-dependent visual disturbances (increased brightness, blurred vision) [76] in one third of treated patients, elevated hepatic transaminases with increasing doses [77,78], and occasional skin reactions likely secondary to photosensitization [41,69,79]. Drug interactions also can be problematic. Concomitant use with sirolimus is contraindicated because concentrations of the immunosuppressant can be increased 2-fold to 10-fold [80,81].

Clinical experience and pediatric data

Voriconazole is statistically superior to amphotericin B deoxycholate in the therapy of aspergillosis. In a prospective clinical trial of 392 patients with invasive aspergillosis, more than 50% of patients initially treated with voriconazole compared with only about 30% of patients treated with amphotericin B had complete or partial responses. Improved survival also was observed among patients initially treated with voriconazole [82]. Similar positive experience with voriconazole was noted in an open-label multicenter study of 116 patients with invasive aspergillosis treated with voriconazole as either primary (60 patients) or salvage (56 patients) therapy [83]. These data have led clinicians to conclude that voriconazole is the preferred agent for treatment of invasive aspergillosis.

Voriconazole also is effective in the treatment of *Candida* infections. In a multicenter evaluation of the therapy of esophageal candidiasis in 391 immunocompromised patients, voriconazole was successful in 98.3%, and fluconazole was successful in 95.1% [84]. In another study of 422 patients with invasive candidiasis, approximately 40% of patients were treated successfully with voriconazole. This success rate was virtually identical to that of amphotericin B therapy, followed by oral fluconazole [85]. Voriconazole also has been evaluated in the management of febrile neutropenic patients. In one large study of more than 800 episodes of fever and neutropenia, voriconazole was slightly inferior to L-amphotericin B. Voriconazole was effective in 26% of 415 subjects, and L-amphotericin B was effective in 30% of 422 subjects. There were more breakthrough infections in the L-amphotericin B recipients, however, including 13 cases of invasive aspergillosis versus 4 cases in the voriconazole recipients [86].

The largest pediatric report of voriconazole is an open-label, compassionate-use evaluation of the drug in 58 children with proven or probable invasive fungal infection refractory to or intolerant of conventional antifungal therapy [87]. Almost three quarters of the patients had aspergillosis. After a mean of 3 months of therapy, 45% of the children had a complete or partial response. Only 7% of the subjects could not tolerate the drug. Stratifying outcome by pathogen revealed a complete or partial response of 43% against aspergillosis, 50% against candidemia, and 63% against scedosporiosis.

Experimental azoles: posaconazole and ravuconazole

Posaconazole is a second-generation triazole that is closely related to itraconazole. It is fungicidal in vitro against *Aspergillus* and has a half-life of at least 18 to 24 hours in humans [41,88]. Presently, only an oral formulation of posaconazole is available. Posaconazole was found to be effective and well tolerated in a multicenter study in patients refractory to other antifungal agents [89]. Experience with posaconazole in children is limited. In an open-label study, two of seven patients with chronic granulmonatous disease and invasive fungal infection were younger than 18 years old [90]. Six patients had a complete response. Similarly, two patients were younger than 18 years old in another open-label study of 23 patients with zygomycosis. The overall success rate of therapy in this study was 70% [91]. Poscaonazole is likely to play a role in antifungal management as an excellent oral agent, but detailed pediatric studies have yet to be performed.

Ravuconazole is structurally similar to fluconazole and voriconazole. It is fungicidal [92,93], has 47% to 74% bioavailability with linear pharmacokinetics [41], and has a long half-life of approximately 100 hours [94]. Of 76 patients with esophageal candidiasis, 76% were cured with 7 days of therapy with ravuconazole. The drug's safety profile was similar to that of fluconazole [95]. Ravuconazole's long half-life could lead to potentially intermittent dosing. No pediatric data are available.

Echinocandins

Mechanism of action

For years, development of new systemic antifungals focused on chemically modifying existing classes. More recently, an entirely new class of antifungals, the echinocandins, has been discovered. These agents interfere with cell wall biosynthesis by noncompetitive inhibition of 1,3-β-D-glucan synthase, an enzyme present in fungi but absent in mammalian cells [41,88]. This 1,3-β-glucan, an essential cell wall polysaccharide, forms a fibril of three helically entwined linear polysaccharides and provides structural integrity to the fungal cell wall [96,97]. Echinocandins are fungicidal against *Candida* but fungistatic against *Aspergillus* [98]. These agents are not metabolized through the cytochrome enzyme system, but through a presumed O-methyltransferase, lessening some of the drug interactions and side effects seen with the azoles.

Caspofungin

Pharmacology and toxicities

Caspofungin (Cancidas) is a fungicidal semisynthetic derivative of the natural product pneumocandin B_0. It has linear pharmacokinetics [99], is excreted primarily by the liver, has a beta-phase half-life of 9 to10 hours [100], and is well tolerated [101–104]. It is not metabolized by the cytochrome isoenzyme system [105], and at present there is no known maximal tolerated dose and no toxicity-defined maximal length of therapy. Elevations of caspofungin plasma concentrations are observed in patients with mild hepatic insufficiency, and a dose reduction in adults from 50 mg to 35 mg daily after the standard 70-mg loading dose is recommended in this setting [77].

A pharmacokinetic study conducted in children evaluated 39 patients between ages 2 and 17 years. Data were analyzed on the basis of weight (1 mg/kg/d) and body surface area (50 mg/m^2/d or 70 mg/m^2/d) [106]. Compared with plasma concentrations attained in adults treated with 50 mg/d, the weight-based approach resulted in suboptimal plasma concentrations, whereas the 50 mg/m^2/d dose yielded similar plasma concentrations in the children. Caspofungin's half-life is approximately one third less in children than in adults.

Because 1,3-β-glucan is a selective target present only in fungal cell walls and not in mammalian cells, caspofungin has few adverse effects [96]. The drug has no apparent myelotoxicity or nephrotoxicity [107]. Plasma concentrations of tacrolimus are reduced by about 20% when coadministered with caspofungin, but tacrolimus does not alter the pharmacokinetics of caspofungin [108]. Cyclosporine increases the concentration of caspofungin by about 35%, but plasma concentrations of cyclosporine are not altered by coadministration of caspofungin [109]. A retrospective analysis of the compassionate use of caspofungin in 25 children, most of whom also received other antifungals, noted that only 3 (12%) had a possible drug-related adverse event [110].

Clinical experience and pediatric data

In the pivotal clinical study that led to FDA approval, 56 adults with acute invasive aspergillosis received caspofungin as "salvage" therapy after failing primary therapy for more than 1 week or developing significant nephrotoxicity. More than 40% of the patients had a favorable response to therapy [111]. Additional patients have been enrolled in this trial, and to date, 45% (37 of 83) have had a complete or partial response, including 50% (32 of 64) with pulmonary aspergillosis and 23% (3 of 13) with disseminated infection [112]. Caspofungin has not been studied for use in primary therapy against invasive aspergillosis.

A study comparing caspofungin and amphotericin B in 224 adults with invasive candidiasis has been conducted. Response to caspofungin (n = 104; 73.4%) was slightly better than response to amphotericin B (n = 115; 61.7%) [113]. Caspofungin was as effective as amphotericin B against all the major species of *Candida*. Mortality was similar in both groups, and the proportion of patients with drug-related adverse events was substantially higher in the amphotericin B group. More recently, caspofungin (n = 556) was compared with L-amphotericin B (n = 539) in febrile neutropenic patients, and overall success was virtually identical (approximately 33%) [114].

Experimental echinocandins: micafungin and anidulafungin

Micafungin is an echinocandin lipopeptide compound [41,115,116] with a half-life of approximately 12 hours. As with other echinocandins, it is fungicidal against *Candida* and fungistatic against *Aspergillus* [117]. The highest drug concentrations of this agent are detected in the lung, followed by the liver, spleen, and kidney. Micafungin was undetectable in the CSF, but low levels were detected in the brain tissue, choroidal layer, and vitreous humor, but not the aqueous humor of the eye [99].

Several pediatric studies of micafungin have been completed. A phase I single-dose, multicenter, open-label study evaluated three dosages (0.75 mg/kg/d, 1.5 mg/kg/d, and 3 mg/kg/d) in two infant weight groups (500–1000 g and >1000 g). The mean serum concentration of micafungin was lower in the smaller infants, the serum half-life was shorter, and clearance was more rapid. In the neonates weighing 500 to 1000 g, the half-life was 5.5 hours with a clearance of 97.3 mL/h/kg. In the neonates weighing more than 1000 g, the haf-life increased to 8 hours, whereas clearance decreased to 55.9 mL/h/kg. These findings compare with the findings in children (age 2–8 years), where half-life was 12 hours, and clearance was slowest at 32.2 mL/h/kg [118].

A study of micafungin in combination with a second antifungal agent in pediatric and adult bone marrow transplant recipients with invasive aspergillosis revealed an overall complete or partial response of approximately 40% [119]. A study comparing prophylaxis in 882 stem cell transplant recipients found that micafungin was more effective in preventing yeast and mold infections (80%) than fluconazole (73.5%) [120]. Other studies have shown the efficacy of micafungin in the primary therapy of esophageal candidiasis [121] and as rescue therapy in patients failing to respond to first-line antifungals [122].

Anidulafungin is a semisynthetic terphenyl-substituted antifungal derived from echinocandin B, a lipopeptide fungal product [123]. It has linear pharmacokinetics [88] with the longest half-life of all the echinocandins (approximately 18 hours) [101,124]. Its in vitro activity is similar to that of the other echinocandins [125]. Neither end-stage renal impairment nor dialysis substantially alters the pharmacokinetics of anidulafungin [126]. Tissue concentrations after multiple dosing were highest in lung and liver, followed by spleen and kidney, with measurable concentrations in the brain tissue. The pharmacokinetics showed approximately sixfold lower mean peak concentrations in plasma and twofold lower area under the concentration-time curve values compared with values with similar doses of capsofungin and micafungin. A study of 601 patients with esophageal candidiasis compared anidulafungin with oral fluconazole and found endoscopic similar success rates exceeding 95% [127]. A phase I/II dose escalation study of anidulafungin involving five centers that enrolled children age 2 to 17 years old with persistent neutropenia who were at risk for invasive fungal infection is now complete, but results have not yet been presented.

Summary

Since the 1960s, there has been limited progress in the treatment of invasive fungal infections, and the field of pediatric antifungal therapy has been largely ignored. Although conventional amphotericin B was the drug of choice for many invasive fungal infections, its clinical utility was thwarted by nephrotoxicity and infusion-related toxicity. Lipid formulations have reduced the toxicity of amphotericin B, and these agents have a role in the management of several specific diseases, such as zygomycosis and others.

The preferred treatment for invasive aspergillosis has shifted to voriconazole, with present debates centering on the possible use of combination antifungal therapy. A reason for failure of therapy in children may be the use of an inadequate dose of voriconazole, originally based on data derived from adults. A knowledge of the differences in the pharmacokinetics of the drug in children and adults results in more optimal dosing. Although voriconazole is a tremendous mold-active agent, gaps in coverage, such as the emerging zygomycosis and non-*albicans Candida* species, are important to address. Presently, investigational posaconazole seems to have better activity against zygomycosis, but no parenteral formulation of this drug is available. Although the extended half-life of ravuconazole could play a role in prophylaxis or long-term intermittent therapy, the drug is not yet available.

The echinocandin class presents one of the best options for therapy of candidiasis, combining an excellent safety profile with an effective fungicidal agent. Although caspofungin likely has some role in salvage therapy for recalcitrant invasive aspergillosis, it may prove to be most valuable as an anti-

Candida drug or possibly as part of combination therapy for invasive aspergillosis. Micafungin and anidulafungin have begun to acquire initial pediatric dosing data, and these drugs may prove to be useful in children.

Few antifungal studies have been conducted in children. Although there have been many phase III antifungal clinical trials in adults, there has never been a large phase III antifungal clinical trial dedicated to pediatric patients. Consequently, most information for the pediatrician has been extrapolated from adult data. Through dedicated clinicians and collaboration, pediatric indications and dosing strategies eventually will be discovered that will benefit pediatric patients directly.

References

[1] Groll AH, Piscitelli SC, Walsh TJ. Antifungal pharmacodynamics: concentration-effect relationships in vitro and in vivo. Pharmacotherapy 2001;21:133S–48S.

[2] Christensen KJ, Bernard EM, Gold JWM, Armstrong D. Distribution and activity of amphotericin B in humans. J Infect Dis 1985;152:1037–43.

[3] Denning DW, Stevens DA. Antifungal and surgical treatment of invasive aspergillosis: review of 2,121 published cases. Rev Infect Dis 1990;12:1147–200.

[4] Ellis M. Amphotericin B preparations: a maximum tolerated dose in severe invasive fungal infections? Transplant Infect Dis 2000;2:51–61.

[5] Luna B, Drew RH, Perfect JR. Agents for treatment of invasive fungal infections. Otolaryngol Clin North Am 2000;33:277–99.

[6] de Pauw BE. New antifungal agents and preparations. Int J Antimicrob Agents 2000;16: 147–50.

[7] Hiemenz JW, Walsh TJ. Lipid formulations of amphotericin B: recent progress and future directions. Clin Infect Dis 1996;22:S133–44.

[8] Schmitt HJ. New methods of delivery of amphotericin B. Clin Infect Dis 1993;17:S501–6.

[9] Wasan KM, Rosenblum MG, Cheung L, Lopez-Berestein G. Influence of lipoproteins on renal cytotoxicity and antifungal activity of amphotericin B. Antimicrob Agents Chemother 1994; 38:223–7.

[10] Dismukes WE. Introduction to antifungal agents. Clin Infect Dis 2000;30:653–7.

[11] Proffitt RT, Satorius A, Chiang SM, Sullivan L, Adler-Moore JP. Pharmacology and toxicology of a liposomal formulation of amphotericin B (AmBisome) in rodents. J Antimicrob Chemother 1991;28:49–61.

[12] Wong-Beringer A, Jacobs RA, Guglielmo BJ. Lipid formulations of amphotericin B: clinical efficiacy and toxicities. Clin Infect Dis 1998;27:603–18.

[13] Luke RG, Boyle JA. Renal effects of amphotericin B lipid complex. Am J Kidney Dis 1998;31:780–5.

[14] Walsh TJ, Goodman JL, Pappas P, et al. Safety, tolerance, and pharmacokinetics of high-dose liposomal amphotericin B (AmBisome) in patients infected with *Aspergillus* species and other filamentous fungi: maximum tolerate dose study. Antimicrob Agents Chemother 2001;45: 3487–96.

[15] Sandler ES, Mustafa MM, Tkaczewski I, et al. Use of amphotericin B colloidal dispersion in children. J Pediatr Hematol Oncol 2000;22:242–6.

[16] Walsh TJ, Seibel NL, Arndt C, et al. Amphotericin B lipid complex in pediatric patients with invasive fungal infections. Pediatr Infect Dis J 1998;18:702–8.

[17] Al Arishi H, Frayha HH, Kalloghlian A, Al Alaiyan S. Liposomal amphotericin B in neonates with invasive candidiasis. Am J Perinatol 1998;15:643–8.

[18] Anak S. Safety and efficacy of ambisome in patients with fungal infections: a post marketing

multicentre surveillance study in Turkey. In: Focus on fungal infections 14. New Orleans: Imedex; 2004 [Abstract 2].

[19] Denning DW. Invasive aspergillosis. Clin Infect Dis 1998;26:781–805.

[20] Graybill JR, Tollemar J, Torres-Rodriguez JM, Walsh TJ, Roilides E, Farmaki E. Antifungal compounds: controversies, queries and conclusions. Med Mycol 2000;38:323–33.

[21] Dix SP, Andriole VT. Lipid formulations of amphotericin B. Curr Clin Top Infect Dis 2000; 20:1–23.

[22] Walsh TJ, Hiemenz JW, Seibel NL, et al. Amphotericin B lipid complex for invasive fungal infections: analysis of safety and efficacy in 556 cases. Clin Infect Dis 1998;26:1383–96.

[23] Linder N, Klinger G, Shalit I, et al. Treatment of candidaemia in premature infants: comparison of three amphotericin B products. J Antimicrob Chemother 2003;52:663–7.

[24] Herbrecht R, Auvrignon A, Andres E, et al. Efficacy of amphotericin B lipid complex in the treatment of invasive fungal infections in immunocompromised paediatric patients. Eur J Clin Microbiol Infect Dis 2001;20:77–82.

[25] Scarcella A, Pasquariello MB, Guigliano B, Vendemmia M, de Lucia A. Liposomal amphotericin B treatment for neonatal fungal infections. Pediatr Infect Dis J 1998;17:146–8.

[26] Weitkamp JH, Poets CF, Sievers R, et al. Candida infection in very low birth-weight infants: outcome and nephrotoxicity of treatment with liposomal amphotericin B (AmBisome). Infection 1998;26:11–5.

[27] Juster-Reicher A, Flidel-Rimon O, Amitay M, Even-Tov S, Shinwell E, Leibovitz E. High-dose liposomal amphotericin B in the therapy of systemic candidiasis in neonates. Eur J Clin Microbiol Infect Dis 2003;22:603–7.

[28] Juster-Reicher A, Leibovitz E, Linder N, et al. Liposomal amphotericin B (AmBisome) in the treatment of neonatal candidiasis in very low birthweight infants. Infection 2000;28:223–6.

[29] Bennett JE. Flucytosine. Ann Intern Med 1977;86:319–21.

[30] Vermes A, Guchelaar H-J, Dankert J. Flucytosine: a review of its pharmacology, clinical indications, pharmacokinetics, toxicity and drug interactions. J Antimicrob Chemother 2000; 46:171–9.

[31] Firkin FC. Therapy of deep-seated fungal infections with 5-fluorocytosine. Aust N Z J Med 1974;4:462–7.

[32] Young RC, Bennett JE, Vogel CL, Carbone PP, DeVita VT. Aspergillosis: the spectrum of the disease in 98 patients. Medicine 1970;49:147–73.

[33] Warnock DW. Amphotericin B: an introduction. J Antimicrob Chemother 1991;28:27–38.

[34] Diasio RB, Lakings DE, Bennett JE. Evidence for conversion of 5-fluorocytosine to 5-fluorouracil in humans: possible factor in 5-fluorocytosine clinical toxicity. Antimicrob Agents Chemother 1978;14:903–8.

[35] Stamm AM, Diasio RB, Dismukes WE, et al. Toxicity of amphotericin B plus flucytosine in 194 patients with cryptococcal meningitis. Am J Med 1987;83:236–42.

[36] Bennett JE, Dismukes WE, Duma RJ, et al. A comparison of amphotericin B alone and combined with flucytosine in the treatment of cryptococcal meningitis. N Engl J Med 1979; 301:126–8.

[37] Dismukes WE, Cloud G, Gallis HA, et al. Treatment of cryptococcal meningitis with combination amphotericin B and flucytosine for four as compared with six weeks. N Engl J Med 1987;317:334–41.

[38] Saag MS, Graybill JR, Larsen RA, et al. Practice guidelines for the management of cryptococcal disease. Infectious Diseases Society of America. Clin Infect Dis 2000;30:710–8.

[39] Pappas PG, Rex JH, Sobel JD, et al. Guidelines for treatment of candidiasis. Clin Infect Dis 2004;38:161–89.

[40] Smego Jr RA, Perfect JR, Durack DT. Combined therapy with amphotericin B and 5-fluorocytosine for *Candida* meningitis. Rev Infect Dis 1984;6:791–801.

[41] Walsh TJ, Viviani MA, Arathoon E, et al. New targets and delivery systems for antifungal therapy. Med Mycol 2000;38:335–47.

[42] De Beule K, Van Gestel J. Pharmacology of itraconazole. Drugs 2001;61:27–37.

[43] Klepser ME, Wolfe EJ, Jones RN, Nightingale CH, Pfaller MA. Antifungal pharmacodynamic characteristics of fluconazole and amphotericin B tested against *Candida albicans*. Antimicrob Agents Chemother 1997;41:1392–5.

[44] Brammer KW, Coates PE. Pharmacokinetics of fluconazole in pediatric patients. Eur J Clin Microbiol Infect Dis 1994;13:325–9.

[45] Wildfeuer A, Laufen H, Schmalreck AF, Yeates RA, Zimmerman T. Fluconazole: comparison of pharmacokinetics, therapy, and in vitro susceptibility. Mycoses 1997;40:259–65.

[46] Debruyne D. Clinical pharmacokinetics of fluconazole in superficial and systemic mycoses. Clin Pharmacokinet 1997;33:52–77.

[47] Vscoli CE, Castagnola M, Fioredda B, Ciravegna G, Barigione G, Terragna A. Fluconazole in the treatment of candidiasis in immunocompromised children. Antimicrob Agents Chemother 1991;35:365–7.

[48] Novelli V, Holzel H. Safety and tolerability of fluconazole in children. Antimicrob Agents Chemother 1999;43:1955–60.

[49] Rex JH, Bennett JE, Sugar AM, et al. A randomized trial comparing fluconazole with amphotericin B for the treatment of candidemia in patients without neutropenia. N Engl J Med 1994;331:1325–30.

[50] Rex JH, Pappas PG, Karchmer AW, et al. A randomized and blinded multicenter trial of high-dose fluconazole + placebo vs. fluconazole + amphotericin B as therapy for candidemia and its consequences in nonneutropenic subjects. Clin Infect Dis 2003;36(10):1221–8.

[51] Fasano C, O'Keeffe J, Gibbs D. Fluconazole treament of neonates and infants with severe fungal infections not treatable with conventional agents. Eur J Clin Microbiol Infect Dis 1994; 13:325–54.

[52] Huttova M, Hartmanova I, Kralinsjy K, et al. *Candida* fungemia in neonates treated with fluconazole: report of forty cases, including eight with meningitis. Pediatr Infect Dis J 1998;17:1012–5.

[53] Driessen M, Ellis JB, Cooper PA, et al. Fluconazole vs. amphotericin B for the treatment of neonatal fungal septicemia: a prospective randomized trial. Pediatr Infect Dis J 1996;15: 1107–12.

[54] Marr KA, Seidel K, Slavin MA, et al. Prolonged fluconazole prophylaxis is associated with persistent protection against candidiasis-related death in allogeneic marrow transplant recipients: long-term follow-up of a randomized, placebo-controlled trial. Blood 2000;96:2055–61.

[55] Koh LP, Kurup A, Goh YT, Fook-Chong SMC, Tan PHC. Randomized trial of fluconazole versus low-dose amphotericin B in prophylaxis against fungal infections in patients undergoing hematopoietic stem cell transplantation. Am J Hematol 2002;71:260–7.

[56] MacMillan ML, Goodman JL, DeFor TE, Weisdorf DJ. Fluconazole to prevent yeast infections in bone marrow transplantation patients: a randomized trial of high versus reduced dose, and determination of the value of maintenace therapy. Am J Med 2002;112:369–79.

[57] Kaufman D, Boyle R, Hazen KC, Patrie JT, Robinson M, Donowitz LG. Fluconazole prophylaxis against fungal colonization and infection in preterm infants. N Engl J Med 2001; 345:1660–6.

[58] Manavathu EK, Cutright JL, Chandrasekar PH. Organism-dependent fungicidal activity of azoles. Antimicrob Agents Chemother 1998;42:3018–21.

[59] Anonymous. Itraconazole. Med Lett Drugs Ther 1993;35:7–9.

[60] de Repentigny L, Ratelle J, Leclerc J-M, et al. Repeated-dose pharmacokinetic of an oral solution of itraconazole in infants and children. Antimicrob Agents Chemother 1998;42: 404–8.

[61] Schmitt C, Perel Y, Harousseau JL, et al. Pharmacokinetics of itraconazole oral solution in neutropenic children during long-term prophylaxis. Antimicrob Agents Chemother 2001;45: 1561–4.

[62] Groll AH, Wood L, Roden M, et al. Safety, pharmacokinetics, and pharmacodynamics of cyclodextrin itraconazole in pediatric patients with oropharyngeal candidiasis. Antimicrob Agents Chemother 2002;46:2554–63.

[63] Tucker RM, Haq Y, Denning DW, Stevens DA. Adverse events associated with itraconazole in 189 patients on chronic therapy. J Antimicrob Chemother 1990;26:561–6.
[64] Marr KA, Leisenring W, Crippa F, et al. Cyclophoshamide metabolism is affected by azole antifungals. Blood 2004;103:1557–9.
[65] Katz HI. Drug interactions of the newer oral antifungal agents. Br J Dermatol 1999;141:26–32.
[66] Morgenstern GR, Prentice AG, Prentice HG, Ropner JE, Schey SA, Warnock DW. A randomized controlled trial of itraconazole versus fluconazole for the prevention of fungal infections in patients with haematological malignancies. Br J Haematol 1999;105:901–11.
[67] Winston DJ, Busuttil RW. Randomized controlled trial of oral itraconazole solution versus intravenous/oral fluconazole for prevention of fungal infections in liver transplant recipients. Transplantation 2002;74:688–94.
[68] Chariyalertsak S, Supparatpinyo K, Sirisanthana T, Nelson KE. A controlled trial of itraconazole as primary prophylaxis for systemic fungal infections in patients wiht advanced human immunodeficiency virus infection in Thailand. Clin Infect Dis 2002;34:277–84.
[69] Sabo JA, Abdel-Rahman SM. Voriconazole: a new triazole antifungal. Ann Pharmacother 2000;34:1032–43.
[70] Johnson EM, Szekely A, Warnock DW. In-vitro activity of voriconazole, itraconazole and amphotericin B against filamentous fungi. J Antimicrob Chemother 1998;42:741–5.
[71] Manavathu EK, Cutright JL, Loebenberg D, Chandrasekar PH. A comparative study of the in vitro susceptibilities of clinical and laboratory-selected resistant isolates of Aspergillus ssp. to amphotericin B, itraconazole, voriconazole and posaconazole (SCH 56592). J Antimicrob Chemother 2000;46:229–34.
[72] Walsh TJ, Karlsson MO, Driscoll T, et al. Pharmacokinetics and safety of intravenous voriconazole in children after single- or multiple-dose administration. Antimicrob Agents Chemother 2004;48:2166–72.
[73] Goldstein JA, deMorais SMF. Biochemistry and molecular biology of the human CYP2C subfamily. Pharmacogenetics 1994;4:285–99.
[74] Purkins L, Wood N, Ghahramani P, Greenhalgh K, Allen MJ, Kleinermans D. Pharmacokinetics and safety of voriconazole following intravenous- to oral-dose escalation regimens. Antimicrob Agents Chemother 2002;46:2546–53.
[75] Johnson LB, Kauffman CA. Voriconazole: a new triazole antifungal agent. Clin Infect Dis 2003;36:630–7.
[76] Lazarus HM, Blummer JL, Yanovich S, Schlamm H, Romero A. Safety and pharmacokinetics of oral voriconazole in patients at risk of fungal infection: a dose escalation study. J Clin Pharmacol 2002;42:395–402.
[77] Stone J, Holland S, Li S, et al. Effect of hepatic insufficiency on the pharmacokinetics of caspofungin. In: Program and abstracts of the 41st Interscience Conference on Antimicrobial Agents and Chemotherapy. Chicago, IL, 2001. Abstract A-14. p. 45.
[78] Tan KKC, Brayshaw N, Oakes M. Investigation of the relationship between plasma voriconazole concentrations and liver function test abnormalities in therapeutic trials. In: Program and abstracts of the 41st Annual Interscience Conference on Antimicrobial Agents and Chemotherapy. Chicago, 2001. Abstract A-18. p. 46.
[79] Denning DW, Griffiths CEM. Muco-cutaneous retinoid-effects and facial erythema related to the novel triazole antifungal agent voriconazole. Clin Dermatol 2001;26:648–53.
[80] Venkataramanan R, Zang S, Gayowski T, Singh N. Voriconazole inhibition of the metabolism of tacrolimus in a liver transplant recipient and in human liver microsomes. Antimicrob Agents Chemother 2002;46:3091–3.
[81] Wood N, Tan K, Allan R, Fielding A, Nichols DJ. Effect of voriconazole on pharmacokinetics of tacrolimus. In: Program and abstracts of the 41st Interscience Conference on Antimicrobial Agents and Chemotherapy. Chicago, 2001. Abstract A-20.
[82] Herbrecht R, Denning DW, Patterson TF, et al. Voriconazole versus amphotericin B for primary therapy of invasive aspergillosis. N Engl J Med 2002;347:408–15.
[83] Denning DW, Ribaud P, Milpied N, et al. Efficacy and safety of voriconazole in the treatment of acute invasive aspergillosis. Clin Infect Dis 2002;34:563–71.

[84] Ally R, Schurmann D, Kreisel W, et al. A randomized, double-blind, double-dummy, multicenter trial of voriconazole and fluconazole in the treatment of esophageal candidiasis in immunocumpromised patients. Clin Infect Dis 2001;33:1447–54.

[85] Kullberg BJ. Voriconazole compared with a strategy of amphotericin B followed by fluconazole for treatment of candidaemia in non-neutropenic patients. In: 14th European Congress of Clinical Microbiology and Infectious Diseases. Prague, Czech Republic, 2004. Abstract 10.111.

[86] Walsh TJ, Pappas P, Winston DJ, et al. Voriconazole compared with liposomal amphotericin B for empirical antifungal therapy in patients with neutropenia and persistent fever. N Engl J Med 2002;346:225–34.

[87] Walsh TJ, Lutsar I, Driscoll T, et al. Voriconazole in the treatment of aspergillosis, scedosporiosis and other invasive fungal infections in children. Pediatr Infect Dis J 2002; 21:240–8.

[88] Ernst EJ. Investigational antifungal agents. Pharmacotherapy 2001;21:165S–75S.

[89] Hachem RY, Raad II, Afif CM, et al. An open, non-comparative multicenter study to evaluate efficacy and safety of posaconazole (SCH 56592) in the treatment of invasive fungal infections refractory to or intolerant to standard therapy. In: Program and abstracts of the 40th Interscience Conference on Antimicrobial Agents and Chemotherapy. Toronto, Ontario, 2000. Abstract 1109.

[90] Segal BH, Barnhart LA, Anderson VL, Malech HL. Posaconazole in salvage therapy in patients with chronic granulomatous disease with invasive fungal infections. In: Program and abstracts of the 43rd Annual Interscience Conference on Antimicrobial Agents and Chemotherapy. Chicago, 2003. Abstract M-1756.

[91] Greenberg RN, Anstead G, Herbrecht R, et al. Posaconazole experience in the treatment of zygomycosis. In: Program and abstracts of the 43rd Annual Interscience Conference on Antimicrobial Agents and Chemotherapy. Chicago, 2003. Abstract M-1757.

[92] Moore CB, Walls CM, Denning DW. In vitro activity of the new triazole BMS-207147 against *Aspergillus* species in comparison with itraconazole and amphotericin B. Antimicrob Agents Chemother 2000;44:441–3.

[93] Arikan S, Rex JH. Ravuconazole. Curr Opin Invest Drugs 2002;3:555–61.

[94] Olsen SJ, Mummaneni V, Rolan P, Norton J, Grasela DM. Ravuconazole single ascending oral dose study in healthy subjects. In: Program and abstracts of the 40th Interscience Conference on Antimicrobial Agents and Chemotherapy. Toronto, Ontario, 2000. Abstract 838.

[95] Beale M, Queiroz-Telles F, Banhegyi D, Li N, Pierce PF. Randomized, double-blind study of the safety and antifungal activity of ravuconazole relative to fluconazole in esophageal candidiasis. In: Program and abstracts of the 41st Interscience Conference on Antimicrobial Agents and Chemotherapy. Chicago, 2001. Abstract J-1621.

[96] Bartizal K, Gill CJ, Abruzzo GK, et al. In vitro preclinical evaluation studies with the echinocandin antifungal MK-0991 (L-743,872). Antimicrob Agents Chemother 1997;41: 2326–32.

[97] Kurtz MB, Douglas CM. Lipopeptide inhibitors of fungal glucan synthase. J Med Vet Mycol 1997;35:79–86.

[98] Graybill JR. The echinocandins, first novel class of antifungals in two decades: will they live up to their promise? Int J Clin Pract 2001;55:633–8.

[99] Groll AH, Gullick BM, Petraitiene R, et al. Compartmental pharmacokinetics of the antifungal echinocandin caspofungin (MK-0991) in rabbits. Antimicrob Agents Chemother 2001; 45:596–600.

[100] Stone JA, Holland SD, Wickersham PJ, et al. Single- and multiple-dose pharmacokinetics of caspofungin in healthy men. Antimicrob Agents Chemother 2002;46:739–45.

[101] Chiou CC, Groll AH, Walsh TJ. New drugs and novel targets for treatment of invasive fungal infections in patients with cancer. Oncologist 2000;5:120–35.

[102] Hajdu R, Thompson R, Sundelof JG, et al. Preliminary animal pharmokinetics of the parenteral antifungal agent MK-0991 (L-743,872). Antimicrob Agents Chemother 1997;41: 2339–44.

[103] Abruzzo GK, Flattery AM, Gill CJ, et al. Evaluation of the echinocandin antifungal MK-0991 (L-743,872): efficacies in mouse models of disseminated aspergillosis, candidiasis, and cryptococcosis. Antimicrob Agents Chemother 1997;41:2333–8.

[104] Stone EA, Fung HB, Kirschenbaum HL. Caspofungin: an echinocandin antifungal agent. Clin Ther 2002;24:351–77.

[105] Hoang A. Caspofungin acetate: an antifungal agent. Am J Health-Syst Pharm 2001;58: 1206–14.

[106] Walsh TJ, Adamson PC, Seibel NL, et al. Pharmacokinetics of caspofungin in pediatric patients. In: Program and abstracts of the 42nd Interscience Conference on Antimicrobial Agents and Chemotherapy. San Diego, 2002. Abstract M-896.

[107] Sable CA, Nguyen B-YT, Chodakewitz JA, DiNubile MJ. Safety and tolerability of caspofungin acetate in the treatment of fungal infections. Transplant Infect Dis 2002;4:25–30.

[108] Stone J, Holland S, Wickersham P, et al. Drug interactions between caspofungin and tacrolimus. In: Program and abstracts of the 41st Interscience Conference on Antimicrobial Agents and Chemotherapy. Chicago, 2001. Abstract A-13.

[109] Keating GM, Jarvis B. Caspofungin. Drugs 2001;61:1121–9.

[110] Franklin JA, McCormick J, Flynn PM. Retrospective study of the safety of caspofungin in immunocompromised pediatric patients. Pediatr Infect Dis J 2003;22:747–9.

[111] Maertens J, Raad I, Sable C, et al. Multicenter, noncomparative study to evaluate safety and efficacy of caspofungin in adults with invasive aspergillosis refractory or intolerant to amphotericin, amphotericin B lipid formulations, or azoles. In: Program and abstracts of the 40th Interscience Conference on Antimicrobial Agents and Chemotherapy. Toronto, Ontario, 2000. Abstract J-1103.

[112] Maertens J, Raad I, Petrikkos G, et al. Efficacy and safety of caspofungin for treatment of invasive aspergillosis in patients refractory to or intolerant of conventional antifungal therapy. Clin Infect Dis 2004;39(11):1563–71.

[113] Mora-Duarte J, Betts R, Rotstein C, et al. Comparison of caspofungin and amphotericin B for invasive candidiasis. N Engl J Med 2002;347:2020–9.

[114] Walsh TJ, Teppler H, Donowitz GR, et al. Caspofungin versus liposomal amphotericin B for empirical antifungal therapy in patients with persistent fever and neutropenia. N Engl J Med 2004;351:1391–402.

[115] Mikamo H, Sato Y, Tamaya T. In vitro antifungal activity of FK463, a new water-soluble echinocandin-like lipopeptide. J Antimicrob Chemother 2000;46:485–7.

[116] Hatano K, Morishita Y, Nakai T, Ikeda F. Antifungal mechanism of FK463 against *Candida albicans* and *Aspergillus fumigatus*. J Antibiot (Tokyo) 2002;55:219–22.

[117] Tawara S, Ikeda F, Maki K, et al. In vitro activities of a new lipopeptide antifungal agent, FK463, against a variety of clinically important fungi. Antimicrob Agents Chemother 2000;44:57–62.

[118] Heresi GP, Gerstmann DR, Blumer JL, et al. Pharmacokinetic study of micafungin in premature neonates. Presented at: Pediatric Academic Society Meeting. Seattle, 2003. Abstract 83.

[119] Ratanatharathorn V, Flynn P, Van Burik JA, McSweeney P, Niederwieser D, Kontoyannis D. Micafungin in combination with systemic antifungal agents in the treatment of refractory aspergillosis in bone marrow transplant patients. In: Program and abstracts of the American Society of Hematology 44th Annual Meeting. Philadelphia, 2002. Abstract 2472.

[120] van Burik JA, Ratanatharathorn V, Stepan DE, et al. Micafungin versus fluconazole for prophylaxis against invasive fungal infections during neutropenia in patients undergoing hematopoietic stem cell transplantation. Clin Infect Dis 2004;39:1407–16.

[121] Suleiman J, Della Negra M, Llanos-Cuentas A, Ticona E, Rex JH, Buell DN. Open label study of micafungin in the treatment of esophageal candidiasis. In: Program and abstracts of the 42nd Interscience Conference on Antimicrobial Agents and Chemotherapy. San Diego, 2002. Abstract M-892.

[122] Ullmann AJ, Van Burik JA, McSweeney P, et al. An open phase II study of the efficacy of micafungin (FK463) alone and in combination for the treatment of invasive aspergillosis

in adults and children. In: 13th European Congress of Clinical Microbiology and Infectious Diseases. Glasgow, UK, 2003. Abstract O-400.

[123] Zhanel GG, Karlowsky JA, Harding GA, et al. In vitro activity of a new semisynthetic echinocandin, LY-303366, against syemstic isolates of *Candida* species, *Cryptococcus neoformans*, *Blastomyces dermatitidis*, and *Aspergillus* species. Antimicrob Agents Chemother 1997;41:863–5.

[124] Lucas R, De Sante K, Hatcher B, et al. LY303366 single dose pharmacokinetics and safety in healthy volunteers. In: Program and abstracts of the 36th Annual Interscience Conference on Antimicrobial Agents and Chemotherapy. New Orleans, 1996. Abstract F-50.

[125] Petraitis V, Petraitiene R, Groll AH, et al. Antifungal efficacy, safety, and single-dose pharmokinetics of LY303366, a novel echinocandin B, in experimental pulmonary aspergillosis in persistently neutropenic rabbits. Antimicrob Agents Chemother 1998;42:2898–905.

[126] Thye D, Marbury T, Kilfoil G, Henkel T. Anidulafungin: pharmacokinetics in subjects receiving hemodialysis. In: Program and abstracts of the 42nd Annual Interscience Conference on Antimicrobial Agents and Chemotherapy. San Diego, 2002. Abstract A-1390.

[127] Krause DS, Simjee AE, van Rensburg C, et al. A randomized, double-blind trial of anidulafungin versus fluconazole for the treatment of esophageal candidiasis. Clin Infect Dis 2004;39:770–5.

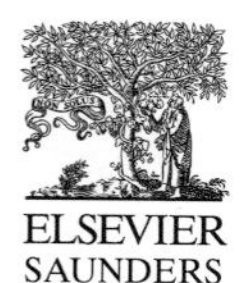
ELSEVIER
SAUNDERS

PEDIATRIC CLINICS
OF NORTH AMERICA

Pediatr Clin N Am 52 (2005) 917–948

Antiparasitic Therapy in Children

Troy D. Moon, MD, MPH[a,*], Richard A. Oberhelman, MD[b]

[a]*Department of Pediatrics, TB-8, Tulane University School of Medicine, 1430 Tulane Avenue, New Orleans, LA 70112, USA*

[b]*Department of Tropical Medicine, SL-29, Tulane School of Public Health and Tropical Medicine, 1440 Canal Street, Suite 2210, New Orleans, LA 70112, USA*

Although parasitic infections are ubiquitous on a worldwide basis, with an estimated 1 billion persons infected with intestinal helminthes alone, physicians in the United States and other developed countries are often unfamiliar with the management of these diseases. Children are traveling internationally in larger numbers than ever before, however, and emigration from developing countries to the United States and other Western countries is increasing, so clinicians in these countries are confronted more frequently with parasitic diseases from the tropics. Treatment of parasitic infections presents many challenges for the clinician. One challenge is the markedly different therapy needed for some parasites that are genetically and morphologically similar. The coccidian protozoan, *Cyclospora cayetanensis* responds well to treatment with trimethoprim-sulfamethoxazole (TMP-SMX), whereas the morphologically similar protozoan, *Cryptosporidium parvum,* is resistant to most commonly used antimicrobial agents. Morphologically similar *Entamoeba* species also can complicate decisions regarding treatment. *Entamoeba histolytica* often causes invasive disease requiring treatment, but *Entamoeba dispar* is a benign commensal that can be ignored. Another challenge is the need to treat some parasites, such as the trypanosomes, with prolonged courses of highly toxic drugs. Optimal treatment of other parasitic organisms, such as malaria, requires an understanding of their complex life cycles. Finally, treatment of some parasitic infections requires special precautions because of the potential for serious adverse clinical reactions. If cysticerci in the brain are treated with antiparasitic agents, without concurrent steroid therapy, the resulting inflammatory response can precipitate seizures. The therapy of

* Corresponding author.
E-mail address: tmoon@tulane.edu (T.D. Moon).

0031-3955/05/$ – see front matter
doi:10.1016/j.pcl.2005.02.012

pediatric.theclinics.com

parasitic diseases requires careful attention to diagnostic studies and pathogen-specific therapy.

Parasites are defined as eukaryotic single-celled or multicellular micro-organisms that differ from fungi in cell membrane structure. Parasites often are classified into two groups, single-celled parasites or protozoa and multicellular parasites or helminthes, including parasitic "worms." Parasites are often host specific, and many parasites found in humans are nonpathogenic.

This article is organized into three main sections, based on parasite structure and disease epidemiology: (1) protozoan infections found primarily in developing countries, (2) protozoan infections distributed globally and infections in immuno-compromised hosts, and (3) helminth infections. Drugs used in the treatment of more than one type of parasite are presented once in detail, with reference to the detailed description in subsequent sections.

Treatment of protozoan infections found primarily in developing countries

Table 1 provides a quick reference to drugs of choice and dosages.

Malaria

Malaria is one of the most prevalent parasitic infections worldwide, and it is among the greatest health and development challenges facing developing countries today [1]. Nearly 2 billion people, a third of the world's population, live in malaria-endemic areas [2]. Each year, approximately 100 million people are infected with malaria, and mortality estimates range from 500,000 to 3 million people annually [2–4]. Ninety percent of deaths occur in Africa, where severe malaria and malaria-related mortality disproportionately affect children, pregnant women, and immunocompromised persons. Travelers without prior immunity visiting endemic areas also are at increased risk [5].

There are four *Plasmodium* species that cause human disease. Most cases of severe disease and death are caused by *P. falciparum,* whereas *P. vivax, P. ovale,* and *P. malariae* cause less severe disease [6]. Drug resistance is one of the major obstacles to effective disease control. It is estimated that in some areas, resistance to chloroquine exceeds 25%, and that other first-line drugs are losing their efficacy quickly [7]. It is estimated that chloroquine resistance results in a fourfold to eightfold increase in mortality rate [8].

Strategies for effective treatment depend on the species of malaria, drug resistance patterns where infection was acquired, and severity of disease [6,9]. Physicians should consult the Centers for Disease Control and Prevention website (www.cdc.gov) or a travel medicine service to identify areas where chloroquine is the recommended therapy. In the following sections, discussion is limited to treatment of disease only. Malaria prophylaxis is beyond the scope of this article.

Plasmodium falciparum

A 3-day course of chloroquine is the recommended first-line treatment of uncomplicated *P. falciparum,* in areas where sensitivity to chloroquine predominates [6,9]. Chloroquine is relatively inexpensive and well tolerated. Side effects include pruritus, dizziness, headache, diplopia, nausea, and malaise. Chloroquine-induced pruritus is accentuated in patients with concomitant filarial infection. These side effects are typically minor and transient. Serious side effects, such as hypotension and ECG abnormalities, can occur at high concentrations [6,7,9]. Chloroquine is the safest of the antimalarial drugs for use during pregnancy [3].

One of the most confusing aspects of choloquine therapy is the frequent reporting of dosages in terms of chloroquine "base" and chloroquine "salt." Calculation of chloroquine doses in terms of milligrams of base is relevant only when there are different salt preparations, as in some countries where there are sulfate, phosphate, and hydrochloride salts available. When several chloroquine salts are available, milligram dosages of these preparations providing equivalent amounts of chloroquine base vary with the molecular weight of the compound. Chloroquine phosphate (eg, Aralen) is the most common chloroquine salt preparation in pharmacies worldwide, and unless preparations other than choroquine phosphate are available, dosage calculations should be made based on chloroquine phosphate salt. Dosages of chloroquine base should be multiplied by 1.6 to determine the corresponding dose of chloroquine phosphate salt.

Quinine sulfate given three times daily and atovaquone-proguanil given once daily are the drugs of choice in areas with chloroquine resistance. Quinine sulfate can be used alone in a 7-day course or combined with doxycycline or clindamycin for a 3-day course. Alternatively, pyrimethamine-sulfadoxine can be given in one dose at the end of quinine treatment. Quinine combined with clindamycin is the recommended first-line treatment regimen for pregnant women with chloroquine-resistant malaria. Quinine sulfate is a relatively safe drug, although it may produce a syndrome known as *cinchonism* (name derived from the cinchona tree, from which quinine is extracted). Cinchonism is a symptom complex including tinnitus, high-tone hearing impairment, nausea, and vomiting. These side effects often interfere with completion of therapy. In large doses, side effects of quinine include hypotension, arrhythmias, visual impairment, and seizures [3,7]. Hyperinsulinemic hypoglycemia is an important complication of quinine therapy in pregnant women, who should have careful blood glucose monitoring during treatment.

Atovaquone-proguanil (Malarone) is an alternative to quinine sulfate. It is given once daily for 3 days. Absorption from the gastrointestinal tract increases when taken with food. Atovaquone-proguanil is generally well tolerated. The most common side effects include rash, fever, gastrointestinal upset, and CNS disturbances. This drug is contraindicated during pregnancy (category C) [7].

Alternative drugs for uncomplicated *P. falciparum* include mefloquine alone or in combination with one of the arteminisins—artesunate or artemether. Mefloquine is often used as a third-line drug because of its rare but significant

Table 1
Treatment of protozoan infections found primarily in developing countries

Parasite	Drug	Pediatric dosage	Adult dosage
Malaria			
P. falciparum (uncomplicated)			
Chloroquine-sensitive			
Drug of choice	Chloroquine phosphate (chloroquine salt, containing 60% chloroquine base by weight)*	16 mg/kg salt (10 mg/kg base), then 8.3 mg/kg salt (5 mg/kg base) at 6, 24, and 48 h	1 g salt (600 mg base), then 500 mg salt (300 mg base) at 6, 24, and 48 h
Chloroquine-resistant			
Drug of choice	Quinine sulfate	10 mg/kg three times daily × 3–7 d	650 mg three times daily × 3–7 d
	plus one of		
	doxycycline	2 mg/kg twice daily × 7 d	100 mg twice daily × 7 d
	or		
	clindamycin	5 mg/kg three times daily × 7 d	300 mg four times daily × 7 d
	or		
	pyrimethamine-sulfadoxine	<5 kg: ¼ tab once 5–10 kg: ½ tab once 11–20 kg: 1 tab once 21–30 kg: 1½ tab once 31–40 kg: 2 tabs once >40 kg: 3 tabs once on the last day of quinine	3 tabs once on the last day of quinine
Alternatives	Atovaquone-proguanil	5–8 kg: 2 peds tabs once daily × 3 d 9–10 kg: 3 peds tabs once daily × 3 d 11–20 kg: 1 adult tabs once daily × 3 d 21–30 kg: 2 adult tabs once daily × 3 d 31–40 kg: 3 adult tabs once daily × 3 d >40 kg: 4 adult tabs once daily × 3 d	4 adult tabs daily × 3 d
	Mefloquine	15 mg/kg once, then 10 mg/kg after 12 h	750 mg once, then 500 mg after 12 h

	Artesunate	4 mg/kg/d × 3 d	4 mg/kg/d × 3 d
	plus mefloquine	15 mg/kg once, then 10 mg/kg after 12 h	750 mg once, then 500 mg after 12 h
P. falciparum (severe disease)			
Drugs of choice	Quinine sulfate	20 mg/kg load over 4 h, then 10 mg/kg over 2–4 h q8 h	20 mg/kg load over 4 h, then 10 mg/kg over 2–4 hrs q8 h
	Quinidine	10 mg/kg load over 1–2 h, then 0.02 mg/kg/min continuous infusion	10 mg/kg load over 1–2 h, then 0.02 mg/kg/min continuous infusion
Alternative	Artemether	3.2 mg/kg IM, then 1.6 mg/kg daily × 7 d	3.2 mg/kg IM, then 1.6 mg/kg daily × 7 d
P. vivax/P. ovale			
Drug of choice	Chloroquine phosphate (chloroquine salt, containing 60% chloroquine base by weight)*	16 mg/kg salt (10 mg/kg base), then 8.3 mg/kg salt (5 mg/kg base) at 6, 24, and 48 h	1 g salt (600 mg base), then 500 mg salt (300 mg base) at 6, 24, and 48 h
	plus primaquine	0.5 mg/kg × 14 d	30 mg once daily × 14 d
P. malariae			
Drug of choice	Chloroquine phosphate (chloroquine salt, containing 60% chloroquine base by weight)*	16 mg/kg salt (10 mg/kg base), then 8.3 mg/kg salt (5 mg/kg base) at 6, 24, and 48 h	1 g salt (600 mg base), then 500 mg salt (300 mg base) at 6, 24, and 48 h
Trypanosomiasis			
T.cruzi (Chagas disease)			
Drugs of choice	Benznidazole	<12 y: 10 mg/kg/day in twice daily × 30–90 d	5–7 mg/kg/d divided twice daily × 30–90 d
	Nifurtimox	1–10 y: 15–20 mg/kg/d 4 times daily × 90 d 11–16 y: 12.5–15 mg/kg/day 4 times daily × 90 d	8–10 mg/kg/d 4 times daily × 90 d
T.brucei gambiense (sleeping sickness)			
Hemolymphatic stage			
Drugs of choice	Pentamidine isethionate	4 mg/kg/day IM × 10 d	4 mg/kg/day × 10 d
	Suramin sodium	5 mg/kg (test dose) IV, then after 48 h 20 mg/kg/day on day 1, 3, 7, 14, and 21	100–200 mg (test dose) IV, then 1 g IV on day 1, 3, 7, 14, and 21

(continued on next page)

Table 1 (*continued*)

Parameter	Drug	Pediatric dosage	Adult dosage
Trypanosomiasis			
T.brucei gambiense (sleeping sickness)			
CNS involvement			
Drugs of choice	Melarsoprol	2.2 mg/kg daily × 10 d	2.2 mg/kg daily × 10 d
	Eflornithine	400 mg/kg 4 times daily × 14 d	400 mg/kg 4 times daily × 14 d
T.brucei rhodesiense			
Hemolymphatic stage			
Drug of choice	Suramin sodium	5 mg/kg (test dose) IV, then after 48 h 20 mg/kg/day IV on day 1, 3, 7, 14, and 21	100–200 mg (test dose) IV, then 1 g IV on day 1, 3, 7, 14, and 21
CNS involvement			
Drug of choice	Melarsoprol	2–3.6 mg/kg/d × 3 d, then after 7 d 3.6 mg/kg/d × 3 d, then repeat after 7 d	2–3.6 mg/kg/d × 3 d, then after 7 d 3.6 mg/kg/d × 3 d, then repeat after 7 d
Leishmaniasis			
Visceral			
Drugs of choice	Sodium stibogluconate	20 mg Sb[†] /kg/d IV/IM × 28 d	20 mg Sb[†] /kg/d IV/IM × 28 d
	Meglumine antimonate	20 mg Sb[†] /kg/d IV/IM × 28 d	20 mg Sb[†] /kg/d IV/IM × 28 d
	Amphotericin B	0.5–1 mg/kg IV daily or every other day for 8 wk	0.5–1 mg/kg IV daily or every other day for 8 wk
	Liposomal amphotericin B	3 mg/kg/d IV for 1–5 d, then 3 mg/kg/d on day 14 and 21	3 mg/kg/d IV for 1–5 d, then 3/mg/kg/d on day 14 and 21
Alternate	Pentamidine	4 mg/kg IV/IM daily or every other day for 15–30 doses	4 mg/kg IV/IM daily or every other day for 15–30 doses

Cutaneous			
Drugs of choice	Sodium stibogluconate	20 mg Sb[†] /kg/d IV/IM × 20 d	20 mg Sb[†] /kg/d IV/IM × 20 d
	Meglumine antimonate	20 mg Sb[†] /kg/d IV/IM × 20 d	20 mg Sb[†] /kg/d IV/IM × 20 d
Alternative	Pentamidine	2–3 mg/kg IV/IM daily or every other day for 4–7 doses	2–3 mg/kg IV/IM daily or every other day for 4–7 doses
	Paromomycin	2x/d topically × 10–20 d	2x/d topically × 10–20 d
Mucosal			
Drugs of choice	Sodium stibogluconate	20 mg Sb[†] /kg/d IV/IM × 28 d	20 mg Sb[†] /kg/d IV/IM × 28 d
	Meglumine antimonate	20 mg Sb[†] /kg/d IV/IM × 28 d	20 mg Sb[†] /kg/d IV/IM × 28 d
	Amphotericin B	0.5–1 mg/kg IV daily or every other day for 8 wk	0.5–1 mg/kg IV daily or every other day for 8 wk
Amebiasis			
Entomoeba histolytica			
Drugs of choice	Metronidazole	30–50 mg/kg/d 3 times daily × 7–10 d	500–750 mg 3 times daily × 7–10 d
Noninvasive disease	Iodoquinol	30–40 mg/kg/d 3 times daily × 20 d	650 mg 3 times daily × 20 d
	Paromomycin	25–35 mg/kg/d 3 times daily × 7 d	25–35 mg/kg/d 3 times daily × 7 d
	Diloxanide furoate	20 mg/kg/d 3 times daily × 10 d	500 mg 3 times daily × 10 d

* Chloroquine salt (chloroquine phosphate) is the preparation available in pharmacies, and dosage calculations should be made based on chloroquine salt rather than chloroquine base, even though the latter is often used for describing dosages.

† Sb, antimony. Dosing of pentavalent antimonials should be done in consultation with infectious disease experts.

side effects, including life-threatening skin reactions, aplastic anemia, psychosis, seizures, and encephalopathy [7]. Although children are more likely than adults to vomit immediately after taking mefloquine, in general they tolerate the drug better than adults. Self-limited neuropsychiatric reactions, such as convulsions and psychosis, occur in about 1 in every 15,000 individuals receiving mefloquine for malaria prophylaxis, but the rate of these reactions in patients receiving antimalarial treatment dosages is about 10 times higher. Mefloquine should not be used in conjunction with quinine or quinidine because it can potentiate their cardiac toxicities, especially arrhythmias [9]. Mefloquine can be used during pregnancy, but should be used with caution in the first trimester (category C) [3]. Side effects for the arteminisins include mild gastrointestinal upset and rash. Serious CNS side effects, although rare, have been reported [7].

For the treatment of severe *P. falciparum,* intravenous quinine and quinidine are the drugs of choice. Both should begin with a loading dose to achieve therapeutic concentrations quickly. Both agents should be diluted in a crystalloid solution such as 5% dextrose. If intravenous administration is not possible, quinine can be given intramuscularly. When the patient can swallow, he or she should be switched to oral tablets to complete a 7-day course of therapy [7,9].

Another alternative drug for severe *P. falciparum* is intramuscular artemether. A loading dose should be given followed by daily injections for 7 days. If tolerated, oral therapy can instituted after 3 days of parenteral treatment and continued to complete a 7-day course [7,9].

Plasmodium vivax *and* Plasmodium ovale

Neither *P. vivax* nor *P. ovale* typically causes severe disease. The drug of choice for both is chloroquine for 3 days, followed by primaquine once daily for 14 days [6,9]. Primaquine is used to eradicate the dormant parasites within the liver (hypnozoites), which could cause relapse. Although typically well tolerated, primaquine is associated with severe hemolysis in patients with glucose-6 phosphate dehydrogenase (G6PD) deficiency. Screening for this deficiency, before using primaquine therapy, is recommended.

Plasmodium malariae

P. malariae is treated with a 3-day course of chloroquine alone. Chloroquine resistance has been reported in Indonesia [6].

Kinetoplastids (trypanosomiasis and leishmaniasis)

American Trypanosomiasis

American trypanosomiasis, also known as Chagas' disease, is caused by the flagellated protozoan *Trypanosoma cruzi.* Transmission is from the bite of a triatomine bug, which contaminates abraded skin or mucous membranes with feces containing trypomastigotes. Chagas' disease is the most important parasitic disease of Latin America, infecting roughly 10 million people [10,11]. The clinical course is characterized by an acute phase, which is often asymptomatic, and a chronic phase. Children are more likely than adults to exhibit symptoms. Typically a chagoma, or red nodule, develops at the site of inoculation. Often inoculation occurs at the eyelid, causing unilateral periorbital edema. This is known as Romaña's sign, when accompanied by conjunctivitis and preauricular lymphadenitis. Infection is followed by fever, malaise, and lymphadenopathy, and complications include myocarditis, hepatosplenomegaly, and meningoencephalitis [10,12]. Manifestations of chronic Chagas' disease, including cardiac aneurysms, megaesophagus, and megacolon, are found almost exclusively in adults with long-standing infections. These late manifestations do not respond to antiparasitic therapy.

Treatment for acute Chagas' disease consists of benznidazole twice daily for 30 to 90 days or nifurtimox four times daily for 90 days. Benznidazole has greater trypanocidal activity than nifurtimox and has been associated with greater improvement in ECG abnormalities. Side effects of both drugs are common. For benznidazole, allergic dermopathy occurs in approximately 50% of patients. Peripheral neuropathy and granulocytopenia also are frequent. Side effects tend to disappear with interruptions in treatment. Patients receiving nifurtimox often experience nausea, vomiting, and weakness. Therapy also can lead to toxic hepatitis and CNS symptoms, such as seizures [13,14].

African Trypanosomiasis

African trypanosomiasis, also known as sleeping sickness, is caused by two morphologically identical protozoa—*Trypanosoma brucei gambiense* and *Trypanosoma brucei rhodesiense*. Both protozoa are transmitted by the bites of tsetse flies. *T. brucei gambiense* typically causes a mild chronic illness occurring months to years after inoculation. Early manifestations of infection include intermittent fever, malaise, and lymphadenopathy, particularly in the posterior cervical chain. Signs and symptoms of meningoencephalitis, including behavior changes, somnolence, severe headaches, and coma, and death may follow. *T. brucei rhodesiense* typically causes an acute, severe, often fatal, generalized illness within weeks of inoculation; CNS symptoms are uncommon [15].

Treatment for sleeping sickness is highly toxic, and parasitic resistance is common [12,15,16]. Four drugs are available to treat sleeping sickness, and selection is based in part on CNS involvement. Suramin sodium can be used for infection with either *T. brucei gambiense* or *T. brucei rhodesiense,* but because it does not cross the blood-brain barrier, it is useful only during the hemolymphatic stages of infection. It is given intravenously in a test dose of 5 mg/kg, followed 48 hours later by 20 mg/kg on days 1, 3, 7, 14, and 21 [12,17]. Severe side effects, including anaphylaxis, neurotoxicity, and nephrotoxicity, have been reported.

Pentamidine isethionate, given in daily intramuscular injections for 10 days, is the recommended treatment for the hemolymphatic stage of *T. brucei gambiense*. This treatment is typically well tolerated, but hypotension and hypoglycemia may occur [15].

Melarsoprol is a highly toxic drug that is indicated for infections involving the CNS. It contains arsenic and can only be given intravenously. For *T. brucei gambiense,* the treatment course consists of daily intravenous injections for 10 days. The treatment course for *T. brucei rhodesiense* consists of a daily infusion on 3 consecutive days, repeated three times, each separated by 1 week [15]. Approximately 5% to 10% of patients develop an encephalopathic syndrome requiring the coadministration of steroids [15,18]. Other side effects reported include abdominal pain, vomiting, fever, and joint pain [19].

Eflornithine is the recommended drug of choice for patients who fail therapy with melarsoprol. Eflornithine treatment requires four infusions daily for 14 days followed by oral administration for 2 to 4 weeks [15,20]. Therapy is typically well tolerated, but side effects include seizures, abdominal complaints, granulocytopenia, and alopecia. Adverse reactions tend to be associated with length of treatment and are reversible when treatment is completed [15,20].

Leishmaniasis

Leishmaniasis is caused by a variety of different species of *Leishmania* parasites, which are transmitted by the bite of an infected sandfly. Infection is characterized by three major clinical syndromes: cutaneous, mucocutaneous, and visceral leishmaniasis [21,22]. Cutaneous disease is divided further into Old World and New World disease by their differing causal species of parasite and geographic distribution; however, the clinical manifestations are similar. Both diseases consist of ulcerative lesions that present on exposed areas of the face and extremities. Infection is often self-limited, and specific therapy is not required [12,21]. Mucocutaneous disease is caused most often by infection from *L. braziliensis*, presenting several months to years after an initial cutaneous lesion. Inflammation of mucosal tissue is followed by potentially disfiguring ulceration and death if disease results in compromise of the respiratory system [21]. Visceral disease results when parasites spread from skin macrophages to local lymph nodes and concentrate in the liver, spleen, and bone marrow. Illness is characterized by fever, weight loss, marked hepatosplenomegaly, and anemia, and death usually occurs within several years as a result of secondary bacterial infections or progressive emaciation [23].

Antimonial drugs, such as sodium stibogluconate and meglumine antimonite, are the mainstays of treatment for leishmaniasis, but the incidence of side effects is high. Dosing is based on antimony concentration in each drug, and treatment should be done in consultation with infectious disease experts. Currently, only sodium stibogluconate is available in the United States from the Centers for Disease Control and Prevention [24]. Treatment often requires a prolonged hospital stay with daily intramuscular or intravenous infusions for 20 to 28 days depending on location and species of leishmania [22]. Retreatment is commonly necessary. Side effects include abdominal pain, nausea, and arthralgias [12]. Prolonged treatment courses can lead to ECG abnormalities, including fatal arrhythmias. HIV-infected persons are prone to clinical pancreatitis [21,23,25,26]. Use of antimonials is becoming compromised because of parasitic resistance.

Reports from India show resistant disease in 65% of infections [27,28]. These drugs are greater than 90% effective in children with Mediterranean visceral leishmaniasis [25,26].

Amphotericin B is the drug of choice for treatment failures with antimonial drugs and is now first-line therapy in areas with high rates of drug resistance, such as India. Cure rates reach 97%, but cost is often a limiting factor. Side effects are common and include hypokalemia; anemia; renal impairment; and infusion-related side effects, such as fever, chills, bone pain, and thrombophlebitis. This regimen is given intravenously daily or every other day for 8 weeks. Liposomal preparations of amphotericin B have been shown to be highly effective and have better tolerance [21,23,25,29].

Pentamidine is an alternative second-line treatment. It is given intravenously or intramuscularly daily or every other day for 4 to 7 doses in cutaneous disease and for 15 to 30 doses in visceral disease. The use of pentamidine is limited because of side effects and the development of resistance [21,23].

Allopurinol in combination with antimonials has shown some usefulness when traditional therapy has failed. It is not recommended currently, however, because of lack of adequate clinical trials [23,30]. Topical paromomycin has shown benefit in cutaneous disease, but should be used only in geographic areas where mucocutaneous disease is rare [17].

Entamoeba histolytica

Entamoeba are pseudo–pod-forming, nonflagellated protozoa that can cause gastrointestinal disease, including amebic dysentery. Most are commensal organisms that do not cause disease in humans. *E. histolytica*, the organism that causes amebic colitis and liver abscess [31], is transmitted by the fecal-oral route. *E. histolytica* is most prevalent in tropical and developing countries, and in the United States it is most frequently found in travelers to endemic areas and recent immigrants [32]. The clinical spectrum of illness in patients with amebic colitis ranges from 1 to 3 weeks of mild diarrhea to grossly bloody dysentery with abdominal pain and tenesmus [31,33]. Often, amebic colitis is mistaken for inflammatory bowel disease [12]. The most common form of extraintestinal disease resulting from *E. histolytica* infection is liver abscess.

Four drugs are useful for the therapy of amebiasis. The recommended management strategy is to treat the invasive disease first, followed by the eradication of intestinal carriage of the organism with agents active in the intestinal lumen [31]. Oral metronidazole, three times daily for 7 to 10 days, is the mainstay for treatment of invasive disease. It is fairly well tolerated with common side effects, including nausea, vomiting, diarrhea, and metallic taste. Less frequently, patients experience neurotoxic effects, such as seizures, confusion, and irritability. Patients receiving metronidazole should avoid alcohol because of its disulfiram-like intolerance [31,32]. Other nitroimidazoles, such as tinidazole and ornidazole, seem to be as effective as metronidazole, but are unavailable in the United States [31,34].

After completion of treatment for invasive disease, a luminal drug is recommended for clearance of intestinal organisms. Three drugs are currently recommended: iodoquinol, paromomycin, and diloxanide furoate [31,32,35,36]. Iodoquinol is given orally three times daily for 20 days. Side effects include nausea, vomiting, diarrhea, and abdominal pain; iodoquinol is contraindicated in patients with allergy to iodine [32]. Paromomycin is given orally three times daily for 7 days. Side effects include diarrhea and gastrointestinal upset. Diloxanide furoate is given three times daily for 10 days. Side effects include gastrointestinal symptoms, such as nausea, vomiting, and flatulence [31,32].

Drainage or surgical removal of amebic liver abscess generally is not recommended. Drainage may be indicated, however, when abscesses are sufficiently large and rupture is of concern; in left lobe abscesses, which hold a higher risk for mortality; and in persons who fail to respond to medical therapy within 5 to 7 days [32].

Treatment of protozoan infections distributed globally and infections in immunocompromised hosts

Table 2 provides a quick reference to drugs of choice and dosages.

*Lumenal Flagellates (*Giardia *and* Trichomonas)

Giardiasis

Giardia lamblia, also known as *Giardia intestinalis* or *Giardia duodenalis*, is a flagellated protozoan that infects the gastrointestinal tract. It is the most frequent parasitic cause of enteritis in the United States and has a worldwide distribution. In industrialized countries, *Giardia* has a prevalence of 2% to 5%, and in developing countries prevalence is 20% to 30%. High-risk groups include children, previously uninfected adults and travelers, and immunocompromised persons. Rates of infection are highest in areas of poor sanitation and where water is unfiltered [37–39]. Clinical presentations of *Giardia* have a bimodal distribution with peaks at 0 to 5 years and 30 to 40 years [39].

Several drugs are effective in the treatment of giardiasis. The drug of choice is oral metronidazole. It usually is given three times daily for 5 to 7 days [40]. It has a cure rate of 80% to 95% [37,40,41]. An oral formulation of metronidazole is not marketed; however, a suspension can be prepared by thoroughly crushing the tablet and suspending it in cherry syrup [40]. Nitazoxanide, which is available as a tablet and an oral suspension, is approved by the Food and Drug Administration for treatment of *Giardia*. Dosing is usually twice daily for 3 days. Nitazoxanide is as effective as metronidazole for the treatment of *Giardia* and the treatment of metronidazole-resistant *Giardia* [17,42,43]. Nitazoxanide is well tolerated [44,45]. Alternative treatments include furazolidone, tinidazole, albendazole, and paromomycin [37,38]. Furazolidone is given four times daily for 7 to 10 days and is available in an oral solution, an advantage for pediatric patients. Side effects include nausea, vomiting, and diarrhea. Cure rates are lower (about 70%) than rates for other options. This drug should be avoided in patients with G6PD deficiency because of hemolysis. Children younger than 1 month old also can experience hemolytic anemia owing to glutathione instability [40]. Single-dose tinidazole, a nitroimidazole, is another effective agent [37,40]. Albendazole has been shown to be safe and effective in treatment of helminth infections (see section on helminthes) and equally as effective as metronidazole in treating giardiasis in children [46]. This broad activity makes it ideal for treating patients with mixed infections [40]. Paromomycin, a poorly absorbed aminoglycoside, is recommended for the treatment of pregnant women. It is given three times daily for 7 days and has an efficacy of 50% to 70%. If systemically absorbed, it may cause ototoxicity and nephrotoxicity, and it should be used with caution in patients with renal impairment [37,40].

Trichomonas

Trichomonas vaginalis is a sexually transmitted flagellated protozoan that causes 3 to 4 million infections annually in the United States [47]. It is the most common nonviral sexually transmitted disease worldwide [48]. Most men who are infected are asymptomatic or have mild urethral discharge. Women often experience symptoms characterized by a malodorous yellow-green vaginal discharge with vulvar irritation [49]. The health consequences of these infections are substantial and include complications of pregnancy, association with cervical cancer, and predisposition to HIV infection [48]. Metronidazole is the drug of choice, resulting in a cure rate of approximately 95%. Sexual partners should be treated concurrently, even if asymptomatic. In older adolescents and adults, treatment can be given as a single large dose or alternatively in a twice-daily regimen for 7 days [48]. Children should receive three-times-daily dosing for 7 days [17]. Symptomatic pregnant women should be treated with the single-dose regimen [49].

Apicomplexa Infections (Coccidians [including Cryptosporidium*],* Babesia, and Toxoplasma*)*

Cryptosporidiosis

C. parvum is a coccidian parasite that infects the epithelial cells of the gastrointestinal and respiratory tracts of vertebrates [48,50]. Transmission is through ingestion of fecally contaminated food and water and direct person-to-person or animal-to-person spread [50]. This disease has been associated with diarrheal illness worldwide with severity of symptoms dependent on the host characteristics. High-risk populations include children in tropical developing areas and immunocompromised individuals [48,50]. Outbreaks secondary to food-borne transmission occur in more affluent countries. Cryptosporidiosis is characterized by profuse watery diarrhea, fever, anorexia, abdominal cramps, and vomiting. Infection is typically self-limited in immunocompetent hosts; diarrhea lasts approximately 10 to 14 days without therapy. Immunocompromised hosts often

Table 2
Treatment of protozoan infections distributed globally and infections in immunocompromised hosts

Parasite	Drug	Pediatric dosage	Adult dosage
Lumenal flagellates			
Giardia duodenalis			
Drugs of choice	Metronidazole	15 mg/kg/d 3 times daily × 5–7 d	250 mg 3 times daily × 5–7 d
	Nitazoxanide	1–3 y: 100 mg twice daily × 3 d 4–11 y: 200 mg twice daily × 3 d	500 mg twice daily × 3 d
Alternatives:	Furazolidone	6 mg/kg/d 4 times daily × 7–10 d	100 mg 4 times daily × 7–10 d
	Tinidazole	50 mg/kg × 1 dose	2 g × 1 dose
	Albendazole	15 mg/kg once daily × 5 d	400 mg once daily × 5 d
	Paromomycin	25–35 mg/kg/d 3 times daily × 7 d	25–35 mg/kg/d 3 times daily × 7 d
Trichomonas vaginalis			
Drug of choice	Metronidazole	15 mg/kg/d 3 times daily × 7 d	500 mg twice daily × 7 d; or 2 g × 1 dose
Apicomplexa infections			
Cryptosporidium parvum			
Drug of choice	Nitazoxanide	1–3 ys: 100 mg twice daily × 3 d 4–11 ys: 200 mg twice daily × 3 d	500 mg twice daily × 3 d
Alternative	Paromomycin		
Isospora belli			
Drug of choice	Trimethoprim-sulfmethoxazole	TMP 5 mg/kg, SMX 25 mg/kg twice daily × 10 d	TMP 160 mg, SMX 800 mg twice daily × 10 d
Prophylaxis in AIDS		TMP 5 mg/kg, SMX 25 mg/kg daily 3 times per wk	TMP 160 mg, SMX 800 mg daily 3 times per wk
Cyclospora cayetanensis			
Drug of choice	Trimethoprim-sulfmethoxazole	TMP 5 mg/kg, SMX 25 mg/kg twice daily × 10 d	TMP 160 mg, SMX 800 mg twice daily × 10 d
Prophylaxis in AIDS		TMP 5 mg/kg, SMX 25 mg/kg daily 3 times per wk	TMP 160 mg, SMX 800 mg daily 3 times per wk

Babesia microti			
Drug of choice	Quinine *plus* clindamycin	25 mg/kg/d 3 times daily × 7–10 d plus 20–40 mg/kg/d 3 times daily × 7–10 d	650 mg 3 times daily × 7–10 d plus 1.2 g IV 2 times daily or 600 mg 3 times daily × 7–10 d
	Atovaquone *plus* azithromycin	20 mg/kg twice daily × 7–10 d *plus* 12 mg/kg once daily × 7–10 d	750 mg twice daily × 7–10 d *plus* 600 mg once daily × 7–10 d
Toxoplasma gondii			
Pregnant female			
Drug of choice	Spiramycin		1 g three times daily until term or fetal infection
Alternative after first trimester if in utero transmission	Pyrimethamine *plus* sulfadiazine		50 mg twice daily × 2 d, then 50 mg once daily *plus* 50 mg/kg twice daily until term
Congenital infection			
Drugs of choice	Pyrimethamine *plus* sulfadiazine	2 mg/kg × 2 d; then 1 mg/kg × 6 mo, then once every M, W, F × 1 y *plus* 50 mg/kg twice daily × 1 y	
Immunocompromised host			
Drugs of choice	Pyrimethamine *plus* sulfadiazine	2 mg/kg × 3 d; then 1 mg/kg *plus* 50 mg/kg twice daily × 4 wk	25–100 mg/d plus 1–1.5 g 4 times daily × 4 wk
Alternative	Trimethoprim-sulfamethoxazole	TMP 5 mg/kg, SMX 25 mg/kg twice daily × 4 wk	TMP 160 mg, SMX 800 mg twice daily × 4 wk
AIDS-related pathogens			
Pneumocyctis jiroveci (formerly *P. carinii*)			
Drugs of choice	Trimethoprim-sulfamethoxazole	TMP 15 mg/kg/d, SMX 75 mg/kg/d IV/PO 4 times daily × 21 d	TMP 15 mg/kg/d, SMX 75 mg/kg/d IV/PO 4 times daily × 21 d
	Pentamidine	3–4 mg/kg/d IV once daily × 21 d	3–4 mg/kg/d IV once daily × 21 d
Prophylaxis			
Drug of choice	Trimethoprim-sulfamethoxazole	TMP 15 mg/m^2, SMX 750 mg/m^2 twice daily on 3 consecutive days per wk	1 tab (single or double strength) daily on 3 consecutive days per week
Alternatives	Dapsone	2 mg/kg/d or 4 mg/kg each week	50 mg twice daily or 100 mg once daily
	Pentamidine	>5 y: 300 mg IV/inhaled monthly	300 mg IV/inhaled monthly

(continued on next page)

Table 2 (*continued*)

Parasite	Drug	Pediatric dosage	Adult dosage
AIDS-related pathogens			
Prophylaxis			
Alternatives	Atovaquone	1–3 mo: 30 mg/kg once daily 4–24 mo: 45 mg/kg once daily >24 mo: 30 mg/kg once daily	1500 mg once daily
Microsporidiosis			
Drugs of choice	Albendazole		400 mg twice daily × 21 d
	Fumagillin		60 mg once daily × 14 d
Free-living ameba			
Naegleria fowleri			
Drug of choice	Amphotericin B	1.5 mg/kg twice daily × 3 d, then 1/mg/kg once daily × 6 d	1.5 mg/kg twice daily × 3 d, then 1/mg/kg once daily × 6 d
Acanthamoeba			
Drug of choice	See text		

have a prolonged course with chronic diarrhea and wasting and involvement of the biliary and pancreatic ducts [50].

Because cryptosporidiosis is self-limiting in most cases, treatment consists of maintaining adequate hydration and supportive care. In severe cases and in immunocompromised patients, however, several treatment options could be considered. Nitazoxanide is the drug of choice. It is available as a tablet and oral suspension and should be given twice daily for 3 days. In a study in Zambia, malnourished children treated with nitazoxanide showed clinical and microbiologic improvements and improved survival [51]. Paromomycin, a nonabsorbed aminoglycoside, has been shown to decrease stool excretion of oocytes in several trials. There are conflicting results with regards to its efficacy in treatment of cryptosporidiosis in patients with AIDS, however [52,53]. When used as a single therapy, treatment regimens have included two to four doses daily from 14 to 28 days. Paromomycin also has been used in combination with azithromycin for 4 weeks, followed by paromomycin alone for another 8 weeks with some improvement in clinical symptoms and decrease in oocyte passage [54].

Isospora *and* Cyclospora

Isospora belli and *C. cayetanensis* are coccidian protozoa that can infect the small intestines and cause human disease. Both cause diarrheal diseases similar to cryptosporidiosis. *Cyclospora* has a worldwide distribution and is endemic in Nepal, Peru, and Haiti. Both infections are a common source of travel-related diarrhea, and both are spread by the fecal-oral routes through food and water [37]. In immunocompetent hosts, both produce self-limiting infections, but in immunocompromised hosts chronic diarrhea and anorexia can cause serious sequelae. The treatment for both infections is TMP-SMX twice daily for 7 to 10 days. In patients with AIDS, treatment should be the continuation of TMP-SMX three times per week as prophylaxis [37,55]. Formulations of TMP-SMX include tablet and oral suspension. Serious reactions include Stevens-Johnson syndrome, aplastic anemia, anaphylactoid and allergic reactions, hepatotoxicity, and nephrotoxicity. Daily pyrimethamine, with or without folinic acid, is an effective alternative for patients who cannot tolerate TMP-SMX [56].

Babesia

Babesia are tick-borne protozoa classified in the Apicomplexa phylum. Human disease is found almost exclusively in the United States and Europe. The most common species in northeastern United States is *B. microti,* transmitted mainly by *Ixodes scapularis* ticks, which are also the main vectors for Lyme disease [57,58]. *Babesia* manifestations range from asymptomatic disease to mild flulike symptoms to more severe symptoms mimicking malaria to death. The most common symptoms include fever, malaise, night sweats, and headache.

The drugs of choice are either oral quinine three times daily plus intravenous/oral clindamycin three times daily for 7 to 10 days or oral atovaquone twice daily plus oral azithromycin once daily for 7 to 10 days [57]. In a study comparing the two treatment regimens in adults, both were similar with regards to clearing symptoms and parasitemia. Clindamycin and quinine were associated with a higher rate of adverse events, however [59].

Toxoplasma

Toxoplasma gondii is an obligate intracellular protozoan with a worldwide distribution. Cats are the definitive host, but *T. gondii* can infect most species of warm-blooded animals. Transmission can occur in-utero, by ingestion of food and water contaminated by cat feces, or by ingestion of undercooked meats infected with *T. gondii* oocysts [48,60]. In most healthy, immunocompetent individuals, infection with *T. gondii* is asymptomatic and resolves spontaneously without treatment. Treatment is indicated, however, for three populations of special concern: pregnant mothers, neonates, and immunocompromised persons.

Infection acquired early in the pregnancy can result in severe congenital toxoplasmosis, in utero fetal demise, or spontaneous abortion. Maternal infections contracted late in pregnancy are associated with a high frequency of vertical transmission, but most resulting congenital infections are asymptomatic. Treatment of pregnant women is aimed at decreasing vertical transmission and the frequency and severity of adverse outcomes for the fetus [60]. The drug of choice for acute toxoplasmosis in a pregnant woman is spiramycin three times a day. If, after the first trimester, there is no evidence of transmission to the fetus, spiramycin can be continued for the length of the pregnancy. If the fetus shows evidence of infection, pyrimethamine and sulfadiazine should be initiated. Pyrimethamine cannot be used in the first trimester because of its teratogenic effects [48,60,61].

Neonates with congenital toxoplasmosis usually are asymptomatic at birth. When present, clinical manifestations may include microcephaly, hydrocephalus, seizures, blindness, petechiae, and anemia. Infected infants should be treated with pyrimethamine once daily for 6 months, then three times weekly to complete 1 year, plus sulfadiazine twice daily for 1 year. While taking pyrimethamine, patients should receive leucovorin three times daily to prevent bone marrow suppression [60,62].

CNS disease is a common complication of toxoplasmosis in HIV-infected adults and children. Focal neurologic deficits include seizures, hemiparesis, cranial nerve palsies, and ataxia. Treatment consists of pyrimethamine plus sulfadiazine plus leucovorin acutely and for a minimum of 4 weeks after symptoms have resolved [60,63]. Clindamycin may be substituted for sulfadiazine if the patient is intolerant of sulfa drugs. TMP-SMX seems to have equal efficacy to pyrimethamine plus sulfadiazine in patients with AIDS and represents an alternative therapy [64]. When the acute therapy is complete, secondary prophylaxis, usually at half the treating dose, should be continued until the patient is no longer severely immunocompromised [60].

*AIDS-related pathogens (*Pneumocystis *and* Microsporidia*)*

Pneumocystis

Pneumocystis jiroveci, formerly known as *Pneumocystis carinii,* is the most common opportunistic infection in children with advanced HIV infection. It is classified as a fungus based on DNA sequence analysis, but retains several morphologic and biologic similarities to protozoa [63]. *P. jiroveci* is ubiquitous in mammals, and most humans have acquired antibody by 4 years of age. Most cases in industrialized countries occur in persons lacking cell-mediated immunity, especially HIV-infected persons. *Pneumocystis* is an extracellular parasite that infects the lungs, resulting in the classic tetrad of symptoms: tachypnea, dyspnea, cough, and fever. Rapidly progressing hypoxemia and subsequent respiratory failure follow [63,65].

The treatment of choice of *Pneumocystis* in HIV-infected children is intravenous TMP-SMX, steroids, and respiratory support. TMP-SMX is given in higher than normal dosages, divided into four daily doses for 21 days. Treatment can be switched to oral formulations when the patient's clinical status has improved [66]. Rates of adverse reactions to TMP-SMX are generally higher for HIV-infected children compared with normal children. Pentamidine, in a single daily intravenous dose for 21 days, is an alternative for patients who are intolerant of TMP-SMX. Pentamidine is similar in efficacy to TMP-SMX. Adverse effects of pentamidine include pancreatitis, hypoglycemia or hyperglycemia, hypotension, fever, rash, and neutropenia [67]. Atovaquone has been approved for the oral treatment of mild-to-moderate *Pneumocystis* in adult patients who are intolerant to TMP-SMX. Experience with this agent in children is limited. Common side effects include rash, fever, nausea, diarrhea, hyperglycemia, and elevated amylase levels [68]. Several other regimens (clindamycin plus primaquine, dapsone plus trimethoprim, and trimetrexate plus leucovorin) have been approved for use in adults, but have not been evaluated in children [69–71].

Guidelines for *Pneumocystis* prophylaxis in HIV-positive and HIV-exposed children were revised in 1995 and are shown in Box 1 [72]. TMP-SMX is the

Box 1. Guidelines for *Pneumocystis* prophylaxis in HIV-positive and HIV-exposed children

1. All HIV-infected and indeterminate children from 4 weeks to 12 months of life (prophylaxis can be stopped if HIV infection has been excluded after 4 months of age)
2. HIV-infected children aged:
   1–5 years: $CD4^+$ count <500/μL, CD4 percentage <15%
   6–12 years: $CD4^+$ count <200/μL, CD4 percentage <15%
3. All HIV-infected children treated for *P. jiroveci* pneumonia

prophylactic medication of choice, given once daily on 3 consecutive days per week. For persons intolerant of TMP-SMX, alternatives include daily oral dapsone, monthly aerosolized or intravenous pentamidine, or daily atovaquone. Dapsone has been associated with hemolytic anemia and is contraindicated in persons with G6PD deficiency [66].

Microsporida

Microsporida are obligate, intracellular protozoa that are ubiquitous in nature and infect numerous animals, including humans. Transmission occurs when spores are ingested, then organisms disseminate into host tissue, such as liver and kidneys, with excretion back into the environment through feces [73]. Before the HIV epidemic, there were few reported human cases of infection. More recently, the incidence of infection has increased dramatically, with most cases reported in immunocompetent persons [74,75]. Clinical features of disease caused by *Microsporida* include diarrhea, corneal infections, cholecystitis, hepatitis, nephritis, and peritonitis [73,75–77]. The drugs of choice for treatment of *Microsporida* are albendazole twice daily for 21 days and fumagillin once daily for 14 days. Albendazole has been shown to improve symptoms of diarrhea, but not to eradicate the organism. Albendazole usually is effective against *Encephalitozoon intestinalis,* but infections with *E. bienuesi* are more difficult to treat [78]. Fumagillin was effective at alleviating symptoms and eliminating the organism from stools in a study conducted in 10 patients with AIDS and 2 organ transplant recipients. Severe neutropenia and thrombocytopenia occurred in several patients [79].

*Free-Living Amebae (*Naegleria, Acanthamoeba*)*

Naegleria *and* Acanthamoeba

Naegleria fowleri and *Acanthamoeba* species are "free-living" amebic organisms because they do not need a secondary host to complete their life cycle. These organisms have a worldwide distribution and are found in soil, freshwater ponds, streams, rivers, and pools. Infection can result in primary amebic meningoencephalitis, an extremely rare and almost uniformly fatal infection [80]. *N. fowleri* causes an acute amebic meningoencephalitis, which initially is indistinguishable from primary bacterial meningitis, whereas *Acanthamoeba* causes a more indolent and subacute granulomatous amebic encephalitis [81].

The drug of choice for treatment of *N. fowleri* is amphotericin B. There have been reports of successful combinations of treatments with amphotericin B, rifampin, and chloramphenicol; amphotericin B and rifampin; amphotericin B, rifampin, and ketoconazole; and combinations of intravenous and intrathecal amphotericin B [82–84]. Outcome of treatment of *Acanthamoeba* infection usually is poor, although several cases have been treated successfully with the combination use of TMP-SMX, rifampin, and ketaconazole [85,86]. Other reports describe use of fluconazole, sulfadiazine, and pyrimethamine in combination with surgical resection of the CNS lesion [87].

Treatment of helminthic infections

Table 3 provides a quick reference to drugs of choice and dosages.

*Intestinal nematodes (*Ascaris, Trichuris, Enterobius, *and Hookworms) and Strongyloides species*

Helminth infections affect more than one quarter of the world's population, making them a major health priority. Campaigns for deworming, launched by the World Health Organization, are targeting high-risk groups, such as school-age children, preschool children, and women of childbearing age in the developing world. In the United States, high-risk groups include international travelers, refugees, recent immigrants, and international adoptees [88–90].

Five antihelminthic drugs are considered the drugs of choice against intestinal nematodes. The benzamidazoles, such as albendazole (single dose) and mebendazole (twice a day for 3 days), are effective first-line treatments against *Ascaris lumbricoides* (roundworm), *Trichuris trichiura* (whipworm), *Ancylostoma duodenale,* and *Necator americanus* (hookworms). Albendazole administered twice a day for 2 days is the drug of choice against *Strongyloides stercoralis*. Albendazole and mebendazole are available as chewable tablets, and both are available as oral solutions [90,91]. Mebendazole is poorly absorbed by the gastrointestinal tract and exerts its action directly on the worms themselves. For extraluminal infections, appropriate tissue levels can be attained if the drug is taken with fatty foods. Side effects for both drugs are typically mild and transient. In a few cases, gastrointestinal symptoms (epigastric pain, nausea, diarrhea, and vomiting), CNS symptoms (dizziness, headache), migration of worms through the mouth, and rare allergic conditions have been reported [90]. Because of their teratogenic potential in animals, benzamidazoles are not recommended for children younger than 2 years of age. Side effects in infants 12 months old are similar to those of older children [92,93].

Pyrantel pamoate, available as an oral solution given as a single dose, is the drug of choice for *Enterobius vermicularis* (pinworm). Single-dose albendazole and mebendazole are effective alternatives. Regardless of the drug used, a second dose is required after 2 weeks. Pyrantel pamoate, as a single dose, is an effective alternative for *A. lumbricoides,* and once-daily dosing for 3 days is an alternative for *A. duodenale* and *N. americanus* [90]. Pyrantel pamoate should be used with caution in patients with hepatic dysfunction. No data exist for use in children younger than 2 years of age, but no age-related problems have been reported [94].

Cutaneous larva migrans, or creeping eruption, usually is caused by the larvae of *Ancylostoma brasiliense* and *Uncinaria stenocephala* (dog and cat hookworms). This infection can be treated topically with thiabendazole cream, two to three times daily for 5 to 10 days. In most cases, pruritus and larval migration resolve within 48 hours. Alternative treatments include albendazole (daily for 3 days) or ivermectin (daily for 1–2 days). Other topical treatments, such as

Table 3
Treatment of helminthic infections

Parasite	Drug	Pediatric dosage	Adult dosage
Intestinal nematode			
Roundworm *Ascaris lumbricoides*			
Drugs of choice	Albendazole	400 mg × 1 dose	400 mg × 1 dose
	Mebendazole	100 mg twice daily × 3 d	100 mg twice daily × 3 d
	Pyrantel pamoate	11 mg/kg once; repeat in 2 wk	11 mg/kg once; repeat in 2 wk
	Ivermectin	150–200 μg/kg × 1 dose	150–200 μg/kg × 1 dose
Whipworm: *Trichuris trichiura*			
Drugs of choice	Albendazole	400 mg × 1 dose	400 mg × 1 dose
	Mebendazole	100 mg twice daily × 3 d	100 mg twice daily × 3 d
	Ivermectin	150–200 μg/kg × 1 dose	150–200 μg/kg × 1 dose
Hookworm: *Ancylostoma duodenale* and *Necator americanus*			
Drugs of choice	Albendazole	400 mg × 1 dose	400 mg × 1 dose
	Mebendazole	100 mg twice daily × 3 d	100 mg twice daily × 3 d
	Pyrantel pamoate	11 mg/kg once daily × 3 d	11 mg/kg once daily × 3 d
Pinworm: *Enterobius vermicularis*			
Drugs of choice	Pyrantel pamoate	11 mg/kg once; repeat in 2 wk	11 mg/kg once; repeat in 2 wk
Alternatives	Albendazole	400 mg once; repeat in 2 wk	400 mg once; repeat in 2 wk
	Mebendazole	100 mg once; repeat in 2 wk	100 mg once; repeat in 2 wk
	Ivermectin	150–200 μg/kg × 1 dose	150–200 μg/kg × 1 dose
Strongyloides stercoralis			
Drugs of choice	Albendazole	400 mg twice daily × 2 d	400 mg twice daily × 2 d
Alternatives	Ivermectin	200 μg/kg once daily × 2 d	200 μg/kg once daily × 2 d
	Thiabendazole	50 mg/kg twice daily × 2 d	50 mg/kg twice daily × 2 d
Cutaneous larva migrans: *Ancylostoma brasiliense* and *Uncinaria stenocephala*			
Drugs of choice	Thiabendazole	Topically 2–3 times daily for 5–10 d	Topically 2–3 times daily for 5–10 d
	Albendazole	400 mg once daily × 3 d	400 mg once daily × 3 d
	Ivermectin	200 μg/kg once daily × 1–2 d	200 μg/kg once daily × 1–2 d

Blood and tissue nematodes			
Filariasis: *Onchocerca volvulus*			
Drug of choice	Ivermectin	150 μg/kg once monthly × 6–12 mo	150 μg/kg once monthly × 6–12 mo
Lymphatic filariasis: *Wuchereria bancrofti, Brugia malayi, Brugia timori*			
Drug of choice	Diethylcarbamazine	6 mg/kg × 1 dose	6 mg/kg × 1 dose
Visceral larva migrans: *Toxocara cari*			
Drug of choice	Albendazole	400 mg twice daily × 5 d	400 mg twice daily × 5 d
	Mebendazole	100–200 mg twice daily × 5 d	100–200 mg twice daily × 5 d
Cestodes			
Tapeworms			
Taeniasis: *T.saginata/T. solium*			
Drugs of choice	Niclosamide	50 mg/kg × 1 dose	2 g × 1 dose
	Praziquantel	5–10 mg/kg × 1 dose	5–10 mg/kg × 1 dose
Cysticercosis: *T.solium*			
Drug of choice	Albendazole	15 mg/kg twice daily × 15–30 d	400 mg twice daily × 15–30 d
Alternative	Praziquantel	50–100 mg/kg 3 times daily × 30 d	50–100 mg/kg 3 times daily × 30 d
Hydatid disease: *Echinococcus granulosus* and *E. multilocularis*			
Drugs of choice	Albendazole	15 mg/kg once daily for 1–6 mo	400 mg twice daily × 1–6 mo
Diphyllobothrium latum, Dipylidium caninum			
Drug of choice	Praziquantel	5–10 mg/kg × 1 dose	5–10 mg/kg × 1 dose
Hymenolepsis nana			
Drug of choice	Praziquantel	25 mg/kg × 1 dose	25 mg/kg × 1 dose
Trematodes			
Schistosomiasis			
Drug of choice	Praziquantel	40–60 mg/kg 2–3 times daily × 1 dose	40–60 mg/kg 2–3 times daily × 1 dose
Liver flukes: *Clonorchis sinesis*, *Opisthorchis viverrini*, and *Opisthorchis felineus*			
Drug of choice	Praziquantel	75 mg/kg 3 times daily × 1 dose	75 mg/kg 3 times daily × 1 dose
Alternative: (*C. sinesis*)	Albendazole	10 mg/kg once daily × 7 d	10 mg/kg once daily × 7 d
Lung fluke: *Paragonimus westermani*			
Drug of choice	Praziquantel	75 mg/kg 3 times daily × 2 d	75 mg/kg 3 times daily × 2 d

freezing the leading edge of the cutaneous trail, have been tried in the past, but are no longer recommended because of blistering and ulceration [91,103].

Ivermectin (single dose for 1–2 days) and thiabendazole (twice daily for 2 days) are acceptable alternatives to albendazole for the treatment of *S. stercoralis* [90, 95,96]. Ivermectin, as a single dose for the treatment of ascariasis, trichuriasis, and enterobiasis, is equal in efficacy to other agents, but it has limited activity against hookworms [94]. Studies suggest that giving a single combination dose of ivermectin plus albendazole produces superior cure rates and egg reduction for trichuriasis than with either drug used alone [97]. Neither ivermectin nor thiabendazole has been studied extensively in children, and safety profiles have not been established for children weighing less than 15 kg. Neither drug is recommended during pregnancy, but if treatment of heavy worm burden during pregnancy is required, ivermectin should be used because of its low risk of adverse events [90]. Thiabendazole is available in chewable tablets and oral solution. It is well absorbed and associated with side effects such as dizziness, nausea, diarrhea, and anorexia [96,98].

Blood and tissue nematodes (filarial parasites, Toxocara, *and visceral larva migrans)*

As with the intestinal nematodes, tissue and blood nematodes are a serious global public health problem. Currently, several World Health Organization–sponsored campaigns are geared toward the eradication of some severe nematode infections. These campaigns are based on antivector measures to decrease environmental exposure and are supplemented with mass treatment campaigns when appropriate.

Ivermectin, as a single dose repeated monthly for 6 to 12 months, is currently recommended for international campaigns against *Onchocerca volvulus* (the agent causing river blindness). It is microfilaricidal and results in approximately 95% reduction in dermal microfilariae after one dose. This drug has been shown to reduce or limit dramatically the transmission of filarial disease when used in community-based disease control programs. On an individual basis, this drug is not completely curative, however, because of its lack of effect on the adult parasite. Side effects of ivermectin are infrequent and often due to the inflammatory responses to the dead microfilariae. The frequency of common symptoms accompanying treatment, including rash, pruritus, and myalgias, is less with each subsequent treatment as the number of microfilariae decreases [99,100].

Lymphatic filariasis is caused by three different filariae species (*Wuchereria bancrofti, Brugia malayi*, and *Brugia timori*) and accounts for approximately 120 million infections per year globally [101]. Most cases of lymphatic filariasis are asymptomatic. Children frequently present with lymphadenopathy secondary to worm infestation of the lymph nodes, most commonly in the legs, arms, and scrotum. Tropical pulmonary eosinophilia, thought to result from immune responses to filarial antigens, rarely occurs in children [102]. Single-dose ivermectin given annually is an effective supplement to community-based control programs, but treatment is not curative [100]. The drug of choice for treatment of lymphatic filariasis is single-dose diethylcarbamazine, which is available in tablet form. A 21-day course of diethylcarbamazine may be required for patients with tropical pulmonary eosinophilia. Although diethylcarbamazine is effective at clearing infection; there is little evidence to suggest that it reverses lymphatic damage or pulmonary fibrosis. Side effects of diethylcarbamazine include pruritus, maculopapular rash, fever, edema, and headache. Data in children are limited, but no other adverse events have been reported [94]. Diethylcarbamazine is effective in vitro against *Onchocerca volvulus*, but it cannot be used clinically because of the intense inflammatory response it causes with rapid killing of microfilariae.

Visceral larva migrans and ocular larva migrans usually are caused by infection most commonly resulting from *Toxocara cani*. Often the disease course for *Toxocara* is subclinical and self-limited, and treatment is controversial. For symptomatic disease, either albendazole or mebendazole twice daily for 5 days is recommended. For patients with ocular or neurologic manifestations, combination therapy with albendazole and corticosteroids is recommended [103,104].

Cestodes (tapeworms [including taeniasis and cysticercosis] and hydatid disease)

Cestodes, or tapeworms, are segmented worms that have two life cycle stages, the adult stage and larval stage, both of which cause disease in humans. Ingestion of undercooked meats containing larvae of *Taenia solium* (pork) or *Taenia saginata* (beef) results in taeniasis when the larvae mature into adult tapeworms. Taeniasis is characterized by mild symptoms of abdominal pain, bloating, nausea, and diarrhea [105]. Niclosamide and praziquantel are the drugs of choice for therapy. Niclosamide, as a single dose, is preferred because it is not absorbed from the intestinal tract, but it is currently not available in the United States. Praziquantel, as a single dose, is available in a scored tablet form [105,106]. Side effects of praziquantel include malaise, abdominal discomfort, headache, dizziness, and rarely urticaria. Safety profiles have not been established in children younger than 4 years old [94].

Cysticercosis and neurocysticercosis are caused by the larval stage of *T. solium,* but not *T. saginata*. In adults, the disease is characterized by symptoms related to increased intracranial pressure and immune-mediated inflammation. The disease differs in children, with generalized seizures a common initial sign, secondary to the cystic mass lesion itself or granuloma formation after cyst destruction [105,107]. Albendazole is the drug of choice for therapy; it is effective and relatively inexpensive. It is administered twice daily for 15 to 30 days and can be repeated as necessary. Praziquantel given three times daily for 15 to 30 days is an alternative. Although effective anticysticercal treatment is available, the decision to treat is controversial because symptoms related to neurocysticercosis are thought to result from the inflammatory response accompanying the death of the organism [105,107]. Studies confirm that neurologic symptoms increase early in the course of treatment. Persons who are not treated, however, have a higher frequency and persistence of neurologic symptoms. These neurologic symptoms can be ameliorated by the concomitant use of dexamethasone and anticonvulsants [108].

Hydatid disease is caused by the larval forms of the dog tapeworms, *Echinococcus granulosus* and *Echinococcus multilocularis* [90,109]. In adults, dissemination of cysts to multiple different tissue sites, especially the liver and lungs, can follow ingestion. Echinococcus is the most common cause of liver cysts worldwide. Symptoms may be mild for many years or result in serious complications, including death. Dissemination to the brain and eyes in more common in childhood. The mainstay of treatment, when possible, is surgical removal of any cysts. In some cases, such as uncomplicated liver cysts, percutaneous aspiration and injection of a protoscolicidal agent is effective. In other cases, either in conjunction with surgery or when surgery is contraindicated, chemotherapy with oral benzimadoles is warranted. Albendazole and mebendazole have been shown to be beneficial, but albendazole is preferred because of poor tissue penetration of mebendazole. Treatment may need to continue for 6 months [17,110]. *Diphyllobothrium* species (fish tapeworm), *Dipylidium caninum* (dog and cat tapeworm), *Hymenolepsis nana* (dwarf tapeworm), and *Hymenolepsis diminuta* (rodent tapeworm) are other tapeworms that cause human disease, which can be treated with single-dose praziquantel [111].

Trematodes (schistosomes, lung and liver flukes)

Schistosomiasis, also known as *bilharziasis,* is caused by the parasitic blood flukes called *schistosomes*. The World Health Organization estimates that approximately 200 million people are infested worldwide, ranking it second to malaria in terms of global public health importance [112,113]. Numerous schistosome species can affect many different animals, with almost all human cases resulting from *S. mansoni, S. haematobium, S. japonicum, S. mekongi,* and *S. intercalatum*. These different species have differing global distributions and differing predilections for sites of residence within the host [112]. These parasites have a complex life cycle that involves snails as the intermediate host. Prevention efforts are geared toward mass chemotherapy, improved sanitation, and snail control through environmental engineering or molluscacides [114,115].

The drug of choice for treatment of all schistosome species is praziquantel, given in either two or three doses for 1 day [112,116]. Praziquantel is one of the safest antihelminthic medications with minimal side effects. It has not been tested in pregnant and lactating women, however, and is classified as Pregnancy category B. Currently, countries such as Ghana, China, Egypt, and the Philippines have adopted the routine treatment of pregnant women with praziquantel because of a presumed disproportionate risk from infection compared with treatment [116].

Clonorchis sinesis, Opisthorchis viverrini, and *Opisthorchis felineus* constitute a group of trematodes termed *liver flukes,* which reside in the human biliary tract. Infections are caused by ingestion of uncooked fish that have been infested with larval cysts. Praziquantel, given in three doses for 1 day, is the drug of choice for the three trematodes. Albendazole, given daily for 7 days, is an alternative for *C. sinesis* [17].

Paragonimus westermani, the lung fluke, is a trematode commonly causing human disease in eastern Asia. After ingestion of uncooked crabs or crayfish, the larvae penetrate through the diaphragm into the pleural space and migrate through lung tissue into the bronchi. Approximately 1% of infections result in cerebral disease, which is more common among children [117]. Praziquantel, given three times daily for 2 days, is the drug of choice. For patients developing cerebral disease, corticosteroids given concurrently with praziquantel can reduce symptoms of inflammation caused by dying flukes [17].

Summary

Parasitic infections in children present many challenges for the pediatrician. These complex diseases are often difficult to diagnose and require pathogen-specific treatment with drugs that are unfamiliar to many clinicians. International travel and immunodeficiency states, such as AIDS, have been factors in the increasing prevalence and clinical importance of these infections in children. As in bacterial and viral infections, the emergence of drug resistance is a continuing potential threat. From endemic malaria in persons in sub-Saharan Africa to giardiasis in children US daycare centers to *Pneumocystis* infections in AIDS patients, it is likely that parasitic infections will remain a persistent challenge for public health and infectious disease specialists for many years to come.

References

[1] Sachs J. Helping the world's poorest. Economist 1999;14:17–20.

[2] Guerin PJ, Olliaro P, Nosten F, et al. Malaria: current status of control, diagnosis, treatment, and a proposed agenda for research and development. Lancet Infect Dis 2002;2:564–73.

[3] Alecrim WD, Espinosa FEM, Alecrim MGC. Emerging and re-emerging diseases in Latin America: *Plasmodium falciparum* infection in the pregnant patient. Infect Dis Clin North Am 2000;14:83–95.

[4] Shann F. The management of severe malaria. Pediatr Crit Care Med 2003;4:489–90.

[5] World Health Organization. World malaria situation in 1994. Parts I–III. Wkly Epidemiol Rec 1997;72:269–90.

[6] Suh KN, Kain KC, Keystone JS. Malaria. Can Med Assoc J 2004;170:1693–702.

[7] Winstanley P. Modern chemotherapeutic options for malaria. Lancet Infect Dis 2001;1:242–50.

[8] Trape JF, Pison G, Preziosi MP, et al. Impact of chloroquine resistance on malaria mortality. C R Acad Sci III 1998;321:689–97.

[9] John CC. Drug treatment of malaria in children. Pediatr Infect Dis J 2003;22:649–50.

[10] Miles MA. The discovery of Chagas disease: progress and prejudice. Infect Dis Clin North Am 2004;18:247–60.

[11] Prata A. Clinical and epidemiological aspects of Chagas disease. Lancet Infect Dis 2001;1:92–100.

[12] American Academy of Pediatrics. Summaries of infectious diseases. In: Pickering LK, editor. Red book: 2003 report of the Committee on Infectious Diseases. 26th ed. Elk Grove Village (IL): American Academy of Pediatrics; 2003.
[13] Estani SS, Segura EL, Ruiz AM, Velazquez E, Porcel BM, Yampotis C. Efficacy of chemotherapy with benznidazole in children in the indeterminate phase of Chagas' disease. Am J Trop Med Hyg 1998;59:526–9.
[14] Viotti R, Vigliano C, Armenti H, Segura E. Treatment of chronic Chagas' disease with benznidazole: clinical and serological evolution with long-term follow-up. Am Heart J 1994;127: 151–62.
[15] Legros D, Ollivier G, Gastellu-Etchegorry M, et al. Treatment of human African trypanosomiasis—present situation and needs for research and development. Lancet Infect Dis 2002;2:437–40.
[16] Burchman RJ, Ogbunude PO, Enanza B, Barrett MP. Chemotherapy of African trypanosomiasis. Curr Pharm Des 2002;8:256–67.
[17] Drugs for parasitic infections. Med Lett Drugs Ther. Available at: www.medletter.com/. Accessed November 4, 2004.
[18] Pepin J, Milord F, Khonde AN, et al. Risk factors for encephalopathy and mortality during melarsoprol treatment of *trypanosoma brucei gambiense* sleeping sickness. Trans R Soc Trop Med Hyg 1995;89:92–7.
[19] Ortega-Barria E. Trypanosoma species (trypanosomiasis). In: Long SS, Pickering LK, Prober CG, editors. Principles and practice of pediatric infectious diseases. 2nd ed. New York: Churchill Livingstone; 2003. p. 1324–30.
[20] Burri C. Eflornithine for the treatment of human African trypanosomiasis. Parasitol Res 2003; 90:S49–52.
[21] Markle WH, Makhoul K. Cutaneous leishmaniasis: recognition and treatment. Clin Infect Dis 1997;25:677–84.
[22] Zuckerman A, Lainson R. *Leishmania*. In: Kreier JP, editor. Parasitic protozoa, vol 1. New York: Academic Press; 1977. p. 77–87.
[23] Guerin PJ, Olliero P, Sundar S, et al. Visceral leishmaniasis: current status of control, diagnosis and treatment, and a proposed research and development agenda. J Infect Dis 1999;180:564–7.
[24] Kafetzis DA, Maltezou HC. Visceral leishmaniasis in paediatrics. Curr Opin Infect Dis 2002; 15:289–94.
[25] Kafetzis DA. An overview of paediatric leishmaniasis. J Postgrad Med 2003;49:31–8.
[26] Herwaldt BL, Berman JD. Recommendations for treating leishmaniasis with sodium stibogluconate (Pentostam) and review of pertinent clinical studies. Am J Trop Med Hyg 1992; 46:296–306.
[27] Sundar S, Pai K, Kumar R, et al. Resistance to treatment in Kala-azar: speciation of isolates from northeast India. Am J Trop Med Hyg 2001;65:193–6.
[28] Lira R, Sundar S, Makharia A, et al. Evidence that the high incidence of treatment failures in Indian Kala-azar is due to the emergence of antimony-resistant strains of leishmania donovani. J Infect Dis 1999;180:564–7.
[29] Meyerhoff A. US Food and Drug Administration approval of Ambisome (liposomal amphoteracin B) for treatment of visceral leishmaniasis. Clin Infect Dis 1999;28:42–8.
[30] Di Martino L, Mantovani MP, Gradoni L. Low dosage combination of meglumine antimoniate plus allopurinol as first choice treatment of infantile visceral leishmaniasis in Italy. Trans Soc Trop Med Hyg 1990;84:534–5.
[31] Li E, Stanley SL. Protozoa: amebiasis. Gastroenterol Clin North Am 1996;25:471–92.
[32] Hughes MA, Petri WA. Amebic liver abscess. Infect Dis Clin North Am 2000;14:565–82.
[33] Adams EB, MacLeod IN. Invasive amebiasis: amebic dysentery and its complications. Medicine 1977;56:315–24.
[34] Bassily S, Farid Z, El-Masry A, Mikhail EM. Treatment of intestinal *E. histolytica* and *G. lamblia* with metronidazole, tinidazole, and ornidazole: a comparative study. J Trop Med Hyg 1987;90:9–12.

[35] McAuley JB, Juranek DD. Paromomycin in the treatment of mild-to-moderate intestinal amebiasis. Clin Infect Dis 1992;15:551–2.
[36] McAuley JB, Herwaldt BL, Stokes SL, et al. Diloxinide furoate for treating asymptomatic *Entamoeba histolytica* cyst passers: 14 years' experience in the United States. Clin Infect Dis 1992;15:464–8.
[37] Katz DE, Taylor DN. Parasitic infections of the gastrointestinal tract. Gastroenterol Clin North Am 2001;30:797–815.
[38] Lebwohl B, Deckelbaum RJ, Green PH. Giardiasis. Gastrointest Endosc 2003;57:906–13.
[39] Procop GW. Gastrointestinal infections. Infect Dis Clin North Am 2001;15:1073–108.
[40] Gardner TB, Hill DR. Treatment of giardiasis. Clin Microbiol Rev 2001;14:114–28.
[41] Hill DR, Nash TE. Intestinal flagellate and ciliate infections. In: Guerrant RL, Walker DH, Weller PF, editors. Tropical infectious diseases. Philadelphia: Churchill Livingstone; 1999. p. 703–12.
[42] Ortiz JJ, Ayoub A, Gargala G, Chegne NL, Favennec L. Randomized clinical study of nitazoxanide compared to metronidazole in the treatment of symptomatic giardiasis in children from northern Peru. Aliment Pharmacol Ther 2001;15:1409–15.
[43] Abboud B, Lemee V, Gargala G, et al. Successful treatment of metronidazole and albendazole resistant giardiasis with nitazoxanide in a patient with acquired immunodeficiency syndrome. Clin Infect Dis 2001;32:1792–4.
[44] Diaz E, Mondragon J, Ramirez E, Bernal R. Epidemiology and control of intestinal parasites with nitazoxanide in children in Mexico. Am Trop Med Hyg 2003;68:384–5.
[45] White Jr AC. Nitazoxanide: an important advance in anti-parasitic therapy. Am Trop Med Hyg 2003;68:382–3.
[46] Hall A, Nahar Q. Albendazole as a treatment for infections with *Giardia duodenalis* in children in Bangladesh. Trans R Soc Trop Med Hyg 1993;87:84–6.
[47] Lossick J. Epidemiology of urogenital trichomoniasis. In: Honinberg BM, editor. Trichomonads parasitic in humans. New York: Springer-Verlag; 1989. p. 311–23.
[48] Christie JD, Garcia LS. Emerging parasitic infections. Clin Lab Med 2004;24:737–72.
[49] Centers for Disease Control and Prevention. Sexually transmitted disease treatment guidelines. MMWR Morb Mortal Wkly Rep 2002;51(RR06):1–80.
[50] Kosek M, Alcantara C, Lima A, Guerrant RL. Cryptosporidiosis: a review. Lancet Infect Dis 2001;1:262–9.
[51] Amadi B, Mwiya M, Musuku J, et al. Effect of nitazoxanide on morbidity and mortality in Zambian children with cryptosporidiosis: a randomized controlled trial. Lancet 2002;360: 1375–80.
[52] White Jr AC, Chappell CL, Hayat CS, Kimball KT, Flanigan TP, Goodgame RW. Paromomycin for cryptosporidiosis in AIDS: a prospective, double-blind, placebo-controlled trial. J Infect Dis 1994;170:419–24.
[53] Hewitt RG, Yainnoutsos CT, Higgs ES, Carey JT, Geiseler PJ, Soave R. Paromomycin: no more effective than placebo for treatment of cryptosporidiosis in patients with advanced human immunodeficiency virus infection. Clin Infect Dis 2000;31:1084–92.
[54] Smith NH, Cron S, Valdez LM, Chappell CL, White Jr AC. Combination drug therapy for cryptosporidiosis in AIDS. J Infect Dis 1998;178:900–3.
[55] Pape JW, Verdier RI, Boncy M, Boncy J, Johnson Jr WD. Cyclospora infection in adults infected with HIV: clinical manifestations, treatment and prophylaxis. Ann Intern Med 1994; 121:654–7.
[56] Weiss LM, Perlman DC, Sherman J, Tanowitz H, Wittner M. *Isospora belli* infection: treatment with pryimethamine. Ann Intern Med 1988;109:474–5.
[57] Krause PJ. Babesiosis. Med Clin North Am 2002;86:361–73.
[58] Speilman A. Human babesiosis on Nantucket Island: transmission by nymphal *Ixodes* ticks. Am J Trop Med Hyg 1976;25:784–7.
[59] Krause PJ, Lepore T, Sikand VJ, et al. Atovaquone and azithromycin for the treatment of human babesiosis. N Engl J Med 2000;343:1454–8.

[60] Montoya JG, Liesenfeld O. Toxoplasmosis. Lancet 2004;363:1965–76.

[61] Bale JF. Congenital infections. Neurol Clin North Am 2002;20:1039–60.

[62] Sanchez PJ. Perinatal infections. Clin Perinatol 2002;29:799–826.

[63] Abrams EJ. Opportunistic infections and other clinical manifestations of HIV disease in children. Pediatr Clin North Am 2000;47:79–108.

[64] Torre D, Casari S, Speranza F, et al. Randomized trial of trimethoprim-sulfamethoxazole vs. pyrimethamine-sulfadiazine for therapy of toxoplasmic encephalitis in patients with AIDS. Italian Collaborative Study Group. Antimicrob Agents Chemother 1998;42:1346–9.

[65] Bye MR, Bernstein LJ, Glaser J, Kleid D. *Pneumocystis carinii* pneumonia in young children with AIDS. Pediatr Pulmonol 1990;9:251–3.

[66] Hughes WT. *Pneumocystis carinii* pneumonia: new approaches to diagnosis, treatment and prevention. Pediatr Infect Dis J 1991;10:391–9.

[67] Rieder MJ, King SM, Read S. Adverse reaction to trimethoprim-sulfamethoxazole among children with human immunodeficiency virus infection. Pediatr Infect Dis J 1997;16:1028.

[68] Dohn MN, Weinberg WG, Torres RA, et al. Oral atovaquone compared with intravenous pentamidine for *Pneumocystis carinii* pneumonia in patients with AIDS. Atovaquone study group. Ann Intern Med 1994;121:174–80.

[69] Toma E, Thorne A, Singer J, et al. Clindamycin with primiquine vs. trimethoprim-sulfamethoxazole therapy for mild and moderately severe *Pneumocystis carinii* pneumonia in patients with AIDS: a multicenter, double-blind, randomized trial. Clin Infect Dis 1998;27: 524–30.

[70] Black JR, Feinberg J, Murphy RL, et al. Clindamycin and primiquin therapy for mild-to-moderate episodes of *Pneumocystis carinii* pneumonia in patients with AIDS. AIDS Clinical Trials Group 044. Clin Infect Dis 1994;18:905–13.

[71] Sattler FR, Frame P, Davis R, et al. Trimetrexate with leucovorin versus trimethoprim-sulfamethoxazole for moderate to severe episodes of *Pneumocystis carinii* pneumonia in patients with AIDS: a prospective, controlled multicenter investigation of the AIDS Clinical Trials Group Protocol 029/031. J Infect Dis 1994;170:165–72.

[72] Centers for Disease Control and Prevention. 1995 Revised guidelines for prophylaxis against *Pneumocystis carinii* pneumonia for children infected with or perinatally exposed to human immunodeficiency virus. MMWR Morb Mortal Wkly Rep 1995;44(RR-4):1–11.

[73] Bryan RT, Cali A, Owen RL, Spencer HC. Microsporidia: opportunistic pathogens in patients with AIDS. Prog Clin Parasitol 1991;2:1–26.

[74] Weber R, Bryan RT. Microsporidial infections in immunodeficient and immunocompetent patients. Clin Infect Dis 1994;19:517–21.

[75] Weber R, Bryan RT, Schwartz DA, Owen RL. Human microsporidial infections. Clin Microbiol Rev 1994;7:426–61.

[76] Wittner M, Tanowitz HB, Weiss LM. Parasitic infections in AIDS patients: cryptosporidiosis, isosporiasis, microsporidiosis, cyclosporiasis. Infect Dis Clin North Am 1993;7:569–86.

[77] Orenstein JM, Dieterich DT, Kotler DP. Systemic dissemination by a newly recognized intestinal microsporidia species in AIDS. AIDS 1992;6:1143–50.

[78] Weber R, Sauer B, Spycher MA, et al. Detection of *Septata intestinalis* in stool specimens and coprodiagnostic monitoring of successful treatment with albendazole. Clin Infect Dis 1994; 19:342–5.

[79] Molina JM, Tourneur M, Sarfati C, et al. Fumagillin treatment of intestinal microsporidiosis. N Engl J Med 2002;346:1963–9.

[80] Jain R, Prabhakar S, Modi M, Bhatia R, Sehgal R. Naegleria meningitis: a rare survival. Neurol India 2002;50:470–2.

[81] Galarza M, Cuccia V, Sosa FP, Monges JA. Pediatric granulomatous cerebral amebiasis: a delayed diagnosis. Pediatr Neurol 2002;26:153–6.

[82] Wang A, Kay R, Poon WS. Successful treatment of amoebic meningoencephalitis in a Chinese living in Hong Kong. Clin Neurol Neurosurg 1993;95:249–52.

[83] Poungvarin N, Jariya P. The fifth non-lethal case of primary amebic meningoencephalitis. J Med Assoc Thai 1991;74:112.

[84] Brown RL. Successful treatment of primary amebic meningoencephalitis. Arch Intern Med 1991;151:1201–2.
[85] Singhal T, Bajpai A, Kalra V, et al. Successful treatment of *Acantamoeba* meningitis with combination oral antimicrobials. Pediatr Infect Dis J 2001;20:623–7.
[86] Sison JP, Kemper CA, Loveless M, McShane D, Visvesvara GS, Deresinski SC. Disseminated *Acanthamoeba* infection in patients with AIDS: case reports and reviews. Clin Infect Dis 1995; 20:1207–16.
[87] Seijo Martinez M, Gonzalez-Mediero G, Santiago P, et al. Granulomatous amebic encephalitis in a patient with AIDS: isolation of *Acanthamoeba* sp. group II from brain tissue and successful treatment with sulfadiazine and fluconazole. J Clin Microbiol 2000;38:3892–5.
[88] Muennig P, Pallin D, Sell R, Chan MS. The cost effectiveness of strategies for the treatment of intestinal parasites in immigrants. N Engl J Med 1999;340:773–9.
[89] Crawford FG, Vermund SH. Parasitic infections in day care centers. Pediatr Infect Dis J 1987;6:744–9.
[90] Urbani C, Albonico M. Antihelminthic drug safety and drug administration in the control of soil-transmitted helminthiasis in community campaigns. Acta Trop 2003;86:215–21.
[91] American Academy of Pediatrics. Drugs for parasitic infections. In: Pickering LK, editor. Red book: 2003 report of the Committee on Infectious Diseases. 26th ed. Elk Grove Village (IL): American Academy of Pediatrics; 2003. p. 744–70.
[92] Montresor A, Stoltzfus RJ, Albonico M, et al. Is the exclusion of children under 24 months from antihelmintic treatment justifiable? Trans R Soc Trop Med Hyg 2002;96:197–9.
[93] Montresor A, Awasthi A, Crompton DWT. Use of benzimidoles in children younger than 24 months for the treatment of soil-transmitted helminthiasis. Acta Trop 2003;86:223–32.
[94] Wilson CM, Freedman DO. Antiparasitic agents. In: Long SS, Pickering LK, Prober CG, editors. Principles and practice of pediatric infectious diseases. 2nd ed. New York: Churchill Livingstone; 2003. p. 1547–58.
[95] Naquira C, Jimenez G, Guerra JG, et al. Ivermectin for human strongyloidiasis and other intestinal helminths. Am J Trop Med Hyg 1989;40:304–9.
[96] Schaffel R, Nucci M, Portugal R, et al. Thiabendazole for the treatment of strongyloides in patients with hematologic malignancies. Clin Infect Dis 2000;31:821–2.
[97] Belizario VY, Amarillo ME, de Leon WU, de los Reyes AE, Bugayong MG, Macatangay BJC. A comparison of the efficacy of single doses of albendazole, ivermectin, and diethylcarbamazine alone or in combinations against *Ascaris* and *Trichuris* spp. Bull World Health Organ 2003;81:35–42.
[98] Grove DI. Treatment of strongyloidiasis with thiabendazole: an analysis of toxicity and effectiveness. Trans R Soc Trop Med Hyg 1982;76:114–8.
[99] Elgart GW, Meinking TL. Ivermectin. Dermatol Clin 2003;21:277–82.
[100] Richard-Lenoble D, Chandenier J, Gaxotte P. Ivermectin and filariasis. Fundam Clin Pharm 2003;17:199–203.
[101] Michael E, Bundy DA, Grenfell BT. Re-assessing the global prevalence and distribution of lymphatic filariasis. Parasitology 1996;112:409–28.
[102] Boggild AK, Keystone JS, Kain KC. Tropical pulmonary eosinophilia: a case series in a setting of nonendemicity. Clin Infect Dis 2004;39:1123–8.
[103] Caumes E. Treatment of cutaneous larva migrans and toxocara infection. Fundam Clin Pharm 2003;17:213–6.
[104] Dinning WJ, Gillespie SH, Cooling RI, Maizels RM. Toxocariasis: a practical approach to management of ocular disease. Eye 1988;2:580–2.
[105] Garcia HH, Gonzalez AE, Evans CA, Gilman RH. Taenia solium cysticercosis. Lancet 2003; 362:547–56.
[106] Flisser A, Sarti E, Sarti R, Schantz PM, Valencia S. Effect of praziquantel on protozoan parasites. Lancet 1995;345:316–7.
[107] Maguire JH. Tapeworms and seizures-treatment and prevention. N Engl J Med 2004;350:215–7.
[108] Garcia HH, Pretell EJ, Gilman RH, et al. A trial of antiparasitic treatment to reduce the rate of seizures due to cerebral cysticercosis. N Engl J Med 2004;350:249–58.

[109] Thompson RCA. Biology and systematics of Echinococcus. In: Thompson RCA, Lambery AJ, editors. Echinococcus and hydatid disease. London: CAB International; 1995. p. 1–37.

[110] Yorganci K, Sayek I. Surgical treatment of hydatid cysts of the liver in the era of percutaneous treatment. Am J Surg 2002;184:63–9.

[111] Richards Jr FO. *Diphyllobothrium, Dipylidium, and Hymenolepsis* species. In: Long SS, Pickering LK, Prober CG, editors. Principles and practice of pediatric infectious diseases. 2nd ed. New York: Churchill Livingstone; 2003. p. 1351–4.

[112] Elliott DE. Schistosomiasis. Gastroenterol Clin North Am 1996;25:599–625.

[113] Sturruck R. The parasites and their life cycles. In: Jordan P, Webbe G, Sturruck R, editors. Human schistosomiasis. Wallingford, UK: CAB International; 1993. p. 1–31.

[114] Parraga IM, Assis AM, Prado MS, et al. Gender differences in growth of school-aged children with schistosomiasis and geohelminth infection. Am J Trop Med Hyg 1996;55:150–6.

[115] Capron A. Schistosomiasis: forty years' war on the worm. Parasitol Today 1998;14:379–84.

[116] Olds GR. Administration of praziquantal to pregnant and lactating women. Acta Trop 2003;86: 185–95.

[117] Harinasuta T, Pungpak S, Keystone J. Trematode infections—opisthorchiasis, clonorchiasis, fascioliasis, and paragonimiasis. Infect Dis Clin North Am 1993;7:699–716.

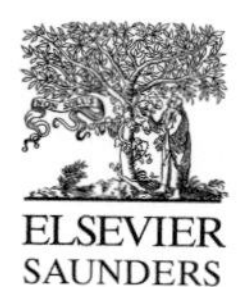

ELSEVIER
SAUNDERS

PEDIATRIC CLINICS
OF NORTH AMERICA

Pediatr Clin N Am 52 (2005) 949–961

Index

Note: Page numbers of article titles are in **boldface** type.

0031-3955/05/$ – see front matter
doi:10.1016/S0031-3955(05)00093-3

B

D

G

H

P

Q

R

S

T

U

V

W

Y

Z

Changing Your Address?

Make sure your subscription changes too! When you notify us of your new address, you can help make our job easier by including an exact copy of your Clinics label number with your old address (see illustration below.) This number identifies you to our computer system and will speed the processing of your address change. Please be sure this label number accompanies your old address and your corrected address—you can send an old Clinics label with your number on it or just copy it exactly and send it to the address listed below.

We appreciate your help in our attempt to give you continuous coverage. Thank you.

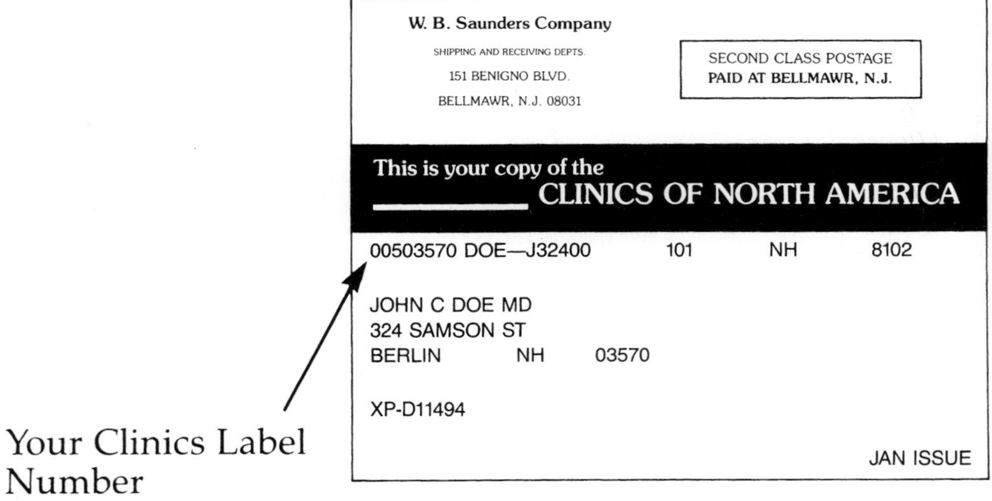

Copy it exactly or send your label along with your address to:
W.B. Saunders Company, Customer Service
Orlando, FL 32887-4800
Call Toll Free 1-800-654-2452

Please allow four to six weeks for delivery of new subscriptions and for processing address changes.

Order your subscription today. Simply complete and detach this card and drop it in the mail to receive the best clinical information in your field.

YES! Please start my subscription to the **CLINICS** checked below with the ❑ first issue of the calendar year or ❑ current issues. If not completely satisfied with my first issue, I may write "cancel" on the invoice and return it within 30 days at no further obligation.

Please Print:

Name ______________________________

Address ______________________________

City ______________ State ______________ ZIP ______________

Method of Payment

❑ Check (payable to **Elsevier**; add the applicable sales tax for your area)

❑ VISA ❑ MasterCard ❑ AmEx ❑ Bill me

Card number ______________ Exp. date ______________

Signature ______________________________

Staple this to your purchase order to expedite delivery

❑ **Adolescent Medicine Clinics**
- ❑ Individual $95
- ❑ Institutions $133
- ❑ *In-training $48

❑ **Anesthesiology**
- ❑ Individual $175
- ❑ Institutions $270
- ❑ *In-training $88

❑ **Cardiology**
- ❑ Individual $170
- ❑ Institutions $266
- ❑ *In-training $85

❑ **Chest Medicine**
- ❑ Individual $185
- ❑ Institutions $285

❑ **Child and Adolescent Psychiatry**
- ❑ Individual $175
- ❑ Institutions $265
- ❑ *In-training $88

❑ **Critical Care**
- ❑ Individual $165
- ❑ Institutions $266
- ❑ *In-training $83

❑ **Dental**
- ❑ Individual $150
- ❑ Institutions $242

❑ **Emergency Medicine**
- ❑ Individual $170
- ❑ Institutions $263
- ❑ *In-training $85
- ❑ Send CME info

❑ **Facial Plastic Surgery**
- ❑ Individual $199
- ❑ Institutions $300

❑ **Foot and Ankle**
- Individual $160
- Institutions $232

❑ **Gastroenterology**
- ❑ Individual $190
- ❑ Institutions $276

❑ **Gastrointestinal Endoscopy**
- ❑ Individual $190
- ❑ Institutions $276

❑ **Hand**
- ❑ Individual $205
- ❑ Institutions $319

❑ **Heart Failure (NEW in 2005!)**
- ❑ Individual $99
- ❑ Institutions $149
- ❑ *In-training $49

❑ **Hematology/ Oncology**
- ❑ Individual $210
- ❑ Institutions $315

❑ **Immunology & Allergy**
- ❑ Individual $165
- ❑ Institutions $266

❑ **Infectious Disease**
- ❑ Individual $165
- ❑ Institutions $272

❑ **Clinics in Liver Disease**
- ❑ Individual $165
- ❑ Institutions $234

❑ **Medical**
- ❑ Individual $140
- ❑ Institutions $244
- ❑ *In-training $70
- ❑ Send CME info

❑ **MRI**
- ❑ Individual $190
- ❑ Institutions $290
- ❑ *In-training $95
- ❑ Send CME info

❑ **Neuroimaging**
- ❑ Individual $190
- ❑ Institutions $290
- ❑ *In-training $95
- ❑ Send CME inf0

❑ **Neurologic**
- ❑ Individual $175
- ❑ Institutions $275

❑ **Obstetrics & Gynecology**
- ❑ Individual $175
- ❑ Institutions $288

❑ **Occupational and Environmental Medicine**
- ❑ Individual $120
- ❑ Institutions $166
- ❑ *In-training $60

❑ **Ophthalmology**
- ❑ Individual $190
- ❑ Institutions $325

❑ **Oral & Maxillofacial Surgery**
- ❑ Individual $180
- ❑ Institutions $280
- ❑ *In-training $90

❑ **Orthopedic**
- ❑ Individual $180
- ❑ Institutions $295
- ❑ *In-training $90

❑ **Otolaryngologic**
- ❑ Individual $199
- ❑ Institutions $350

❑ **Pediatric**
- ❑ Individual $135
- ❑ Institutions $246
- ❑ *In-training $68
- ❑ Send CME info

❑ **Perinatology**
- ❑ Individual $155
- ❑ Institutions $237
- ❑ *In-training $78
- ❑ Send CME inf0

❑ **Plastic Surgery**
- ❑ Individual $245
- ❑ Institutions $370

❑ **Podiatric Medicine & Surgery**
- ❑ Individual $170
- ❑ Institutions $266

❑ **Primary Care**
- ❑ Individual $135
- ❑ Institutions $223

❑ **Psychiatric**
- ❑ Individual $170
- ❑ Institutions $288

❑ **Radiologic**
- ❑ Individual $220
- ❑ Institutions $331
- ❑ *In-training $110
- ❑ Send CME info

❑ **Sports Medicine**
- ❑ Individual $180
- ❑ Institutions $277

❑ **Surgical**
- ❑ Individual $190
- ❑ Institutions $299
- ❑ *In-training $95

❑ **Thoracic Surgery (formerly Chest Surgery)**
- ❑ Individual $175
- ❑ Institutions $255
- ❑ *In-training $88

❑ **Urologic**
- ❑ Individual $195
- ❑ Institutions $307
- ❑ *In-training $98
- ❑ Send CME info

*To receive in-training rate, orders must be accompanied by the name of affiliated institution, dates of residency and signature of coordinator on institution letterhead. Orders will be billed at the individual rate until proof of resident status is received.